THE NATURE OF CLINICAL CARE

VOLUME 1

A Gentle Introduction

by

David Zitner and H. Dominic J. Covvey

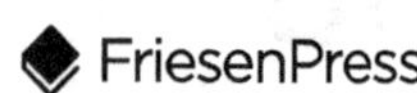

One Printers Way
Altona, MB R0G 0B0
Canada

www.friesenpress.com

First Edition — 2024

ISBN
978-1-03-918003-1 (Hardcover)
978-1-03-918002-4 (Paperback)
978-1-03-918004-8 (eBook)

1. MEDICAL, HEALTH CARE DELIVERY

Distributed to the trade by The Ingram Book Company

Dedications and Credits

DAVID:

My family, patients and students taught me most of what I know. Friends and family motivated me and organized my thinking. Neil Roberts, CEO of the Halifax Infirmary, John Ruedy, Dean of Medicine at Dalhousie, and Brian Lee Crowley, CEO MacDonald Laurier Institute diverted me from clinical practice to research and teaching. My students showed me that people who understand the basic ideas in Medicine as discussed in these books could solve many simple and complex medical problems and more easily collaborate with clinicians.

DOMINIC:

Over 7 years ago, David invited me to co-write a book with him. His success in his Health Informatics course at Dalhousie University motivated his belief that similar material could benefit others. I accepted and enjoyed hundreds of highly stimulating phone discussions that underpin this Compendium. Thank you David! Thanks also to Elisabeth and Henry! I am the lucky dog who got the excellent attention they provide to pets and other animals. Finally, to Natela, Zaza, Lizi and Tina, whom Putin displaced. Слава Україні! Героям слава! You too are heroes!

CREDITS:

Dominic's daughter, Laura S. Thompson, painted the cover image. She and her husband, Frank Rekrut, are artists with an art school in Florence, Italy (www.theflorencestudio.com). Dominic's younger daughter, Beth A. Covvey, illustrated this and the other Volumes. Learn about her work at www.bethcovvey.ca. Beth lives in Yellowknife, Northwest Territory, Canada. Thanks also to Brittany Kraus for addressing the many issues in the books! Brittany, you were a lucky find!

Comment

Our goal in producing these books was affordability. Several publishers quoted well over $100 USD for each volume. So, we opted for less expensive electronic publishing and minimal royalties. We would welcome any error-finds and suggestions regarding content so we can improve the text. You can share with us via we.inform.people@gmail.com.

Table of Contents

Preface

Many books describe the health system. This compendium of books, though, is unique. We commence our story with the nature of the clinical process – what doctors do – and reflect on the clinical process as the source of information that serves as the foundation from which every aspect of health care devolves, from caring for patients to evaluating the value of medical investigations, treatments and the care agencies themselves. We examine many aspects and styles of practice, especially from the perspective of patients. A consistent theme throughout the material is patient engagement in care so the patient is understood to be a crucial operational agent in the system. These books provide the perspectives of both the clinician and the informatician, being strongly shaped by the background of its authors.

What You Have in Hand

Everyone participating in health care must comprehend a set of essential ideas.

There are three books in this series. Volume 1 introduces the ideas related to understanding, diagnosing, treating, and preventing biological problems. Volume 2 applies those ideas to enable the reader to understand Mental Health and Public Health. Volume 3 reflects on important issues that underly the practice of clinical care.

Readers can visit the chapters in each book in order, or it is possible to skip around and read the material relevant to your needs at the time and to your background. However, each chapter is a kind of 'microbook' that can be read on its own. We have attempted to write the chapters so there is little essential dependence on other material. Where we believe that understanding something is enhanced by or dependent on by other material, we have stated such. Though scientific articles are usually written in a highly structured way and build up a story, many scientists read their contents in different orders. Richard Feynman, the famous Nobel Laureate, was known to often read only the introductory abstract of an article, then read the conclusions, then work it all out in his head and only go through the rest if he came to different conclusions. So, you see, to each, your own!

There are 3 books with 85 chapters divided up into the 3 volumes. We will include this same **Introduction** in each of the volumes, thereby assisting in our 'start anywhere- go anywhere' approach!

Note that this material is available printed, in whole or part on request at a nominal charge.

Why Consider these Books

We assume you thought that one or more of these books looked interesting because you picked them from a list, the Web or a shelf and began reading them. Nevertheless, might they really be of value to you or your students?

There are many texts on Medicine or that address various aspects of health care, but this compendium is different. It unseals and unwraps what we call the 'healthcare system' (though many would deny that it is organized enough to be called a 'system'), enabling a deep understanding of its nature, parts, people and functions. In a way, these books describe the anatomy (parts and connections) and physiology (functions) of the health system. They describe the professionals that make the system work and what they do, as well as the strengths, weaknesses and flaws of every important aspect – their pathology.

This compendium of books describes the most important concepts that medical professionals – clinicians (physicians, nurses and allied care providers) – use to assess, diagnose and treat problems. It explains how clinicians think, the kinds of information they use to reach conclusions, how they decide to treat and what they can and cannot do. Those ideas will give readers, including teachers and students in many disciplines, the understanding, skills and confidence to themselves find pertinent health information and will enable non-clinical healthcare professionals and patients to understand the clinical process and to have intelligent conversations with clinicians about their work. It will also help any reader to participate better together in healthcare processes.

The material likely surprises the reader by revealing that not all recommended medical tests or treatments are necessarily good ones that they should accept. It will, on the other hand, also suggest how to decide when it is appropriate to accept or reject suggestions that a problem is not real or is "unimportant" and therefore not requiring tests or treatments. Readers will realize that medical care is powerful but has limits. We try to identify beliefs that lead people to accept useless and possibly harmful care or to agree with incomplete or mistaken diagnostic conclusions.

After reading the books in this series, the reader will know the most important ideas that clinicians use. That will give the reader the confidence and skills to find and understand pertinent health information, converse with and about clinicians, and understand how patients can become active participants in their own and their families' health care.

Beyond all that, these books will help the reader understand what it means to be healthy and how patients can help physicians[1] keep them as healthy as possible. In addition, they will help readers understand the origins of controversies in health services administration and prepare them to contribute to the discussion.

Why Develop Health Literacy and Engage Patients

On September 22nd, 2011, the now-defunct Health Council of Canada released "*How Engaged are Canadians in their Primary Care? Results from the 2010 Commonwealth Fund International Health Policy Survey*" and reported that fewer than half (48%) of all Canadians are active participants in their own health care.[2] We are fairly sure that this is the case in most other jurisdictions.

The Commonwealth Fund study found that engaged patients are happier with their care and more likely to participate in disease prevention, in appropriate screening and in health promoting activities. It has become clear that modern technology enables everyone, clinicians and non-clinicians alike, to work together to achieve better health and better treatment.

The World Health Organization[3] reports that several interventions help non-clinicians (including patients, administrators and regulators) become more health literate and able to play an active role in their own care. This is important, as **health-literate patients feel comfortable in shared decision-making** because they feel

1 Note: We will refer to the role 'physician' throughout these books to avoid cumbersome language and because physicians have a broader scope of practice, including an almost unlimited ability to order tests and treatments. Other clinicians (nurses and allied professionals) might carry out similar functions, but their scope of practice is more limited. We recognize that all members of the healthcare team are vital, and that many clinicians who are not physicians have unique and essential roles and expertise.

2 https://publications.gc.ca/site/eng/9.572779/publication.html. Link from UBC Centre for Health Care Management. Accessed Sept 8, 2023.

3 Self-care interventions for health (who.int). https://www.who.int/health-topics/self-care#tab=tab_1. Accessed July 9, 2022.

confident in evaluating professional suggestions. Health-literate patients are better able to recognize when self-management is appropriate and when they need advice. FIGURE 1.P.1 illustrates a patient working with a clinician.

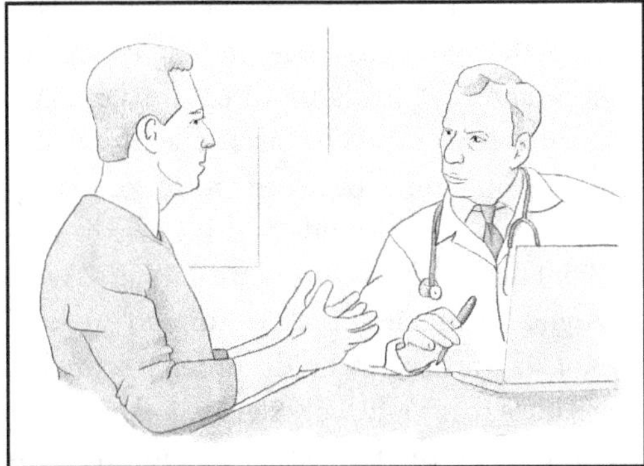

FIGURE 1.P.1: Patient and clinician must work together

Health literacy improves when patients have access to:

- Written information that supplements clinical consultations.
- Web sites and other electronic information sources.
- Personalized computer-based information and virtual support.
- Decision aids for patients.
- Self-management education programs including the ideas in these volumes.

The fact is that ordinary people can easily find information on the causes of many health problems and on the effectiveness of treatments if they know where to look and what questions to ask.

Why Health Professionals Need Similar Information

Health services administrators, health informaticians and other healthcare-interested professionals need the same information as patients and their care providers. Administrators, for instance, need information about the effectiveness of care to evaluate the services that they manage and support. Journalists need that information so they can inform the public. In addition, Health Informatics (See Volume 1 Chapter 19) experts must know about the kinds of information that are or can be produced and collected during care and how clinicians and researchers use or should use it. Clinical information is the essential content of health information systems intended to assess care and inform clinicians and administrators about the benefits and harms of care.

Artificial Intelligence

IBM's Big Blue long ago beat two contestants in *Jeopardy*. Then another computer, using artificial intelligence (AI[4], also called 'Machine Intelligence') defeated an expert in the complicated game *Go*, a game requiring knowledge and strategy. There is the promise that those same artificial intelligence techniques can help clinicians and patients make better choices as they try to diagnose what is wrong with the patient and attempt to decide the best way to treat both common and rare health problems.

Artificial intelligence systems process vast amounts of information and discover the relationships among various pieces of information. People who develop and use artificial intelligence systems to support health care must understand the knowledge base and principles of health care to select meaningful information and to evaluate if the conclusions produced by AI systems are meaningful and correct.

In Volume 1 Chapter 4, we discuss distinctions between the art of Medicine and the science of Medicine. Artificial intelligence methods rely on machines having access to massive amounts of scientific information to

4 The Guardian Wed. Jan 27, 2016. https://www.theguardian.com/technology/2016/jan/27/google-hits-ai-milestone-as-computer-beats-go-grandmaster. Accessed July 11, 2022.

discover relationships among patient characteristics, healthcare activities and results. However, at this stage of development, artificial intelligence systems are less useful when it comes to the art of Medicine. They are impaired in inferring suggestions when the information and research is insufficient to reach a scientific conclusion, although AI systems may help scientists develop testable ideas (hypotheses) that can be supported or rejected by additional research.

Whenever clinicians differ on the approach to problems, patients and clinicians must have the knowledge and tools to help decide among different possibilities, especially when the science backing choices is limited.

The Importance of Health

We all worry, from time to time, about our health, even when we are well. We may worry even more when we do not feel right, when something hurts, or when we are unable to do what we were able to do before.

However, the next most important thing after our general satisfaction with ourselves, our lives and those we love is our health, both physical and mental. Our first thought is for the persons themselves, but the next concern is for how well we and they feel, think, function, and, sometimes, how long we and they are likely to be around. Health is right up there near the top of each of our lists. Like it or not, our health affects every day of our lives and every hour of each of those days. Further, what we do on those days affects our health.

Some of us get through life with few health problems. But that's not true of all of us and we each know of someone not so lucky. A certainty is that all of us will from time to time get sick, sometimes very sick and eventually mortally sick. In other words, we will die.

Regarding our health, there are many questions.

What exactly do we mean by 'being healthy' and what do we mean by 'being sick'? What can be done to keep us healthy and what can be done to help us when we're sick? How can we contribute and help clinical teams help us? Who are those people who do the helping? What are their and our responsibilities related to health both for ourselves and for others? What is the system that tries to help us remain healthy and that treats us when are sick, and how does it work? What is a 'diagnosis' and what information is necessary to make a diagnosis? What are the kinds of things we can do to maintain health, avoid and treat illness? Why do some treatments, that we intend to help us, fail or hurt us? Why do other treatments sometimes magically work? Why is everything the way it is – the human body, the care providers, the healthcare system, the treatments, and the effects they deliver? What information do we need to predict whether a treatment is more likely to help or to harm? Why is mental illness controversial? What are the differences between problems we call 'illnesses' and those labelled 'mental illness'?

We answer all these questions and many more in these volumes.

Most people will find the ideas we present compelling and easy to understand. People who understand the important ideas can better understand most clinical information, accept useful suggestions, and discard harmful ones. People who know the important ideas will also find it easier to access the information they need to guide their professional, personal and political choices for health care.

Eventually, all of us make healthcare choices. Clinicians ask us to opine on healthcare interventions for ourselves, for friends and for family. At the ballot box, politicians ask us to choose the best proposals for organizing health care. Health is an important part of life and touches everyone and everything.

So, we have a lot to learn. What's important is that health knowledge will empower us!

VOLUME 1

Section 1

INTRODUCTION

We all have different senses of humor. Hopefully, though, the humor in this book will at least - like good treatments - do no harm, i.e., offend. The intention is to provide a break from all the serious stuff. Many items are not even relevant to the topics discussed. If needed, blame any negative effects on DC!

SURGEONS VS INTERNISTS

In every profession there are friendly rivalries among specialists. It's the same in health care. We have both had the great privilege of knowing countless physicians of every professional focus and have heard our share of good-natured joshing. Here is one anecdote that illustrates the friendly combat between Internists and Surgeons – the Internist joking that Surgeons do cutting rather than thinking.

There were 3 medical staff rushing for the elevator to get upstairs to the lab. Suddenly, the elevator door started to close. The surgeon was quickest and ran forward to keep the elevator available. Its doors were almost closed when he got there, so he stuck his head between them to prevent that. "My goodness, George," one of the Internists said to the surgeon as they got on the elevator with him, "Why in heaven's name did you use your head that way???" George responded: "Well, I didn't want to injure my hands!"

A Story: Knowledgeable Patient Participation Contributes to Miraculous Cures

Anyone who understands the essential ideas we discuss in these volumes will be able to participate in their own care and thereby increase the speed of diagnosis and the likelihood they will get appropriate treatment. Consider this person's story:

Rose, a 78-year-old woman with little formal education, had nevertheless always been an active participant in her own care and in the care of her adult children. She read widely and understood health and health care far beyond what would have her level of education might lead us to expect.

I learned that Rose had intervened, years ago, when doctors wanted to do an appendix operation on her oldest son. Somehow, she realized that people with appendicitis (an inflammation of the appendix) would have tenderness and inflammation in the abdominal cavity. When the doctor suggested removal of the appendix – an 'appendectomy' – to cure her son's abdominal cramps, she asked her son to jump up and down. When that movement did not cause any pain, she rejected the idea of an appendectomy. Fortunately, it turned out to be fine.

Her youngest son, when he was 11, broke the bone (the Humerus) in his upper arm 3 times over the course of one year. X-rays showed that he had a cyst in the bone. The third time, surgeons wanted to operate. They told her, it was "bad to have a hole in a bone." They proposed taking bone from his hip and using it to fill the hole. She replied, "If it is bad having a hole in a bone what will be used to fill the hole in the hip?" The orthopedic surgeon just walked away! Upset, she took her son from the hospital without signing him out. Instead, she took him to a family doctor who strapped his upper arm to his chest wall, no cast necessary, put his arm in a sling and asked him to return in 6 weeks. The arm was fine, and he had no additional problems for at least 50 years.

Unfortunately, Rose developed a gait disorder with the feeling that her feet were stuck to the floor, and then she developed a resting tremor. Her family doctor and a neurologist told her she had Parkinson's disease. At the time, they did not do brain imaging, as they were certain of the diagnosis. Despite her sophistication, Rose assumed her doctor knew what they were doing. When her gait disorder became so severe that she could not cross the street, she became concerned. Before her next medical visit, she read a little. Based on that she insisted the doctor arrange some kind of head x-ray to see if she had a cancer or anything else that might be visibly wrong with her brain. Reluctantly, certain it was a waste of time and resources to do an imaging test, the doctor arranged one. The image showed she had 'normo-pressure hydrocephalus,' a rare problem that sometimes mimics Parkinson's disease. When doctors inserted a brain shunt – a little tube that drained excess fluid to a vein – this relieved the symptoms and she realized 9 years of quality living before dying at age 87!

When she had her problems, many doctors would not do imaging because, on someone they were sure had Parkinson's symptoms, discovering a different cause would be rare. However, many doctors would be more thorough. In diagnosis and treatment, when the answer is not clear, doctors may disagree on the next step. It is important for doctors and patients to understand when recommendations are based on art and when on science. The ideas we describe will help people navigate when clinicians disagree on what is best for a patient.

Chapter 1: Welcome to Our Readers

KEYWORDS: Welcome, Targeted Reader, Content Description, Book Purpose, Empowerment, Expectations

ABSTRACT: In this book we touch on what people must know to make personal decisions about their care, and what health care itself must do to evaluate health interventions as to their success or failure, allocate resources, base choices on the results of care and decide among competing demands for finite resources. We also have kept in mind what journalists and other writers must understand about the nature and practice of medical care to be able to interpret and report on new research results and claims related to treatment, to care and to health system organization and performance. Readers will understand how to make decisions about submitting to testing or to undertake a treatment. The information will inform good decisions based on real facts about the chances that testing or treatment will help or harm. We help people realize that health care is a 'team sport,' an interactive relationship between knowledgeable care providers and informed patients. Patients and the care providers make up the central team of health care.

Introduction

The material in this compendium is meant for many different groups of readers. The ideas are important for anyone interested in participating in, studying, evaluating, reporting on, administering, or in any other way becoming involved with the healthcare system. The ideas are important but are of a nature that everyone can understand. In fact, many people will already have an intuitive understanding of important ideas in these books, which include:

- The purposes of health care.
- How the impact of health care is measured and assessed (for example, the benefits versus the harms of medical treatment).
- What Preventive Medicine and screening for undiagnosed problems are about.
- What diagnosis involves and how it determines the presence of absence of disease.
- How the results of diagnostic tests and procedures are interpreted and used.
- Why some positive test results for a disease may be false alarms and some negative tests may give misleading reassurance.
- What the value, benefits and harms are of certain treatments, medicines and surgical procedures.
- How tests and treatments are used to avoid illness and maintain health.
- What the purposes of treatment in mental health are and why some problems are labeled as 'mental' illness while other people with similar problems are

just said to be 'ill', without the modifiers 'mental' or 'mentally'.

> How we evaluate treatments of mental health problem.
> What the major healthcare controversies in screening, diagnosis and treatment are.

We wrote these volumes to inform any, particularly non-clinical, professionals who work in or interact with the healthcare system. These include not only patients, but also health informaticians and health information managers (medical records librarians), technicians and technologists, health services administrators, journalists, pharmaceutical company representatives, politicians, lawyers, judges and insurance company leadership and staff. All must know how to do things such as: make personal decisions about their care, evaluate health interventions as to their success or failure, allocate resources, base choices on the results of care and decide among competing demands for finite resources.

'Health informatician' might not be a familiar professional designation to some. These are professionals who must understand every aspect of medical information: the nature of information, how we collect clinical information, what information is normally recorded and how the information is used by patients, clinicians, health services administrators, researchers and regulators. On the other hand, pretty much everyone knows what a lawyer does, but they sometimes interact with patients and the healthcare system – assessing claims of medical damage or injury and then interpreting what the causes and effects of injuries are. They must also understand the clinical results or outcomes that are possible and likely in different circumstances. Judges must address healthcare-related lawsuits and drug and insurance company personnel interact directly with the healthcare system selling or applying their products. Technicians and technologists use equipment in care processes.

Last, but not least, we have kept in mind that journalists and other writers must understand the nature and practice (as well as the vocabulary) of medical care and be able to interpret and report on new research results and claims related to treatment, to health care and to health system organization and performance.

Although clinicians already have a deep knowledge of Medicine, they must work with others to provide the best possible care to patients. To collaborate, clinicians must share compatible understandings of the purposes of care, hold harmonious ideas around general and specific approaches to clinical problems and agree on how to resolve differences of opinion among team members. In other words, they too must understand the key concepts in these books.

The Function of this Compendium

The reader will find that this compendium is like medical care itself. Much of what we discuss is based on scientific evidence, while other things represent what people call the 'art of Medicine,' a necessary and valuable part of clinical care. The reader will learn how to tell the difference between conclusions based on medical science and those which, necessarily, are based on the art of Medicine.

Sometime this art of Medicine relies on luck, sometimes on the nature of the human spirit, sometimes on inferences from scientific principles and sometimes it defies any explanation.

We show how the parts of the healthcare system work (what we called its 'Physiology', which is the science of the function and relationships among the body's cells, organs and the systems that connect them) – and sometimes do not – and what their good and bad effects are. We also will discuss the magic of medical care. And yes, there is magic, sometimes hiding behind the descriptor 'placebo effect.' Some people even call these magical effects "miracles." So, we will approach the material a bit scientifically and a bit artistically. Interestingly, it happens that both the science and the art are crucial, and, in patient care, it is important to understand when conclusions are based on art, and when on established science.

THE MAGIC OF MEDICINE

David Zitner first practiced with Dr. Mendel Burnstein, a thoughtful and caring physician. Dr. Burnstein understood the magic of Medicine and the importance of not doing harm. He recognized that medicines could be helpful or harmful and that haphazard use of potentially harmful drugs was not in the best interest of patients.

To illustrate his philosophy, consider the following.

Fatigue, loss of energy or depressed feelings are common reasons for visits to family doctors. When, even after extensive investigation, the cause cannot be determined, many doctors, then and now, prescribe antidepressant medication, hoping drugs will provide relief. Dr. Burnstein was different. He recognized that many problems are benign and self-limited and that, without a clear diagnosis, drug use should be a last resort. Yet, people often expected something.

Rather than prescribe antidepressants, Dr. Burnstein would recommend an injection of Vitamin B12. He was straightforward with patients and told them that many people feel better following B12 injections, even though no one really knew how the drug worked. It was better to prescribe a benign substance that seemed effective for many people and was side-effect free. Interventions like that can work! Current research suggests that most people with mild or moderate feelings of depression improve with benign placebos or no treatment at all (read: JAMA https://jamanetwork.com/journals/jama/article-abstract/185157)[5]. Dr. Burnstein was just ahead of his time in starting with safe interventions rather than harmful ones when no one knew the biological cause of the problem.

The Expectations on the Reader –

As we have mentioned, we intend these books for many audiences. We have done our best to define every term and present each explanation as clearly and succinctly as we can. We must apologize if any ideas seem obscure; that's probably the result of our own limitations.

There are no truly complicated ideas in these books. The important ideas are easy to understand and do not require sophisticated understanding of Mathematics, Biology, Biochemistry, Pharmacology or Physiology.

If there is any math, it is limited to arithmetic. For those of you who want more, we will refer to appropriate sources. There are a few more challenging sections, such as those related to testing and interpreting test results. Even in this case, readers can understand the important ideas without deep knowledge of the underlying concepts, but some people who want a deeper more theoretical understanding will find these chapters interesting and will see how to go deeper. Again, there are no really complicated ideas, but some might take a bit more mental effort. They are here because they are worth the effort, but you can skip over them at least the first time through.

We have not expected people reading these books to be any more than curious. We expect no background in Medicine, health, health care or illness, other than our own life experiences.

5 Fournier JC, DeRubeis RJ, Hollon SD, et al. Antidepressant Drug Effects and Depression Severity: A Patient-Level Meta-analysis. *JAMA*. 2010;303(1):47–53. doi:10.1001/jama.2009.194. "The magnitude of benefit of antidepressant medication compared with placebo increases with severity of depression symptoms and may be minimal or nonexistent, on average, in patients with mild or moderate symptoms." https://pubmed.ncbi.nlm.nih.gov/20051569/. Accessed Sept 8, 2023.

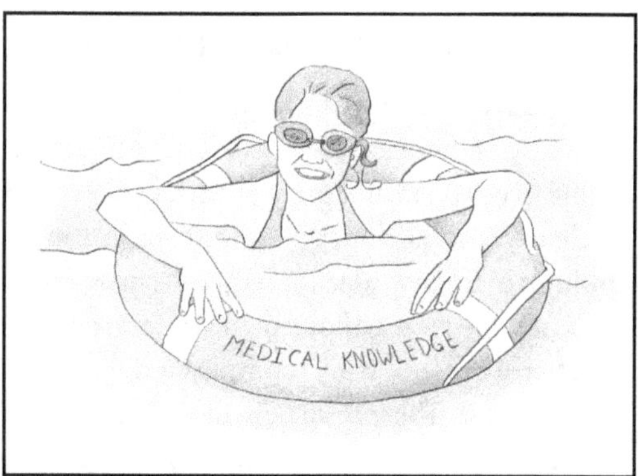

FIGURE 1.1.1: Medical knowledge can be a life preserver

Medical Knowledge as Life Saving

There is another reason these books are important: the ideas in them could save lives. Yes! Save lives! FIGURE 1.1.1 gets that point across!

Delayed and mistaken diagnoses and treatments are important causes of preventable error. Every participant in health care can help to avoid these kinds of mistakes.

Few people realize that some interventions undertaken in health care can have disastrous impacts. Medicines can kill us. Even the best efforts of brilliant and skilled surgeons still leave some patients either permanently injured or no longer among us. The results of screening tests, meant to prevent illness, sometimes initiate a cascade of ill-advised follow-up procedures and treatments. The result can be that people who accepted tests hoping to maintain health and prevent illness experience injury rather than benefit.

Readers will understand how people should make decisions about whether to submit to testing or to undertake a treatment of whatever kind. The information herein will inform good decisions based on real facts about the chances that testing or treatment will help or harm.

When it comes to maintaining health and overcoming illness, the knowledge in these books encourage direct, sensible and appropriate participation in the care process. The buzz-phrase today is 'patient engagement.' What it means is that care providers work **with** their patients in order to make together the best choices (and patients often have many, as FIGURE 1.1.2 shows) that make the most sense for each person. After all, a physician may recommend an intervention, but the patient is the one gambling that the intervention will help, not harm.

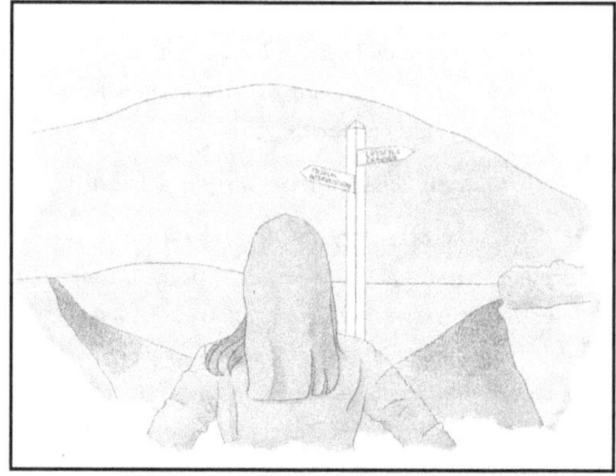

FIGURE 1.1.2: Choosing a treatment – decisions, decisions...

You may have heard in a movie a surgeon saying: "I'm going to take the risk...." However, it's the patient who takes the risk! The patient bears the burden of the effects of the intervention. So, it must be the patient who ultimately decides whether or not to accept a physician's recommendation – in these books we will discuss the real meaning of 'informed consent' to treatment. Physicians don't and can't really do it on their own. Perhaps it would make it clearer if we said that patients are the **CEOs** (Chief Executive Officers) of their own bodies and the physician really is a consultant! The final responsibility is and must be with the patient. The world has been changing about this. It used to be that some people saw the doctor as a kind of demigod, with unique access to medical information, and the patient was supposed to be an obedient disciple. But that's no longer the case, because we all know that godlike power is not imbued by the medical school curriculum, no graduate is endowed with omnipotent competencies and everybody has access to important medical information.

We, as authors, have spent our lives trying to help people realize that health care is a 'team sport', an interactive relationship between knowledgeable care providers and informed patients. The patient and the care providers make up the central team of health care. As in any team, each player, if we can use that word, must have the competence to act independently, as well as to work together.

These books detail what everybody needs to understand to participate in health care. Without the knowledge in them, each of us is left like a clued-out amateur being placed in the middle of a football game without knowledge of what the rules are, how football works, what I can and must do, where I'm supposed to go, what the goals of the game are and just about everything else. It is our objective to bring our readers up to an adequate knowledge of this healthcare 'game' so all can be competent players. As you will see, health care is an exciting game where people often make important wagers whose outcome is crucial to their health and well-being.

Promoting Empowerment is a Major Goal

We believe that readers and those they affect can, armed with these ideas, understand empowerment and become empowered. These books, though, focus their efforts on making readers deeply aware of the nature of health and the health system, as this provides the foundation for empowerment. We think immersing oneself in the content of the books being like entering basic training in the military. There a recruit is put through a series of transitions that are life changing. For example, during military training, identity with one's family is to a degree transformed into an identity with one's fellow soldiers. The recruit learns about the instruments of warfare, the importance of fitness and how to get there and stay there. In boot camp people are transformed into fighting units, where working as a cohesive team to overcome an enemy becomes more important even than staying alive.

The knowledge in these books can effect transitions like this in the reader, albeit for peaceful and defensive purposes. In health care, becoming part of a cohesive team can help people feel better, and improve their function and stay alive.

We guarantee that these books will give a new perception of the healthcare system, of care providers and of what is needed for patient-physician collaboration. They will transform the reader into a competent care team member. They will give every reader the tools to help make good decisions or to teach others how to do that. These decisions are the 'weapons' for dealing with health care and the enterprises and agents that provide that care. We will tell the truth and we are sure that some of the truths will be surprising, and some may even be a bit difficult to swallow. However, it is the truth and with that truth, people can improve and protect their lives.

The Results We Expect

So, we have written what this compendium of books is all about, what the content can do, why people need to absorb it and what they can do with it. We are convinced that the knowledge learned will reduce medical errors, save people from injury and death, reduce the cost of the healthcare system, and give people a potential for a longer, more comfortable life. And, importantly, one with less worry. Read on!

Chapter 2: Our Promises and Overview

KEYWORDS: Medical Knowledge, Self-Sufficiency, Purposes of Health Care, Common and Uncommon Diagnoses, The Patient's Wager, Making Medical Decisions.

ABSTRACT: The chapter describes what reading this book will accomplish. Our promises include providing the information needed to understand the clinical enterprise and how we use health information. We discuss the importance of various ideas including the purposes of health care, how we make diagnoses, how tests are reviewed and interpreted, and how anyone can understand the clinical enterprise.

Introduction

Promises, promises! Here they are.

Promise 1: We wrote that we shall dissect the anatomy and describe the function of healthcare system, define human health and sickness and reveal the nature of medical care (both the art and science thereof). We will do this by reflecting on the nature of the human body and its complexity (see Volume 3), what sickness is all about (Volume 1 Chapter 8), and the nature of the health system (see Volume 1 Chapter 10) that itself must be sufficiently complex to address the needs of complex human beings. Specifically, we look at the components of the health system and how physicians function and deliver medical care (see Volume 1 Section 3).

Promise 2: We have undertaken to define every term and to explain things clearly, at least clearly enough to satisfy all readers. The reader will see that in the text, but we also address terminology when we deal with records and medical vocabulary (see Volume 1 Chapters 29, 29 and 31). When a deeper explanation is required, we address it when we touch on the scientific material throughout.

Promise 3: We pledged that we would offer knowledge that can save lives. We were not kidding about this. Specifically, we will explain how testing can generate results that lead patients to undertake unnecessary further investigation or treatment. We will explain how, sometimes, these investigations or treatments can do you in. We will explain the 'patient's wager' and how patients can get information to estimate how likely treatments are to help or harm. We will give the basis for making decisions and show how to avoid unnecessary risk. Particularly important to this promise are Volume 1 Section3 and Chapter 36.

Promise 4: Our most important promise is to provide sufficient information to facilitate participation in care. This means that people can collaborate with their physicians in decision-making, agree to or avoid undertaking sometimes difficult therapies, find information and become members of their care teams. Topics related to this are discussed in Volume 1 Chapter 3, 37, 40, 43 and elsewhere.

Promise 5: In a way, we have promised to surprise. Things many people think are true, will turn out not to be. Things that people think not to be important, may be. Thinking that there was nothing someone can do, may be incorrect. For those who are not scientists, quite a bit in these books may be counterintuitive. Because of that, we will provide, hopefully, enough information to convince the reader of the validity of certain ideas.

Promise 6: This promise is a new one. We will try to keep your attention, sometimes with anecdotes from our or others' experience. One of us, David, has had a long and rich life of medical practice with probably thousands of stories, a few of which we will share with you. Dominic, on the other hand, has been a medical computing researcher and an informatics consultant and has had surprising experiences with organizations – he was a consultant for hundreds of hospitals. From that background he will share a few stories that should interest you. To do that, we have arranged the material and presented it in ways that should make it memorable. Examples of this include providing illustrations, anecdotes and easy-to-find reference material and how to access it. Lastly, we have worked hard at making this all very readable and interesting.

Hopefully readers will agree that we have delivered on these promises after we finally drag them into the books.

Some of the Key Ideas in this Compendium

if readers ever find themselves taking on a challenge similar to writing books like these, they will probably get sucked into thinking, as I'm sure we have, that every word is important. Unfortunately, for a few readers some words may prove to be too many, too few words or the wrong ones. A consequence of this is that, today, being primarily fed by news organizations, many expect tiny parcels of knowledge and minimalist texts. Some either won't want to read all the way through the books; others will wish for some kind of Reader's Digest-like summary. Therefore, we thought it worthwhile to bring forward some of the key elements of knowledge, which you'll find in Volume 1 Chapter 1. However, our division of the material into topical chapters should help appeal to those seeking a more enjoyable 'tapas' approach to learning.

We intend these books to reach everyone who must interact with the health system at some point.

Summary

After absorbing the messages of this compendium of books, readers of many kinds:

- Will understand the purposes of health care.
- Will understand how we can measure health.
- Will understand how doctors reach common and uncommon diagnoses.
- Will understand issues around preventive medicine and screening.
- Will understand the information necessary to decide whether a test result likely to be misleading – providing false reassurance or creating unnecessary alarm.
- Will understand the patient's wager and how to find information to determine how likely an intervention is to help or harm or to be merely a waste of time and money.
- Will understand the nature of mental health, the purposes of mental health care and how we measure and evaluate mental health.
- Will understand a much more extensive set of possible mental health interventions.
- Will understand the importance of evaluating health interventions.
- Will see the need to intelligently allocate resources – including how to measure results.

- Will have the basis to decide between competing demands for resources.
- These books are also useful for clinical team members who must work together and must be able:
- To generate compatible ideas around the purposes of care.
- To generate compatible ideas around approaches to clinical problems.
- To develop an approach to achieving consensus among professionals working in teams.

Chapter 3: Introduction to Health Care

KEYWORDS: Miraculous Cures, Dangerous Interventions, Medical Error, Patient Engagement, Personal Approach to Health Care.

ABSTRACT: For many people, health care produces miraculous cures, as well as a few disastrous harms. People can avoid harm and maximize benefit if they engage and participate with clinicians in their own care. In the information age, ordinary citizens who understand the ideas we present can find the information they need to meaningfully participate in their care and become the CEOs – the Chief Executive Officers – of their own care.

Health Care Is Sometimes Miraculous, Sometimes Dangerous

Every day, people experience seemingly miraculous benefits from health care. They benefit when treatments delay death and improve comfort and function.

However, American and Canadian health care is also plagued with errors leading to preventable death, discomfort and disability. [6] [7] It is hardly surprising that care providers – themselves people – working in health care, just like people participating in other human activities, will make the occasional mistake. However, patients and administrators who are vigilant and knowledgeable are more likely to detect and avoid mistakes in diagnosis and treatment[8] and to avoid the harmful effects of medical mistakes.

Health care can be dangerous! Reports from the United States[9], Canada[10], and Great Britain[11] suggest that the risk of mistakes makes health care riskier than activities we normally regard as dangerous, such as bungee

6 To Err is Human Building a Safer Health Care System, Kohn, L.T., Corrigan, J.M., Donaldson, M.S., Institute of Medicine, National Academy Press, Washington D.C., 2000. https://nap.nationalacademies.org/catalog/9728/to-err-is-human-building-a-safer-health-system. Accessed Sept 8, 2023.

7 G. Ross Baker, Peter G. Norton, Virginia Flintoft, et. Al., The Canadian Adverse Events Study: the incidence of adverse events among hospital patients in Canada CMAJ May 25, 2004 1seven0:16seven8-1686; doi:10.1503/cmaj.1040498. https://pubmed.ncbi.nlm.nih.gov/15159366/. Accessed Sept 8, 2023.

8 B. C. Johnston, P. Alonso-Coello, Jan O. Friedrich et. Al. Do clinicians understand the size of treatment effects? A randomized survey across 8 countries CMAJ cmaj.150430; published ahead of print October 26, 2015, doi:10.1503/cmaj.150430. July 11, 2022. https://pubmed.ncbi.nlm.nih.gov/26504102/. Accessed Sept 8, 2023

9 Leape LL. Error in Medicine. *JAMA*. 1994;272(23):1851–1857. https://jamanetwork.com/journals/jama/article-abstract/384554. Accessed October 16, 2023.

10 G. Ross Baker, Peter G. Norton, Virginia Flintoft, et. Al., The Canadian Adverse Events Study: the incidence of adverse events among hospital patients in Canada CMAJ May 25, 2004 1seven0:16seven8-1686; doi:10.1503/cmaj.1040498 https://pubmed.ncbi.nlm.nih.gov/15159366/. Accessed Sept 8, 2023.

11 NHS hospitals more dangerous than bungee-jumping, Telegraph, June 29, 2008. Asco Connection, The Professional Networking Site for our Worldwide Oncology Community. Quality of Care: One on One! Dr. Abdul-Rahman Jazieh. https://www.telegraph.co.uk/news/health/2213807/NHS-hospitals-more-dangerous-than-bungee-jumping.html. Accessed July 11, 2022.

jumping, mountain climbing or working near a nuclear reactor. We speculate that one reason for the higher error rate reflects that few healthcare systems have in place the failure-aware attitudes and the redundant systems aviation and other industries implemented. Increasing patient knowledge and participation adds another level of safety because there is another set of eyes, ears and brains evaluating the choices clinicians recommend.

To quantify the danger, take notice of the fact that the Canadian Events Study suggested that 200 people admitted to Canadian teaching hospitals die each year because of preventable mistakes.[12] We don't know if it is higher or lower now because the study has not been repeated. Knowledge about and active participation in health care reduces the chances of harm, including death, from a mistake!

It is also important for everyone who engages with the health system to think like doctors and become active participants in their own care if they are to gain the most benefit from doctors' experience, thoughts and advice.

Patient Engagement

On September 22, 2011, the aforementioned "*How Engaged are Canadians in their Primary Care? Results from the 2010 Commonwealth Fund International Health Policy Survey*" reported that fewer than a disappointing fraction of all Canadians are active participants in their own health care. Remember also that the Commonwealth Fund study found that engaged patients are happier with their care and more participative in major aspects.

More recently, a Canadian research consortium reported, "Ignoring the patient's role on the care team may contribute to fragmented care. However, understanding the team through the patient's lens – and collaborating meaningfully among identified team members – may improve healthcare delivery".[13] The study identified at least 15 clinical disciplines that contribute to the care of a single patient who has complex heart problems. Successful collaboration requires agreement at least on the purposes of care, how to mediate differences among team members, and for all to choose the best from a wide array of clinical alternatives.

Modern technology enables everyone, clinicians and non-clinicians, to work together to achieve better health and better treatment. However, participants must know at least the 10 crucial knowledge elements we identify below and have access to health information and research.

The World Health Organization[14] reports that several interventions help patients understand these important ideas and to become more health literate and able to play an active role in their own care. Health literate patients are better at self-management. Furthermore, health literate patients feel more comfortable in shared decision-making because they feel confident evaluating professional suggestions.

Patients can be better collaborators in care when they:

12 G. Ross Baker, Peter G. Norton, Virginia Flintoft, et. Al., The Canadian Adverse Events Study: the incidence of adverse events among hospital patients in Canada CMAJ May 25, 2004. https://pubmed.ncbi.nlm.nih.gov/15159366/. Accessed Sept 8, 2023.

13 LaDonna KA, Bates J, Tait GR, et al. "Who is on your health-care team?" Asking individuals with heart failure about care team membership and roles. *Health Expectations: An International Journal of Public Participation in Health Care and Health Policy*. 2017;20(2):198-210. doi:10.1111/hex.12447. https://pubmed.ncbi.nlm.nih.gov/26929430/. Accessed Sept 8, 2023.

14 World Health Organization. Regional Office for Europe, Health Evidence Network, European Observatory on Health Systems and Policies, Coulter, Angela, Parsons, Suzanne. et al. (2008). Where are the patients in decision-making about their own care? World Health Organization. Regional Office for Europe.. https://apps.who.int/iris/handle/10665/107980. Accessed Sept 8, 2023.

- Understand what 'health' is, what 'disease' is, what diagnosis is about and its limits, and what 'treatment' is.
- Can access and obtain Web-based and published and validated information from authoritative sources that supplements interactions with clinical professionals.
- Can get personalized computer-based information and virtual support.
- Have a sense of trust in the clinical professionals trying to help them.
- Can ask questions, get clarifications and have discussions with their clinical professionals.
- Have access to decision aids for patients.
- Can participate in self-management education programs.

Richer conversations with clinicians might increase the time for some visits to the doctor. However, more-knowledgeable patients might be able to shorten some visits because they will require less explanation and may be able to avoid other visits entirely.

Today, ordinary citizens can easily find information on the causes and treatment of many health problems, and on the effectiveness of treatments, if they know what to ask for and where to look. Indeed, non-clinical professionals addressing the healthcare system need the same information as patients. As we mentioned, administrators need information about the effectiveness of care so they can evaluate the services they provide, and journalists must understand health care to inform the public. Finally, Health Informatics experts must understand the types and quality of the information clinicians capture and how clinicians and researchers use that information to assess patient health, health care and health outcomes.

It is important to note that we also exist in societies, and, as citizens, we must recognize that knowledge about health services is increasingly important as we all can become involved in the healthcare controversies headlined in print and broadcast media. People who know the important ideas about health and health care can easily find the information necessary to guide their professional, personal and political healthcare choices. Clinicians and communities routinely expect people with non-medical training to make choices about health care and health services delivery. Those people must be able to interpret most clinical information, accept useful suggestions and discard harmful ones. It is a fact of our modern times that, with the technology available, a thoughtful person, with the world's knowledge at hand, can be as or more effective at solving health problems than those trying to manage with only the knowledge they carry in their heads.

Unfortunately, without the type of content of this book, people may lack the knowledge they need to determine if diagnostic and treatment suggestions from friends, relatives and doctors are the right ones. Health services regulators and administrators, who do not know the important ideas you will find in this book may also be poorly informed and impaired in deciding how to evaluate and organize health services.

We designed this book to help everyone think about health and health care, to make informed decisions and to see the importance of and enable participation in healthcare teams.

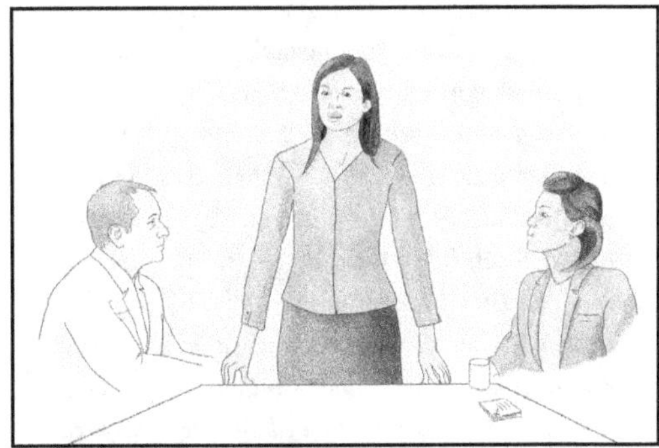

FIGURE 1.3.1: We must be the CEO of our health care

Developing a Personal Approach to Better Health: On Becoming the CEO of Your Health Care

FIGURE 1.3.1 illustrates that this is not hyperbole and is the basis for care that the patient needs and can accept.

Previous generations were forced to rely on experts because only experts knew how and where to find answers or had the nerve to make up answers (that's like informational snake oil!). Now, information tools allow participation in the healthcare system and personal care. Everyone can now find, interpret and employ information that previous generations could only get from an expert or, at times, a charlatan.

However, to benefit, people must know which questions to ask and how to interpret and judge the answers. Only by asking the right question does one have any hope of getting the right answer. Then it is crucial to have at least some sense of the validity of that answer. So, it all revolves around information and understanding. Everybody gets sick from time to time, and everybody needs to learn what caused the problem and understand what that means. Understanding if the suggested treatments make sense and if they are more likely to help or hurt us or merely waste money is essential. With this knowledge patients can recognize and avoid the injurious and deadly mistakes that plague modern health care. It might even be fun to grasp it all.

HEALTH INFORMATICS COURSE

This book is based on a graduate course in the 'Masters of Health Informatics' program at the Dalhousie University Medical School. The program is a collaboration between the Faculties of Medicine and Computer Science that has matured to include collaborators from the Faculties of Law and Management. It fosters the development of students who understand health, health care and the information systems that support clinical care, medical research, healthcare administration and patient education. The program is based on a book inspired and fostered by Dominic Covvey, "Competencies and Curricula in Health Informatics," which outlines the competencies health informaticians need to collaborate in health care. The content also comes from conversations with students, lawyers, health administrators, informatics experts, government policy makers and a variety of health experts, including doctors and nurses, who recommended specific topics and identified the most important ideas. Readers can use the summarized ideas from this course to understand the nature and purposes of health care, how to interpret illness, why being an active participant in decision-making is important and how they can find and evaluate solutions that increase longevity and help them feel better.

Chapter 4: The Art of the Art of Medicine

DIFFERENT STROKES; DIFFERENT FOLKS

Often, patients and administrators become confused when well-intentioned and dedicated doctors offer different solutions for the same problem. In my (DZ's) medical practice, sometimes I found it difficult to know to which specialist to refer a patient. For example, young children with recurrent episodes of tonsillitis could be sent to a nose and throat specialist who was aggressive and was more likely than not going to recommend surgical tonsillectomy. On the other hand, other equally reputable specialists would routinely recommend watchful waiting (giving the time for the body to heal itself). Was it really getting a second opinion when I chose which specialist to refer to? As another example, consider a patient who had a complete blockage of one carotid artery and a partial blockage of the other carotid, the blood vessels that bring blood to the head. I needed advice from a vascular surgeon, someone who deals with problems with blood vessels. However, again, it was clear that some surgeons would recommend aggressive treatment – surgery. However, others would suggest a medical intervention and watchful waiting.

Conflicting opinions about what to do often arise when there isn't clear scientific evidence that one method is better than the other. In those circumstances, the considerate doctor will reflect on the patient's needs, values and tolerance of risk and make a suggestion considered compatible with the patient's preferences.

KEYWORDS: Understanding Medical Uncertainty, How Doctors Differ, the Humanity of Medicine, The Art of Medical Practice, The Science of Medical Practice, Creative Solutions to Medical Problems

ABSTRACT: Here we explore the human elements of clinical practice. We explain why, from time to time, dedicated, well-trained clinicians offer different solutions to the same problem. When scientific research supports a singular conclusion, there is usually widespread agreement between clinicians. When the research is incomplete or absent, different clinicians may present different solutions that differ because they reflect different clinicians' values, experiences, the research they are current on, and what they might do for themselves and their family.

Precis

Thoughtful and knowledgeable clinicians do not always provide the same solutions to identical problems. Where well-controlled scientific studies provide cogent evidence, clinicians usually agree. Where rigorous scientific evidence is lacking, patients must rely on their clinicians' judgement. Sadly, when clinicians disagree on treatments not based on scientific evidence (because none exists) there is often no simple way to decide among those disagreements.

Are doctors artists or scientists or both?

Doctors are human beings that deal with other human beings. They must integrate understanding, compassion and empathy with their care.

Doctors are <u>medical scientists</u>, when they intervene in ways that science indicates is appropriate to patients' problems.

However, they are <u>medical artists</u>, when there is insufficient scientific evidence regarding how to effectively address patients' problems.

They are always medical artists in how they care for their patients. The Hippocratic Oath directs us "to do no harm". Humanity, however, demands doing much better than that.

Introduction

The practice of Medicine should, whenever possible, be based on science, including peer-reviewed evidence that a specific problem exists, and that treatment is appropriate to address a problem. However, there are many instances in clinical practice when the science is uncertain or lacking, or a patient exhibits unusual symptoms and signs that hinder determining a definitive diagnosis or a scientifically validated treatment. How does the physician go about helping the patient when there are gaps in the science meant to provide the basis for deciding and acting? The answer is that the physician must use 'artful' approaches in the attempt to help the patient.

There is also the reality that science is a bit 'cold'. Often the science must be surrounded with words and deeds that make it acceptable. Adding a human dimension to that science is crucial. The art of Medicine also helps here by bringing humanity into the equation – and that can make all the difference in how patients react and if they will accept sometimes challenging therapies.

We will discuss both these aspects of the art of Medicine.

The Humanity of Physician and Patient

We need to realize that physicians are humans like the rest of us. Humans are, fundamentally, subjective beings, not machines. Scientific evidence, while being to some degree mechanistic by nature, is a crucial element in clinical practice. However, it must be understood, appreciated, interpreted, and used in investigation, diagnosis and treatment by subjective beings and applied sensitively to other human beings for it to be 'humanized' – expressed in the context of humanity. Humans always subjectively color, emphasize and apply science according to their subjective leanings, beliefs and emotions. What they do may be analogously described as 'enterically coating' the science – enteric coating is used on drugs to protect the stomach or protect the drugs from being broken down in the stomach. People may do this unconsciously or deliberately – in the latter case perhaps trying to make the science more palatable or digestible.

Sometimes, the science does not fit perfectly with a patient's nature, feelings or state. If this subjective aspect – this humanizing of science applied in care – were absent, a medical visit would be like entering symptoms on a keyboard or by setting switches and having a raw, plastic-sealed intervention pop out from a machine, bereft of warmth or personal consideration. Subjectivity is not a weakness. It is often the best answer we have as a holistic response in our time of need, recognizing the patient's humanity, goals and preferences.

We also all know that nothing on this planet is perfect. People are not perfect and what they produce is surely not. This means that we all must deal with people, problems and interventions that are hard to pin down precisely enough to deal with them with absolute scientific-grade confidence. We live in a world of uncertainties that fill the space around what we believe we know and understand. We have islands of great intellectual clarity, but they are in a sea of the uncertain or even the unknown. Not infrequently we must act despite uncertainty or absent guidance from science. If we were not able to deal with this by applying thoughtfulness, using good personal judgment or falling back on our experiences, we would be paralyzed and ineffective, exhibiting so-called analysis paralysis.

Acting in the Face of Uncertainty

Think about how we act in the face of uncertainty related to nutrition and food preparation. We have firm knowledge that there are certain nutrients that we need to survive and thrive. Foregoing or over-indulging in one of these crucial nutrients can threaten our health. There is science behind that. In fact, there is a great deal of science related to nutrition, though the chefs who produce meals may not be familiar with all of it.

We all must ingest these nutrients, but we want to enjoy eating. This means that we add many flavorings and condiments, as well as use methods of preparation to achieve a tasty meal that we and our guests will appreciate. So, we use our own personal (artful) approach to cooking. The science regarding some of these cuisine-determined additives and processes may be spotty – we may not, at least yet, have the science related to their interactions with the food and with us. Hence there are articles about condiments, artificial flavoring and coloring, sodium levels, fats, raw versus frying and so on. A competent cook produces a meal using cooking art to give us gustatory pleasure, using some science, even though untrained in food science – as most of us are.[15] And, even the best chef does not satisfy every palate.

It's the same with the clinician. Some argue that, when several clinicians treat a patient – something common with complex diseases – we get the equivalent of too many cooks in the kitchen and the result is what artists call "mud" – a 'dog's breakfast'! On the other hand, there are those who claim that many opinions produce a better result.[16] Who knows!

The factors considered in stating a diagnosis even in the face of uncertainty, in choosing a therapeutic course – also in the face of uncertainty – suited for both the problem and the patient, in deciding how to act and speak in a sensitive way, in recommending more or less intrusive treatments, and even in deciding how much to say, all comprise the 'art of Medicine'. These are essential considerations for effective physicians who plan to help people who have different problems, personalities, needs, behaviors, or who come from different cultures.

15 https://www.amazon.ca/Always-Hungry-Conquer-Cravings-Permanently/dp/1455533874. Accessed July 12, 2022.

16 The Benefit of Additional Opinions, June 2006. Current Directions in Psychological Science 13(2), 2022, DOI: 10.1111/j.0963-7214.2004.00278.x, 2022. https://www.researchgate.net/publication/5101230. Yaniv, I, The Benefit of Additional Opinions. Accessed July 12, 2022.

THINKING ABOUT ART FOR A MOMENT

Art comes in many forms. It can be a painting, a sculpture, a musical concert, dancing, a video production, the architecture of a building, a song, acting in a play, poetry, public speaking and so on. Each of these art forms is a type of medium for artists to express themselves, but they each use the medium uniquely. Some artists deliver their expression indirectly – they create a painting or write a poem appreciated later. Other artists deliver their expression directly – we get to watch or interact with them by attending a play or listening to their singing.

Each artist has a style, perhaps indescribable but evident in what the artist produces. Consider a painting. It can be of many subjects, using many styles and many tools. Reflect on what we like in painting. Some prefer, almost photograph-like images; others prefer impressionism – Gauguin might be a good example. Still others are entranced by abstract pieces that portray a feeling or are just a pleasurable visual stimulus.

The key realizations here are that the beauty of art is in the eye of the beholder and different people prefer different artists! C'est la vie! This tells us that to satisfy the widest number of people, we need a variety of artists, art forms, and styles. Human beings aren't just moved by science but are even more affected by perceptions and feelings. Physicians are medical artists, and their patients are medical art appreciators. There must be many different kinds of medical artists and each patient must find the kind that suits.

The Physician as Artist

True, there are many medical professionals highly talented in the arts. Some physicians play classical piano or paint salable art or sculpt tiny netsuke. That is not at all relevant to what we are focusing on here. Our point here is that the physician must be an artist in the practice of Medicine. That is a fundamental requirement! Artistry is essential when dealing with problems where scientific evidence is missing <u>and</u> dealing with patients with differing personal preferences or from different cultures. To get the 'picture', consider FIGURE 1.4.1.

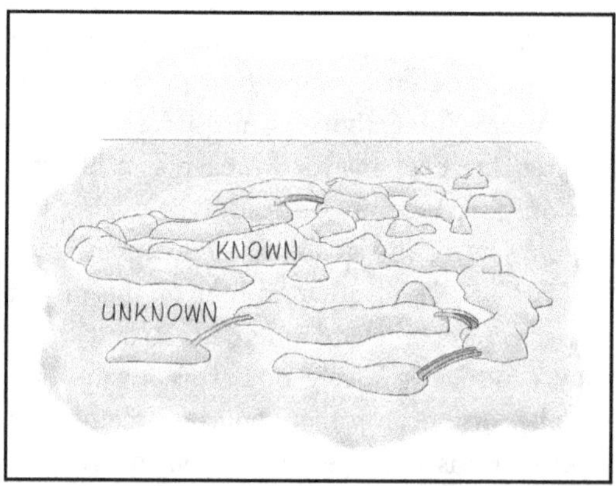

FIGURE 1.4.1: Bridging the gaps and bringing Humanity to health care

Some patients, for example, prefer a highly directive physician who cuts to the chase. Others seek a physician with whom they can engage in a more warm and friendly way. Some patients may change their preferences depending on the problem, preferring discussion of some issues but more directive care for others. Some physicians have naturally directive personalities; others are perhaps more 'Teddy Bearish'. The same can be said about the physician's ability to sense what the patient really needs or the physician's ability to formulate an approach to care management that suits that particular patient. Sometimes the physician will need to project a different persona for different patients.

The artistry of Medicine also depends on <u>the art of thinking when there is uncertainty</u>. If the cause or treatment of the patient's problem is not clear or is difficult to determine, the physician still needs to act to at least provide mental and physical comfort and therapeutic suggestions that might help the patient.

SCIENTISTS AS ARTISTS AND ARTISTS AS SCIENTISTS

All professions balance science and art. Some professions are weighted more heavily towards science, while others are weighted towards art. The most scientific of professions are likely Physics and Chemistry, as they deal entirely with the physical world. Communicating science, though – consider Neil Tyson deGrasse – requires art.

Medical Science and particularly its direct application to people, what we call Medical Care or Medicine, might be considered as sitting somewhere in the middle of the spectrum of professions between those extremes. Its foundations are in science but its superstructure – what patients see and experience – is in the human domain. This makes the art of Medicine a crucial and essential competence of its executors. Physicians' diagnostic and therapeutic methods and tools must be science-based, but how they deliver them must be art-based.

Architecture illustrates these points. Architects often design innovative structures with visual appeal using available methods and tools. The best-known of architects envisioned exciting structures like the Sydney Opera House or the Bilbao Guggenheim Museum. These structures are intentionally impressive and imposing. Imagine, though, if those architects had not considered the physical forces on the structure or the strength of the materials. Science enabled art! Without science only rubble results.

Does this mean that all architects are scientists or engineers? No. However, they must either understand and apply the science or work with those who do, or they would be failures. The same is true of physicians. Architects usually work with experts in materials and forces, or they'd design unstable structures. Physicians do this either by learning the scientific literature and by consulting with medical specialists or researchers when required.

Finally, consider Frank Lloyd Wright, who designed the Guggenheim Museum in New York. Wright was recognized as an architectural genius. However, it is claimed he never designed a roof that did not leak and his beautifully cantilevered roofs – like at Fallingwater – had significant structural problems. Wright did design pillars for what some believed were impossibly heavy roofs, but he did not follow science-based advice at Fallingwater. Rather, the engineers snuck in additional concrete to stabilize it.

So maybe Wright is a comparator for physicians, including related to that aspect of all humans, imperfection!

Practicing Medical Art

Researchers develop medical therapeutics with a target in mind, for example, killing a noxious organism or correcting some physiological dysfunction. The agents they develop hopefully address the targeted problems. Sometimes, therapeutics have different effects from the ones researchers anticipated. Physicians may use these effects – called prescribing a drug 'off label' – to address a problem for which it was not developed or use another therapeutic approach when a scientifically proven problem-specific alternative is not available. If chosen carefully and it works, the patient gets better. If the intervention does not work – assuming it hasn't harmed the patient – then the patient will see that the physician is trying and may feel comfort from that. This is the application of the art of Medicine to therapeutics. Hopefully, clinicians keep track of and report the results of off label treatment.

Realize that prescribing like this is not irrational. The physician will be using concepts of human physiology and the nature of the therapeutic agent and the patient to suggest something that might work or at least ameliorate symptoms. Published evidence of effectiveness might be minimal or lacking, but it is still based on an understanding of biology, physiology and pharmacology. So, this isn't just **any** drug or a shot in the dark. However, in the face of uncertainty, different, knowledgeable, well-meaning and thoughtful clinicians might recommend completely different remedies. This is one reason that second and third opinions might differ. Absent scientific, empirical studies, it becomes very difficult to decide which of the differing opinions based on art is the best.

This aspect of the art of Medicine is crucial. A needy patient is sitting there asking for help. Practicing the art of Medicine enables a physician to think and look more broadly, beyond the standard tools, and to consider a placebo or an intervention that creates a little breathing room perhaps giving the patient time to self-heal. Something like that can also relieve the patient's apprehension about the threat the problem represents. That too is part of the art of Medicine.

Then there is harm avoidance. Sometimes, psychoactive pharmaceuticals exist that alter feelings including depressed feelings and anxiety. However, the physician may recognize that these powerful drugs may not really be necessary as a starting point and might suggest other therapies that have some scientific support including periods of relaxation, diet and exercise (or a distraction like entertainment) to see if those might help. Another possibility is engaging the patient psychotherapeutically as a non-biological remedy for depressed feelings. When benign solutions fail it affirms that innocuous alternatives were not a solution and there is a basis for considering more aggressive, sometimes untested, options.

The patient might come into the office demanding a drug. The art of Medicine involves realizing when NOT to apply an intervention – and this is often based on the confidence developed through experience with like problems. Being steeped in the art of Medicine can give the physician the emotional fortitude and the personal confidence to work in the best interest of the patient and feel comfortable offering hopefully helpful advice when scientific evidence is missing. It can also help the patient to trust the physician and give the suggested approach a chance.

This will enable physicians to communicate the crucial message to patients that someone is there who is trying to help and on whom the patient can depend.

The Artistic Expertise of the Physician

Here's where it might be confusing. Is there such a thing as 'artistic expertise' and, if so, then how can we recognize it?

Artists develop the set of abilities that allow them to express what they want to communicate in the way they want. They live with the hope that someone will like their work or maybe will even experience the intended effect.

Political posters, for example those from the Russian Revolution, project what the viewer should feel and think. During the Revolution, the objective was to motivate the masses to work in industry or on collective farms. They portrayed 'supermen' and 'superwomen' working together using modern, powerful equipment. The same was done by the countries in World War 2, motivating people to buy bonds or forswear their butter and meat to feed the allies.

All art forms are like this. Artists create objects that communicate feelings or impressions – a goal that requires intellectual as well as manual skills. Making a great video requires understanding what people want, how they perceive and what will move them.

What are the types of artful expertise that physicians should develop, noting that not every physician might need to have the same set of capabilities, and some might be better at one than another?

Another message: much like different people appreciate different art forms, different artists or different examples of their work, so patients must think about what they like. What would make them feel the most comfortable and responsive? Some might prefer a 'dragon', others a Teddy Bear, others an Einstein, and still others an entertainer or Joe next door. And even artists differ on what constitutes excellent art.[17]

17 New York Times, October 12, 1997, ART; Is It Art? Is It Good? And Who Says So? By Amei Wallach. https://www.nytimes.com/1997/10/12/arts/art-is-it-art-is-it-good-and-who-says-so.html. Accessed August 24, 2022.

Expertise in the Art of Medicine –

Some of the different characteristics of the art of Medicine include (with no priority intended):

1. **Judgment.** This is the aspect of the art of Medicine that we have emphasized throughout the books. Not all Medicine is science. The consequence is that the gaps between the scientific components of Medicine and the existence of less well-based material must occur quite frequently. The physician must be able to bridge these gaps, based on experience, knowledge of physiology and personal creativity, while helping the patient despite no canonical pathway. The COVID-19 Pandemic required this aptitude because COVID initially presented with a bizarre and highly variable constellation of symptoms and signs. Physicians were often faced with the need to help mortally ill patients and simply had to try things. Only with experience did physicians became better and better at it, meaning that their patients did better and the mortality rate dropped. Experience certainly seems to change behavior and thinking. However, this change can sometimes be for the better, but sometimes for the worse – consider the note below.

> **Note:** *For experience to increase the effectiveness of diagnosis and treatment, there must exist a crucial co-factor: evaluation. Physicians or overseers must document their diagnoses and treatments and review what actually happens to patients over the longer term. To see the importance of this, reflect on blood-letting – the practice of bleeding patients that was common a few centuries ago. Physicians were personally convinced that this practice could help patients and took each experience as 'evidence' of success. Some patients were brought to the edge of the abyss or even over it by the practice. Luckily, some physicians and medical scientists eventually recognized that the practice was both ineffective and dangerous.*[18]

However, judgement is not the only application of the art of Medicine; there are other key artful aspects.

2. **Listening ability.** This type of expertise means that the physician has well-honed social skills and can stop, listen to what the patient is saying, make it clear what was heard and show comprehension. Listening skills are crucial in just about every form of professional relationship.
3. **Empathy.** This is the ability of the physician to palpably relate to what the patient is dealing with. Some people listen, but we may sense that they don't really understand or internalize what we said and its importance to us. The empathetic physician exhibits an evident emotional response that indicates appreciation for the patient's situation.
4. **Control-Adaptivity.** What we mean here is that the physician can understand what the patient needs in terms of forcefulness. Some patients may prefer being told what to do. Others may want options, information and advice and then time to think and decide. Different people prefer different levels of directivity. Sometimes it is comforting to be told what to do; other times we may need to absorb and reflect on what we have heard.
5. **Concern.** The physician may need to express this in a bipolar way, showing deeper concern with this one patient and minimal concern with another so as not to alarm the latter person.
6. **Creativity.** The opposite of the highly experienced physician might be a newbie who takes a 'fresh look' at a difficult situation and sees solutions the others' experiences blinded them to. Sometimes,

18 Greenstone, G., The History of Bloodletting, BCMJ, vol. 52, No. 1, January-February 2010, Pages 12-14. https://bcmj.org/premise/history-bloodletting. Accessed Oct. 8 2023.

the neophyte can make a unique contribution everybody else missed.

7. **Persistence.** If the patient has a complex problem or a vague array of symptoms, sometimes proceeding medically just takes a kind of doggedness. So, an important kind of expertise for physicians is never giving up, suspending frustration and trying harder and harder until, if possible, the solution is found.
8. **Kindness and humanity.** Sometimes the practice of Medicine becomes so grueling and frustrating that it is possible to forget that the patient is a fellow human who needs kindness and TLC. Being able to fight through defeatism, exhaustion, frustration and the pressures of practice and maintain the ability to relate as one human to another becomes crucial.

Of course, being facile in all of these would be somewhere between a dream and a superpower. These artful aspects of the practice of Medicine are in addition to all the factors that comprise medical competence. However, individual physicians will probably find themselves strong in some capabilities and weak in others. In other words, there is a spectrum of capabilities possessed by each physician or that is natural for the person to acquire.

The Message for Patients

Patients need to get a sense of these characteristics related to physicians on whom they depend. It may take a visit or two or it might involve speaking with a previous patient to find out what the physician is like. First, though, patients should think about which of these characteristics is crucial and which they can do without. The idea is finding a physician one can resonate with and achieve a synergistic relationship.

There are many studies indicating that patients have issues complying with therapeutic regimens. Non-compliant patients are those to whom the physician doles out advice or gives a prescription, but who don't fill the prescription or abandon it after a short time. Our hypothesis is that, if patients made assessments of physicians related to their artistry – assuming, of course, medical competence – they would be better able to benefit from their encounters. That might make it easier to be honest with their physicians, more thoughtful about their physicians' advice and recommendations, and more prone to comply with those recommendations or tell the physicians why they rejected them.

This is like art appreciation. The physician's approach to the patient is an art form. The patient's liking it or not is a personal choice. What's more, patients pay for it one way or another. Why should they not determine their preferences for the artistic aspects of physicians who care for them?

Chapter 5: Overview of Crucial Knowledge

KEYWORDS: The Nature of Health, The Purposes of Care, Measuring Health, Understanding Diagnosis, The Usefulness of Tests, Biomarkers, The Patient's Treatment Wager, Mental Health, The Health System, Medical Ethics, Complex Adaptive Systems.

ABSTRACT: This chapter is a brief overview of the key concepts necessary for the patient's participation in care and why that's important. Those concepts include understanding why and how to measure health, what tests are and are not, the patient's treatment choices and the nature and purposes of mental health care. The purposes of health care in general are to improve the patient's comfort, function, and longevity. The specific purposes of all mental health interventions are to influence how people think, feel and behave. We discuss briefly how health care is a complex adaptive system addressing the care of the human body, which is itself a complex adaptive system where minor changes can have major impacts.

The Big-Ten!

We promised to reveal the Big Ten Important Ideas.

There are ten crucial areas of knowledge people must have in order understand health care and to participate in their own care or that of others. These ten concepts are also fundamental to understanding and developing healthcare services and health information systems.

Idea 1: Understanding the Nature of Health and the Purposes of Health Care

People visit doctors for only five reasons. Firstly, they want to feel better, be able to do more and\or to live longer. They also see doctors in order to hear recommendations for actions to maintain and improve their healthiness. Finally, people visit clinicians for administrative reasons – they might need a doctor's note for getting or claiming on insurance, for having missed work, for having been absent from school, for entering a program or for traveling or immigrating to another country or region.

At every visit, doctors collect information about a patient's comfort and function and an objective or subjective estimate of their longevity. Health informaticians develop systems to use these measurements to learn if people were better or worse after treatment, thereby informing health system administrators and other decision-makers about how to improve the efficiency, interventions and results of care. They also develop systems to link health status and changes in health status with clinical or community interventions to help identify services that are appropriate.

Idea 2: Understanding Why and How to Measure Health

Chapters 23 to 25 discuss ways to measure health. We reveal how to systematically capture objective information about a patient's comfort, function, and other physical findings including the results of laboratory and imaging tests. Qualitative and quantitative information about symptoms (what a person feels), signs (objective measures from observing a patient or doing tests such as knee reflexes or walking speed) and findings (numeric and other results) from laboratory tests and diagnostic imaging may be used to estimate a person's current and future health, formulate a diagnosis, determine the chances that an intervention will succeed and what impact it may have on the patient.

Assessing the value of health system interventions on individuals and populations requires systematic collection of information about the health of a person or a population before and after the intervention, along with documentation of the intervention itself. We have to learn if, when and how what we do works: if what we do is good or bad. Health informaticians, information scientists and administrators should have the knowledge and skills required to specify how to capture and process pertinent information about the health of individuals and of communities before and after an intervention. This way they can learn which interventions are helpful, harmful or irrelevant. The information systems they put in place and use must collect data including about patient demographics and about comfort, function, other findings and community context.

Understanding health systems and how we collect and use information is important for communities that want excellent health care. We debated whether to present summary information about health systems first or information about clinical care first. We decided that everyone is familiar with some element of their health system and should have an understanding of the infrastructure that supports all health care in modern societies. However, evaluating the impacts of the healthcare system requires knowledge of the essential elements of clinical care. Therefore, we decided to discuss the clinical issues first. People who understand clinical care and the measurement of health outcomes are better able to understand if the health system they use is suitable or what kinds of changes would improve it.

Idea 3: Understanding Why and How to Make a Diagnosis

A diagnosis is an explanation or interpretation of the cause of a problem. Most problems have many possible diagnoses or interpretations. For example, there are at least 3,000 diagnoses associated with fatigue. The challenge for clinicians is to develop strategies that enable them to recognize not only common causes for a condition but also rare ones. Clinicians should use a variety of techniques to make sure that they have considered all possible causes of a problem before giving up the search. Many lists and computer programs are available that enumerate what might be causing any problem and the additional information necessary to confirm or disprove a cause. They may also suggest the most effective strategies (e.g., specific examinations or testing) to pinpoint the correct diagnosis.

Idea 4: Understanding Why and How to Evaluate the Usefulness of Tests

The observations from the physical examination of the patient and the findings from laboratory tests and imaging produce indicators of a person's health. Usually, these indicators are easy to interpret and suggest a specific health condition or diagnosis. However, occasionally, testing that should signal the presence of a disease does not and instead provides false reassurance that all is well. On the other hand, test results that should be normal might incorrectly suggest the presence of a condition that the patient does not have. False alarms in health care are like false alarms for detecting fire. A false alarm causes needless anxiety and might also result in harm. Just as a fire truck responding to a false fire alarm can be involved in an accident, so a patient can be harmed when a doctor follows up on a false alarm from a medical investigation. For example, a disease-free patient might suffer from a perforated bowel when undergoing a colonoscopy to follow up on an incorrect test result for blood in the stool (feces).

The chances of false reassurance or false alarms relate to the physical characteristics of the tests (sensitivity and specificity – discussed in the chapter on testing) – they are almost never perfectly accurate – and to the prevalence (frequency) of the condition in the population that is tested. This is easily understood by thinking about a fire alarm again. A fire alarm is more likely to be correct when indicating a fire in old dry wooden houses in an arid area than in the case of brick structure in a city with lots of rain. Similarly, a test result is more likely to be correct if it gives a positive result in an area with a high prevalence of the detected condition. To evaluate the predictive value of a test result, it is necessary to know not only the characteristics of the test, but also the frequency of the condition in the population being tested. Informaticians and epidemiologists acquire information about the frequency of diseases in various populations and regions and this helps in test result interpretation.

StatMed is a site that provides information about diagnoses and assists patients and clinicians in finding potential causes of a particular problem, and the tests necessary to confirm or disprove a diagnostic hypothesis.[19]

Idea 5: Knowing About Health Biomarkers

Biomarkers are a set of objective – the key word – findings that provide factual information about a person's health. Chapters 16, 21, 27 and elsewhere discuss various types of biomarkers. These objective indices point to one or more possible problems or diseases.

Idea 6: Understanding that Treatment Choice is a Kind of Wager

By accepting a treatment recommendation, a patient is effectively making a wager that the intervention will more likely be helpful than harmful. Almost every treatment helps many people but also harms some people.

The standard way of portraying risk of a medication, one that is hardly ever revealed to patients, is the combined 'Number Needed to Treat' (NNT) and of the 'Number Needed to Harm' (NNH). In other words, how many people, on average, must receive a treatment until one of those treated has benefitted, and how many people, on average, will receive a treatment until one among them will suffer harm?

The other important ideas are the distinction between relative risk reduction and absolute risk reduction. One way to understand these concepts is to consider pedestrians crossing the street. They can cross either at an intersection or they can jaywalk by crossing mid-block. Although the chances of getting hit by a car are remote, a person might be twice as likely to be hit when jaywalking in the middle of the block. By crossing at the intersection, your relative risk reduction is 50%; you are half as likely to be hit by a car. However, this might mean that for every 100,000 crossings at an intersection one person is struck, while for every 100,000 people jaywalking two people are struck. Your absolute risk reduction is quite

19 https://www.statmed.org/differential_diagnosis. Accessed August 24, 2022.

small! Based on the latter figure, most people would be unlikely to change their behavior. So reported relative risk reduction figures are confusing and likely to mislead…which the authorities may intend in this case. Later in the book we indicate examples of Numbers Needed to Treat, Numbers Needed to Harm, and relative and absolute risk reduction.

Treatments are usually meant to influence a defined condition. However, treatments may have unintended consequences. Consequently, measures of the effectiveness of treatments must include an estimate of how the treatment changes all-cause mortality (death) and morbidity (sickness or injury). A treatment that ablates a headache but is debilitating because it induces drowsiness, might or might not be worthwhile for a patient who operates large equipment. Knee surgery, which successfully cures a knee problem, but is associated with a stroke or other brain problems from the surgery or anesthetic, is not necessarily worthwhile.

Consequently, in evaluating interventions it is important to measure the impact of the treatment on overall health, as well as on the condition that was treated. The website E-HealthMe provides information about the frequency of adverse reactions and other information related to particular drugs.[20]

Idea 6: Understanding the Nature of Mental Health

Mental health has an influence on comfort, function, and lifespan. However, the unique purpose of mental health interventions, including those by psychiatrists, is to help influence the way people think, how they feel and how they behave. There are no other specific goals for mental health interventions.

Mood disorders (for example, depression or mania – excessive or inappropriate excitement or euphoria) describe abnormalities in how a patient feels; behavioral disorders (like psychopathic behavior, personality disorders) describe maladaptive behaviors; and thought disorders (e.g., schizophrenia) describe abnormal or unusual thinking.

Mental health problems can be categorized in 4 ways according to how much we know about the etiology or biological cause of the condition.

> Some mental health problems are caused by known biological abnormalities (for example thyroid or adrenal disease leading to mood disturbance or abnormal brain development leading to psychosis). When the biology is known, there are usually laboratory test results, for example, for thyroid or adrenal hormone or abnormalities revealed by imaging that can indicate the biological abnormality. Drug abuse can also cause biological abnormalities.

> Some mental health problems are hypothesized to be based on biology, but there is no objective evidence of a biological abnormality in the patient. Clinicians may use the term 'biochemical abnormality' or 'imbalance' to describe their belief in the cause of some conditions. When the biology is known the clinician will be able to identify the specific chemical or other biological problem that is causing the imbalance; without this, the belief is dubious at best.

> Some mental health problems are the normal consequence of the person's living conditions or context and lifestyle. For example, someone who eats poorly and never exercises is more likely to feel depressed compared to others who maintain fitness and eat healthy food. Some people may experience emotional turmoil because of the behavior of their community, friends or relatives. People

20 https://www.ehealthme.com/. Accessed July 14, 2022 Insert the name of a drug to get information about the reported frequency of various adverse reactions to the drug.

in these circumstances may develop mental health problems, such as feeling depressed, but there is no need to search for or speculate about a biological cause.

› Finally, there are mental health problems where clinicians do not know enough to even imagine if the causes are contextual, genetic or biologic. They are just in the realm of the unknown.

It is interesting to realize that medical (pharmaceutical) interventions may influence the thoughts feelings and behavior of everyone, including those who do not have any biological abnormalities. Getting a certain effect from a drug does not prove the existence of a specific abnormality.

Idea 7: Understanding Mental Health Treatments

Various medical and non-medical interventions influence thinking, feeling and behavior. Drugs can have these effects in people who have biological abnormalities and in people who have normal health. For example, diazepam is a relaxant, amphetamines usually energize people, and certain drugs, for example LSD, also have a profound influence on how people think and perceive. However, many other interventions, including diet and exercise, training and changing one's community context, also have these effects.

The section on mental health discusses the variety of interventions that humans use to influence the people around them (including friends, clients and patients). They include behavioral therapies that may use rewards and punishments, cognitive therapies, diet, exercise and, yes, drugs.

Idea 8: Understanding the Health System

People and health systems both are complex adaptive systems. An important feature of complex adaptive systems is that when one variable changes, other parts of the system may or may not change in simple ways as an adaptation to the new circumstance.[21 22]

In individual health, one example of an adapting system is the effect of modest amounts of alcohol on the liver. Liver enzymes detoxify poisons, and the same enzymes facilitate the elimination of drugs. People who drink modest amounts of alcohol (but not enough to significantly damage or destroy the liver) have an increased production of detoxifying enzymes. Consequently, and unexpectedly, mild to moderate drinkers also eliminate some drugs more quickly and consequently may require higher doses. The heart also has these characteristics, with multiple redundant components that ensure it keeps beating for many decades.

Idea 9: Understanding Why and How to Become the CEO of Our Health

Teaching and encouraging people how to become the CEOs of their own health is a crucial objective of this book. The reason this is crucial is that maintaining health and getting appropriate health care depends on each individual collaborating with care providers and being responsible for decisions that affect care. This is because health interventions, especially when one is sick but also when one is well, are imperfect and can potentially injure as well as help. The best way to get optimal care is to work with care providers in every aspect of

21 ALipsitz LA. Understanding Health Care as a Complex System: The Foundation for Unintended Consequences. JAMA: the journal of the American Medical Association. 2012;308(3):243-244. doi:10.1001/jama.2012.7551. https://www.ncbi.nlm.nih.gov/pmc/articles/PMC3511782/. Accessed August 24, 2022.

22 Bircher J, Hahn EG. Applying a complex adaptive system's understanding of health to primary care. F1000Research. 2016; 5:1672. doi:10.12688/f1000research.9042.2. https://www.ncbi.nlm.nih.gov/pmc/articles/PMC5043445/. Accessed August 24, 2022.

care. This book will teach about the realities of health, sickness and the interventions intended to return us to a healthy state. Hard decisions are sometimes required, but individual decision-making is always required. We are the masters of our bodies and cannot cede their care entirely to someone else.

Idea 10: Understanding Ethics in Health Care

History is awash with stories of how health maintenance, disease detection, intervention and end-of-life care can be used in ways that are not in people's interests but serve someone else. This can happen in many ways: a drug company may promote a drug it knows to be ineffective; a physician can effectively experiment with a patient without consent; care providers can accept financial or other considerations for prescribing an agent; and, in addition to many other ways, a provider can undertake unnecessary testing and treatment in order to make money. Matters like these are issues of right and wrong. Ethics involves a set of principles and codes of behavior that protect us from those who would take advantage of us.

We need to trust those who care for us and the system within which they work. Therefore, the Russian proverb must apply "doveryay, no proveryay" – "trust, but verify"!

Chapter 6: Misinformation Disease

KEYWORDS: The Nature of Information, Misinformation, Disinformation, Communication, White Lies, Avoiding Deception, Toxic Effects of Misinformation

ABSTRACT: Excellence in health care, including mental health care, relies on the use of accurate information. Sometimes groups have an incentive to fool or manipulate people and give them misleading advice. Insufficient information, for example about chances of benefit and harm from testing and treatment, is a form of information inadequacy.

Misinformation can kill and it has!

Virtually everyone today is concerned about the environment. Many now realize that pollution in the form of factory emissions, herbicides, plastics, x-ray and nuclear radiation and even ultraviolet light either directly cause or potentiate illnesses including breathing problems and cancers and even death. Worse still, their effects can be slow and insidious.

Some are also awakening to the realization that there is another kind of toxic emission that originates from fellow humans and is communicated person-to-person through the eyes and ears. This stuff can poison, cause personal and societal dysfunction and can also lead to early death. It can be a weapon of mass destruction, especially during a pandemic. It is contagious without even requiring personal contact, as its vector can be the telephone, the broadcast media and the Internet. Horribly, we are all vulnerable and there is not a 100%-effective vaccination. This clear and present danger is the contagion: **misinformation**.

Information in the Anthropocene Era

Over the last several decades, we have evolved means of communication that permit rapid and widespread dissemination of information from virtually anyone to anyone. In the past, the sources of information were few and traceable to an individual or organization whose credibility we could, in theory, validate. There were still malicious informers, for example authoritarian leaders and governments, that could emit virtually anything they wished to achieve whatever effect they wanted on their captive populations. It was, however, usually possible to pin down a source and to judge the basis for and quality of the information. Ordinary people had limited access to the channels of communication and rapid replication and dissemination of information was impaired by the nature and limitations of the available media. This is not to say that bad actors could not publish a deceitful book, broadcast propaganda, place fraudulent articles in newspapers or communicate false gossip over the telephone. However, limited access to the instruments of communication restricted the reach of an individual, and the effort and cost of dissemination were somewhat onerous. That is no longer true. Personal computerized devices together with Facebook, Twitter and other social media, the World Wide Web, the Internet and countless other tools have given every person a 'bully pulpit' of sorts. They have removed many of the constraints that previously inhibited the spread of messages and they have enabled almost anyone to reach almost everyone.

Elsewhere in this book, we discuss accessing high quality, professionally vetted health information. In that material we point out that anyone can produce or access information, including what amounts to information manure. Here we wish to emphasize the nature of misinformation and the damage it can inflict on the unwary.

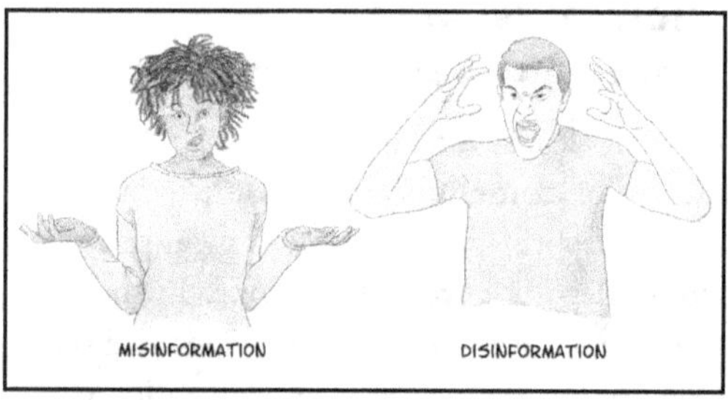

FIGURE 1.6.1: Misinformation may confuse; disinformation manipulates

Types of Misinformation

Misinformation comes in many forms. See FIGURE 1.6.1. Perhaps recognizing the face of evil will help avoid it.

Misinformation can be **Innocent Misstatements**, where people garble fact. It can be unintentionally misquoted data, the unaudited conclusions of a study or just the result of misunderstanding. Innocent Misstatements can also be the unintentional biproduct of confusion – a person or organization might misconstrue material. It can sometimes be in the form of an opinion a bit twisted by bias or a topic 'spun' by a politician. These are the expected and largely inevitable artifacts of ordinary human beings. Generally, they are not malicious, though sometimes manipulative – after all, we do want others to affirm or even adopt our opinions! We are all flawed, so flawed output is not surprising. However, we must be aware of this and always wonder if assertions or claims are valid.

A greater problem avails when someone wishes to pervert another's thinking or acting through **Intentional Misrepresentations** (or **Disinformation**) so as to serve the informant's own interests at the other's expense or jeopardy. Even this has more innocent versions, for example, when a politician or a braggard makes statements to denigrate an opponent or to self-aggrandize...after all, how many times have you seen the word 'aggrandize' without the word 'self'! There are, however, more nasty effects at the extreme of the spectrum. We might think about these further varieties of maliciousness so we understand them and can take steps to avoid their consequences.

Consider deliberately **Mind-altering Misinformation** – the social equivalent of psychoactive drugs. People promulgate this kind of information to cause another individual to think in ways that totally serve the purveyor or ideologically bias the receiver. They are usually at the other's expense and can be injurious or socially damaging to the receiver. These people are taking steps to alter others' thinking or decision-making. One example is when perpetrators deliberately and fraudulently undermine reliable sources of valid information. This can be done by denigrating an agency (for example, the CDC or FDA), a publisher (for example, a recognized peer reviewed journal or a media source) or an individual (for example a respected scientist). The objective may be to destroy confidence in the sources of good information and to permit substituted questionable sources and material ("alternate facts") to reach targeted populations.

Another malicious intervention is to create false information directly: **Manufactured**

Mis-evidence. This is the equivalent of distributing a false medication – one the promises one effect but has another or none. It can involve promoting false concepts, fraudulent misrepresentation of test results or the manufacturing of falsified data. Fraudster companies or scientists have created some misinformation of this type to benefit themselves financially or otherwise. Perhaps the best example is the work of a researcher who claimed to have created an artificial trachea (the swallowing tube) and published falsified data demonstrating success – when, in reality, all implants failed, and the recipients died.[23] Another, non-medical, example is the fraud perpetrated by Volkswagen related to the emissions of their diesel engines.[24] The company installed software that reduced emissions during engine testing. This was a criminal act, and this type of thing does recur from time to time – even scientists are humans and share human foibles.

The more common sources of misinformation are people who traffic in conspiracy theories. We can consider these **Fake Medicine** or **Fake Therapy**. Many have proposed and promoted theories of the causes of disease cause or the effects of treatment with no scientific basis, often claiming that reputable science ignored them because their unconventional schemes would undermine mainstream, legitimate producers' profitability. People of this ilk either harbor fundamental misconceptions or have one or other deeply held position they wish to promote and/or profit from. Of course, they may just be trying to fool people. Whatever their intention or motivation, they either dream up things themselves or build on the bogus edifice of unorthodox predecessors. Medical examples include the 'antivaxxers,' who claim that vaccinations cause injury (such as Autism), represent a means to control people or are an attempt to restrict personal freedom (claimed regarding mandates to wear masks in the COVID pandemic). These theories are often highly intricate – sometimes mixing in genuine science that appears supportive – and shared with a network of like-minded individuals. They thrive in echo chambers and seem to be strengthened by resonance with others. The Internet and the World Wide Web provide an echo chamber without walls!

Misinformation can just be the attractive outer packaging of a commercial product. Let's call that **White Lie Packaging**. Sellers attempt to convince possible buyers to put cash on the barrelhead and buy whatever it is. They make statements intended to catalyze purchasing and they care a little or not at all if their product helps or harms consumers. Sometimes this might be relatively innocent misinformation, like that a product will strengthen your teeth or ablate your wrinkles. At other times, the misinformation can have lethal effects. One needs only to look back a few years to recall that cigarette advertisers claimed smoking would improve lung function – but science proved it can kill. Somewhat longer ago a company used cocaine in their soft drink and, when that became illegal, substituted nearly toxic levels of caffeine.[25] One of the great public health horrors was the dietary supplement (Radiothor[26]) that contained radium and killed or injured many people.

The problem with the latter type of misinformation is that it can be difficult to determine if it results in harm. For example, a company can advertise a product that decreases an unpleasant symptom, like pain, which may be signifying an underlying problem like cancer. Today, the FDA and other agencies demand that pharmaceutical companies at least state some of the major side effects of their products

23 https://www.sciencemag.org/news/2018/06/macchiarini-guilty-misconduct-whistleblowers-share-blame-new-karolinska-institute. Accessed July 22, 2022.

24 https://www.bbc.com/news/business-34324772. Accessed July 22, 2022.

25 https://en.wikipedia.org/wiki/Coca-Cola. Accessed July 22, 2022.

26 https://en.wikipedia.org/wiki/Radithor. Accessed July 22, 2022.

and when using them can cause a problem. Even this can be circumvented in an ad by not specifying the drug's target or by 'creatively' wording a major impact. A good example of the latter is where companies advertising products that suppress the immune system fail to indicate that this exposes patients to the possibility of flourishing infections or even the possible spread of existing cancers.

Perhaps the worst form of misinformation is the promotion of ignorance, or **Ignorance Therapy**. As we are writing this book, senior national leaders are claiming that reducing testing for the SARS-Cov-2 virus would somehow improve the situation, i.e., that lack of information about how many and which people are infected would make the situation look better and reduce public concern. However, many other examples exist where governments, corporations or institutions are silent or downplay information about genuine dangers. Toxic substances have been kept under wraps, known problems (like Lead in the water system[27]) have gone unmentioned, or radioactive radon gas emanating from building foundations[28] has been ignored. All of these and many others leave people uninformed, unaware and unconcerned. They are a kind of mental anesthetic. This is probably the most dangerous and insidious form of malignant misinformation. What is interesting is that that lack of information is the ultimate contagion, as we all are immersed in it and effortlessly and unknowingly share it. It is worse than communicable. It is already in all of us!

It is also worth considering that there can be **Misinformation Epidemics** with the spread of false or biased information within a region or a country and **Misinformation Pandemics** that can circle the world. The R_0 of the misinformation would vary enormously based on its source (e.g., a President or global organization), the transmission method (for example TV) and the susceptibility of the population (like people ravenous for support of their biases). Intervention is challenging and may need to be planet-level! As often is the case, the best intervention would be a prepared mind and critical thinking. Given the plethora of irrational believers and their bizarre beliefs, it is wise to mentally vaccinate yourself now! There are no negative side effects of that vaccine.

Dealing with Misinformation

We have become an information society, founded on agencies, companies and social networks that are information dependent and both copious information sources and information channels. The potential for misinformation is enormous and it easily reaches into our homes and our individual lives. We have embedded, direct and efficient channels for misinformation. If we think that we only get the correct information or that just some of it is wrong or a little-off and won't harm us, we are naïve! Almost any misinformation is a danger, and its effects can be subtle and slow acting. Think heavy metals (like Arsenic or Lead) in your water supply as an analogy. Worse still is the absence of good information. Intentional and malicious information deprivation is akin to depriving a person of a key dietary nutrient... it can impair, injure or kill!

To drive home the latter point, consider the act of breathing. Our atmosphere is about 20% Oxygen and we need it to sustain life. Being deprived of Oxygen, for example during diving or holding our breath, is something we feel viscerally, as the approach of suffocation is a scary experience. However, the body does not feel like it is suffocating if we substitute pure Nitrogen for the normal atmospheric mixture of Oxygen and Nitrogen or if we are in very high-altitude conditions (low Oxygen pressure). A person will only lose consciousness,

27 https://www.nrdc.org/stories/flint-water-crisis-everything-you-need-know. Accessed July 22, 2022.

28 http://www.waterkeeper.ca/blog/2016/11/8/what-you-need-to-know-about-the-port-hope-area-radioactive-waste-cleanup. Accessed July 22, 2022.

feeling nothing and passing out, until oblivion. This is what it is like if we are uninformed. We can die of it!

Solutions for the Information-Threatened

To avoid the threats of all the varieties of misinformation disease, we must become **Information Fit.**

Information is the basis for virtually everything we do, think, feel and decide. It is everywhere and pervades and serves as the foundation for everything. To function and thrive in our information society, we must:

1. **Find and use reliable information sources.** Make sure that information is from reputable, preferably vetted and trustworthy agents, organizations and other authoritative sources.
2. **Always ask questions and get cogent answers** regarding the information that even comes from purportedly reliable sources. An important question is: Does what I have heard, read or seen make sense? Does it comport with what I already know?
3. **Determine if information has been peer reviewed** and by whom. That is a crucial check. Peer review (the careful evaluation of the methods, results and interpretation of research by qualified experts) is the 'good housekeeping seal of approval' for valid information.
4. **Crosscheck or triangulate multiple sources** – trusting only one source or evaluator is risky.
5. **Decide if you actually believe what you have seen or heard**. In other words, can I look at the foundations for the information and use my own thinking to get to the same point? This means more deeply understanding whatever it is and that means becoming knowledgeable. This is the personal quality check and acceptance test.
6. **Always harbor a healthy skepticism!** Never say "uncle" to information or an information source! Only trust after you verify! Don't take assurance as an answer. Always foster a doubt and be curious to find the truth.

HONESTY IS THE BEST POLICY...BUT

How many bakers say: "That bread is stale" (particularly when it is)? How many used car salespeople say: "I wouldn't buy that lemon!" (Especially when it is a post-accident chimera)? How many drug dealers mention: "That hit is contaminated with fentanyl" (even though it is and with other goodies too)? How many TV personalities say: "This isn't worth watching" (right after making fools of themselves)? How many authors say: "Don't believe everything I write" (when that would be proper advice)? This should remind you to apply this to what we state in this book. Find out for yourself! Verify!

Chapter 7: Learning About Health

KEYWORDS: Knowledge, Learning, Just In Time Learning, Just In Case Learning, Comprehension

ABSTRACT: Clinical trainees and the rest of us rely on two types of learning. Just In Time (JIT) learning means understanding basic concepts, the building blocks of knowledge, so that the learner knows what to look for and how to interpret the information they find. Just In Case (JIC) learning, used heavily during medical school training, means hearing about various conditions, trying to learn and remember those conditions, just in case you encounter them at some later date. Unfortunately, over the years clinicians forget rare conditions, ones they heard about in medical school, but seldom see in practice. Just In Time learners look to the literature to find plausible causes and treatments for difficult problems.

Introduction

Some might fear the effort involved in learning about medical subjects. They think of all the seemingly complicated stuff about the body and mind, health and sickness, drugs and other interventions, the nature of the enormous health system and what exactly doctors do. We get it!

Despite any apprehension you might have, we can assure you that your effort in learning about health and health care will not be insuperable or even very challenging. Furthermore, the result will give you pleasure and has the potential to empower you, your students and others you affect. Even more importantly, the effort will bring to light a Fountain of Truth that will protect people, their families and their friends! The reality is that learning about health and health care is simply not difficult. In fact, you will be surprised by how easy it is.

Let's address the effort required. How can we go about what seems like a huge learning task?

Well, the first step is to realize that it isn't daunting! We sometimes see a mountain when what is before us is a set of molehills! It's all perspective! If we perceive ourselves as puny – having inadequate knowledge or ability to acquire it – and being way down there in the grass, a molehill looks like a mountain. The trick is to realize that we are much bigger and more capable. Then the molehills look like, well, molehills.

The topics we address do involve some science and scientific thinking and some may produce a vague sense of discomfort – particularly given all those strange or even exotic words. And, you may have been misinformed that health care is the sole domain of healthcare professionals. Not true!

Perhaps some will even face a barrier because they see the human body as mysterious, find some of its parts somewhat discomfiting and might think that understanding how the body works requires an MD or even a PhD.

Similarly, we might see the healthcare system, despite frequently interacting with it, as an immense and inscrutable enterprise – it is one of the most complex organizations created by homo sapiens – and think that understanding it might require a credential in Healthcare Administration or an MBA.

There is also the problem of getting one's head around the huge human enterprise that makes up the system. It is a diverse ecology of professionals – what the heck is a pediatric oncologist or a cardiothoracic surgeon, anyway – each having individually sophisticated roles and seemingly of a different ilk from anyone familiar. Agreed. It can seem that way, but none of it is beyond a relatively small investment of time and a bit of effort to read. That will clarify everything and reveal its nature, its beauty and its value.

Learning the key stuff is easy. The essential material is in the pages of this book. How can and should we undertake the effort to access that value that will enrich us?

For those harboring a sense or foreboding, we will suggest approaches to learning material like this that will help the reader acquire an asset useful throughout life.

Some Learning Tactics as Parts of a Learning Strategy

Many of us experienced in our formal education the bad effects of the forcing of knowledge into our heads. How often was it that teachers subjected us to learning a lot of what are called 'basics', perhaps for years, before we knew what they applied to and what they would enable us to do? It is unfortunate that our education system tends to make learning overwhelming and even painful by presenting information in a way almost diametrically opposed to efficient learning.

In fact, our education systems would be a lot more capable and effective if they first provided a holistic overview of what it was we were learning about, explained the relevance of the different kinds of knowledge we would need to delve into areas of focus, then explained which basics were crucial, and only then addressed the details. This approach is especially apropos, as the Psychology literature on learning and memory clearly tells us that it is usually easier to remember meaningful material compared with trying to remember seemingly unrelated facts. 'Meaningful material' means new stuff that is correlated with what we already know and that we can integrate with our existing knowledge. That's practically the opposite of what many of us have endured.

A holistic overview of health care would tell us about what 'health' really means and would show how it can be achieved, improved and maintained. This book follows exactly this approach.

To get this holistic overview, all you will need to do is start at the beginning of the book. You do not have to learn Greek and Latin to understand all the words, or to become a doctor to comprehend all the processes we address, including medical thinking and decision-making. And you certainly don't need that to appreciate all the parts of the healthcare system and their functions.

The same is true about the human body and what it's like in sickness and health. It is possible to just read about it to get the entire point. There is no need for memorization, notes, index cards or any of the other paraphernalia of classic learning. It is best to read this kind of material like a novel – none of the accouterments of detailed learning are involved when reading stories. To make the material even more story-like, we have included real-life accounts that should attract your attention and interest you. We have even incorporated some fun stuff – though, admittedly, real comedy is above our pay grade!

We have suggested a strategy for approaching material like this to our students: consider your own health issues or those of family members or friends and pick out topics that you feel are personally relevant. This may work for you too. It is curiosity driven, and curiosity is probably the best stimulant for undertaking the effort of learning.

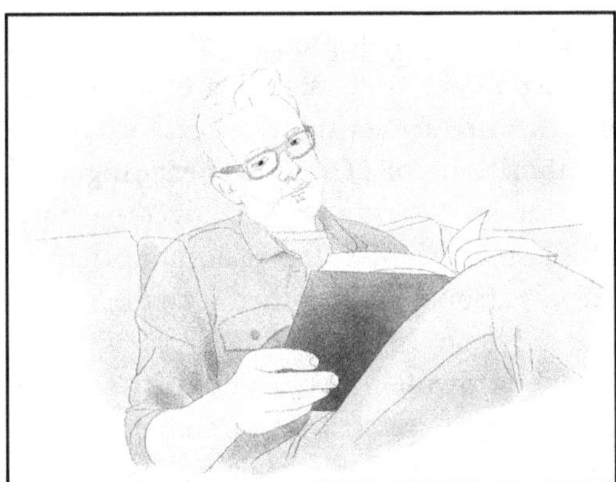

FIGURE 1.7.1: Becoming competent regarding health requires learning

Specific Tactics

To begin learning, we need to be aware of the 'lay of the land,' the major topics and the issues. Learning is crucial – FIGURE 1.7.1 makes that point. This is like looking at the map and getting an idea of what is on it, like cities, towns, rivers, distances and perhaps altitudes. We will call this level of learning **'Awareness-Learning.'** For example, we will try to make you aware of some of the major systems of the body, the significant components of the health system and the key aspects of health, sickness and health care. We will make you conscious of topics such as symptoms, signs and testing; physician-patient inquiry and examination, diagnosis, treatment and the effects of treatment. At various points we will mention some of the details but there is no reason to memorize these.

The point of Awareness-Learning is that you do not need to know the details at this time. Understanding that there is something called diagnosis and having a general idea of what it involves is all you really need. You can just read about the topics, get an idea of what they involve and, later, look at them more carefully when you need to. In other parts of the book, you can find the key details, so there is herein a lot more than a shallow overview. Think of this like enjoying a 'tasting menu' that you can later follow by a meal. The whole meal is there and, of course, there are many other sources of knowledge you can tap into to learn more if you want to or have to.

The next learning tactic we will call **'Osmotic-Learning'** – our term, osmosis being a process of passive perfusion, like through a membrane.[29] The idea is to use this as you pursue awareness of topics.

Osmotic-Learning involves minimizing distractions, reading material without parsing it intimately and simply letting it soak in. Schools tend to make learning more like a discipline, but we see learning more as immersion, like in a hot tub, relaxing and enjoyable. Most of the material in this book is very suited to this approach. Rather than reading this like a classic textbook, you may find it better to skip around driven by a bit of curiosity. You can find topics that turn your crank, that you enjoy or that pique your sense of wonder. Typically, we read textbooks end-to-end. That is not necessary here and it would likely wear most people down. There is not a huge dependence of one section of the book on another and only a loose reliance of certain chapters on each other. So, the book is amenable to this approach. The more you just enjoy it, the more it will soak in!

Another type of learning (addressed briefly elsewhere in the book) is related to when you learn. We define the term **'Just-in-Case Learning,'** which is very typical of the classic approach to teaching, to mean that you learn lots of stuff just in case it might be helpful. However, it may not be helpful for a while, by which time it may be forgotten or hazy at best. Many of us have had that experience with wonderful topics like integral calculus, mechanical advantage, trigonometry or certain philosophical concepts. Our schools are almost entirely dedicated to just-in-case learning, so we expect

29 https://words.usask.ca/gmcte/2013/07/31/learning-through-osmosis/. Accessed July 12, 2022. https://blog.lifescitrc.org/pecop/2015/02/16/is-learning-by-osmosis-real/. Accessed July 12, 2022.

students to shovel in vast amounts of detail. No wonder they need to take notes, as this at least is something they can go back to if they ever find it necessary to recall the details, other than to pass the course exam. That's the problem with Just-in-Case learning. It is just about impossible to undertake that mode of learning related to the topics we will address. Of course, medical schools make a practice of doing precisely that: pre-loading medical students' minds with huge masses of stuff and expecting them to recite it all back and remember it when they need it in practice. The truth is they only really learn most of it when they use it over and over again. They will only fully grasp and make it a part of themselves when they have the time and opportunity to apply it.

There is also **'Just-in-Time Learning.'** JIT (Just In Time) has become a popular tactic in managing the supplies' inventories for manufacturing. It minimizes inventories and therefore is economically sweet. Just-in-time learning means that we learn details when we need them. It is largely the way for all of us to go related to broad and multifaceted topics, like the content of this book. The exception would be those who have to deal with problems on an immediate basis where time is of the essence, like caring for a patient with obstructed breathing, or being responsible for landing an aircraft. That is not the typically case for our readership.

What this means is that we need to learn just enough so we comprehend at least the basic ideas – think of this as learning how to read a map and use it – and then we go into greater depth when the moment for applying or wanting the information is at hand. The wonders of today's technology – computers, workstations, the Internet and the World Wide Web, have made Just-in-Time Learning easy! When we know what to ask, we can find the answers.

The **Learning-Strategy** we suggest for absorbing what's in the book would be to apply these individual tactics in series or in parallel, topic-by-topic towards the goal of getting a deep understanding of health and health care. To start, we suggest using the combination of **Osmotic-Learning** and **Awareness-Learning** to skim over the material, noticing topics that seem important or are of personal interest then tuck them away and move on. In a few of the areas, it probably is worthwhile to use a bit of **Just-in-Case Learning** to create a bit of a mental structure and to understand key points. Finally, when it is appropriate, time is available to go deeper or questions or situations arise, apply the **Just-in-Time** tactic.

THINKING ABOUT THE HUMAN EYE

Is the eye really relevant here? Well, give us a little time and we will make a point.

Evolution is both the great enabler and the great leveler. Species and functionality arise because of an advantage that is gained through biological change and reproduction. As a rule, useful capabilities survive and develop, while useless capabilities disappear like dead leaves or become vestigial features like the bones of the hand in a whale's fins. What evolution has delivered in the human eye may provide a useful lesson to guide how we learn.

The eye is what the brain uses to see. When we look at a scene, we see a lot that is not truly clear and will only become clear if we gaze directly at it, enabling us to see detail. We have 'peripheral vision' that allows us to take in the whole scene, and we have 'central vision' that allows us to see detail. This central portion of the eye is the 'fovea'. We see what surrounds the detail using the rest of the retina – not nearly as high resolution as the fovea. As we look out the window, we may notice motion at the periphery of our vision signaling that a flying creature is there. Then we look in that direction and see that it is a colorful bird with shape and movements that reveal it is a hummingbird and not a butterfly.

In a certain sense, evolution has not 'wasted the effort' of evolving dense arrays of sensor cells throughout the entire retina but has 'economically' produced the fovea. This does require that, on seeing something at the periphery, we must adjust the direction of our gaze to discern what it is.

The entirety of this book is a scene. Each section is a scene, and each chapter is a scene. Switching your attention or gaze to details when something 'catches your eye' of attention, would be optimal. Your mind's eye will notice the equivalent of 'flying creatures' and then you can examine them in detail... and there are lots of 'intellectual hummingbirds' in this tome.

Our suggestion is that you look at the content of this book with a kind of peripheral intellectual vision and then choose those areas of focus that attract your attention.

A Structure for Organizing What You Learn

We mentioned it is worthwhile to create a bit of a structure. We have some suggestions in that regard:

1. **That you conceptualize the parts of the body around the idea of your skeleton.** You can give each part of the skeleton your own name. You don't have to use medical or anatomical terms; it is just useful to be able to recognize them. You can give each organ a name as well. As you think about the parts of the body, think about where they would be relative the skeleton. So, the brain would be in the head, the stomach in the middle of the body called the abdomen, the kidneys also in the abdomen but at the back. It is completely unnecessary to worry about the actual terminology, as we will typically give both versions in the text.
2. **As you think about dysfunction in movement, for example, you don't have to know the Latin words for all of the body parts that can move and how they move.** It's easy enough to consider that almost all joints only flex or extend (except for the shoulder and hip that swing). Abnormal joint function or abnormal movement may result from abnormalities in the joint, in the ligaments that connect the bones, in the muscles around the joint, in the connection (tendons) of the muscles to the bones, in the blood supply or the nerve supply to the muscles, in the skin and other tissues surrounding the muscles or from an infection or other problem in the joint or the tissues around the joint. That's it! You don't need to regurgitate their names for an Anatomy exam!
3. **You can think about the health system in a similar way**, with the physician's office at the top of the healthcare body, hospital below that much like the relationship between the head of the abdomen and all the other components of the health system serve like arms and legs. Within each part of the health system, conceptualize them just like the parts of the body. Psychiatric or mental care corresponds to the brain, Cardiology (the study of the heart) corresponds to the position of the heart, Gastroenterology corresponds to the abdomen, and so on.
4. **We can view what goes on in the clinician's office like water (information) flowing through a pipe or cable.** It comes in from the patient who reports symptoms, moves to the physician who notices signs, does investigations and forms diagnoses, continues with treatment and exits at the results of the treatment (outcomes).
5. **As you learn about specific diseases or problems**, relate them back to the parts of the body and to the loci of where the health system deals with them.
6. **Consider care as a system.** When it does not seem to be working well, consider the incentives that apply to each component. Are those incentives aligned and coordinated? Are parts of the system rewarded for doing unnecessary

or harmful work? Is the system's 'brain' working – do the parts know what each other part is doing, if it's working and is it all working together just like we expect from our body parts? Do the parts of the health system and the community that depends on it know if the health system as a whole is helping people to improve? How many people experience benefit or harm? How long do people have to wait for care and is that appropriate? Just as the body knows if one part is hurting, and the senses provide feedback about how close a runner is to the finish line, so the health system needs sensors and a 'brain' (managers and administrators) to ascertain and assess its actions and accomplishments.

7. **When we deal with mental health in detail, think about the difference between the brain, a physical organ, and the mind, which only exists when the brain is alive.** The mind does not have a separate existence and we cannot properly treat or repair either a damaged brain or a damaged mind without dealing with the other, but each with the interventions appropriate to it. We must address each directly.

8. **Finally, in thinking about either the function of the health system or of the body, recognize that the key is doing things that will help them and not harm them**, measuring what we do to the health system or the body and assessing the effects we have had and whether or not we have improved things. The principle of Hippocrates rules: do no harm! That is the bottom line!

Simplicity is Crucial!

Whatever you do, keep it simple! We have tried to do that with the content of the book. Don't believe that it is difficult to understand, hard to remember or essential that you be able to regurgitate it.

Our objective is for readers to achieve a sense of comfort with the knowledge in the book and a basic understanding of the nature of each topic with which we deal. They should do this with the realization that nothing humans do is perfect and, therefore, it is essential that we measure and assess whatever we do. There are simply no guarantees that the incredible investment in health and health care is actually worth it. We must discover through studies that objectively examine and measure what the investment achieves.

Our primary objective is your understanding and we both trust that you share this objective and will achieve it.

VOLUME 1

Section 2

THE MEANING OF HEALTH

MEDICAL WORDS

There are many unusual and unfamiliar words in Medicine and some may be a little difficult to remember. Here are a few dumb puns to help:

Ophthalmology: Ophthalmologists agree with their patients: they always see eye to eye.

Gastroenterology: (Gastroenterologists specialize in the intestines and stomach, also called the 'alimentary tract.') Dr. Sherlock, a GI Specialist, was asked by Dr. Watson: "That patient is quite sick; what's wrong with him?" Dr. Sherlock replied: "That alimentary, Dr. Watson!"

Dermatology: Dermatologists deal with diseases of the skin. It is a well-established fact that they make many rash judgements.

Psychiatry: Psychiatrists are called "head shrinkers," but they really are mind expanders!

Infectious Disease: What do you think, Dr. Shakespeare? Dr. Shakespeare: "TB or not TB, that is the question."

A Story: Health is in the Mind of the Beholder

Every culture values health. Governments and individuals spend lavishly to alleviate illness, to maintain health and avoid disease. In most communities, healthcare systems, doctors, nurses and other clinical experts devote themselves to helping the sick. In developed societies, and increasingly in developing societies, governments spend large amounts on the determinants of health. Communities try to implement proper sanitation and ensure clean water, provide access to nutritious food, develop adequate housing and avoid air pollution and contaminated food.

All of us who spend lots of time and our hard-earned money on health would like to know if our contributions of time and treasure make a positive difference, harm us, or are merely wasted.

To understand the effect of interventions, it is necessary to assess their impacts on both physical and mental health. The old and classical World Health Organization (WHO) definition claims that health is *"a state of complete physical, mental and social well-being and not merely the absence of disease or infirmity"*. When you read Section 4 on measuring health, you will see why this definition is not particularly useful. However, the WHO definition clearly emphasizes the importance of physical, mental and social well-being as well as disease and infirmity.

Each of us has some limitations in our mental and physical capacities. Consider David:

David, 78-year-old man complains that, despite the absence of pain and reasonable motion for all usual activities, his hip flexibility is insufficient, and he laments that he can no longer easily mount his bike using an efficient scoot and run method. On the other hand, Mary, a 42-year-old former runner, had a below the knee amputation as a consequence of a motor vehicle accident. She has a mild disability, her capabilities affected by the amputation, but a cane and sometimes a wheelchair restore some mobility, and Mary, having adjusted to the amputation, reports that she is in excellent health.

The important lesson is to recognize that isolated elements and measures of illness and disability may be insufficient to make a judgement about overall health. When clinicians suggest an intervention, for example to help a painful or dysfunctional knee, patients must inquire if more aggressive intervention makes sense. More dramatic interventions sometimes include surgery and anaesthesia, and these might have an adverse effect on other body systems. It may be better, depending on the amount of pain and disability, to adjust to being reasonably good than to pursue its enemy: perfection!

Chapter 8: The Meaning of Health

KEYWORDS: Definition of Health, WHO Definition of Health, Meaning of Health, Meaning of Sickness, Physical Health, Emotional Health, The Dimensions of Health

ABSTRACT: The World Health Organization (WHO) definition of health recognizes physical health, emotional health and feelings of well-being. The definition is valuable because it recognizes that health is not just the absence of physical illness. However, the WHO definition is not useful because a strict interpretation implies that no one is healthy. Definitions focusing on the dimensions of health are more useful because they support measuring changes in health associated with care and estimating health at any time, before, during or after care.

Resorting to the Dictionary

Looking up words like health and healthy, sick and sickness in the dictionary will show that these terms are ambiguous and often circular. The Oxford and Merriam-Webster dictionaries define 'health' as the condition of a person's body or mind and the state of being physically and mentally healthy, as well as the condition of being sound in body, mind, or spirit. They define 'Healthy' as having good health and not likely to become ill or being in a good physical or mental condition or in good health. They define 'sick' as being physically or mentally ill, affected with disease or ill health or being mentally or emotionally unsound or disordered. 'Sickness' is illness, bad health or an unhealthy condition of body or mind.

We discuss later that the World Health Organization (WHO) defines health as "*a state of complete physical, mental and social well-being and not merely the absence of disease or* infirmity."

The problem is that all these definitions are quite uninformative, as, after all, what does "the condition of being sound in body, mind or spirit" mean? How can we use it to learn if treatments help or harm?

Moreover, all too often people disagree about whether to call someone sick or healthy. Is an amputee who has full function with the aid of a prosthetic or a wheelchair healthy or sick? Is an elite athlete with mild kidney disease healthy or sick? Does it matter? Does defining someone as healthy or sick help solve particular mental or physical problems or do the labels sidetrack us from identifying and treating the problem? What matters is what people seek and, generally, that is comfort, function and longer lives. Labels can be a problem and don't necessarily help.

Throughout this book we oft repeat that the dimensions of health are comfort, function and lifespan. This is a useful and easily remembered mantra, but let's analyze what it means.

Sensing our Health

We have a feeling or sense of our health in each moment of life. It is an existential aspect of all our lives. Whenever we reflect on how we feel, or we hear those around us say how bad or how well they feel, it reinforces this. It is crucial to recognize that we all experience our health holistically (as a total integrated being) and seem to do it instantaneously, sometimes with only moments separating "I feel good" from "I feel awful."

It helps to note that our sense of our health is relativistic. If we have felt good and suddenly have a headache or crush a toe, we immediately go from feeling well to feeling badly. A person experiencing the throes of chemotherapy might one day say: "I feel bad" and another day say: "I feel good" or "I feel better," referencing the surround of the unpleasant effects of treatment.

What confounds things is that feeling healthy is different from being healthy. It's somewhat obvious that a person with an undetected cancerous tumor may feel perfectly fine. On the other hand, a person enduring a serious illness may feel fine today but didn't feel okay yesterday or won't tomorrow. Feeling healthy does not mean being healthy!

What Does it Mean to be Healthy Versus to be Sick?

Is being healthy just the opposite of feeling sick? Well, the answer is no! We can have something physically wrong with our bodies without knowing it. So, we aren't healthy, but we don't feel sick. Sick is, to all of us, a state of feeling badly. It can be that when something is bodily wrong, we feel it – like an intestinal infection that causes abdominal cramps or pain. But we can actually be sick and feel totally well. Even more confusing, is that we can feel badly (sick) even if nothing is physically wrong – we are suffering from mental or emotional discomfort or even just a fear that something is wrong.

The fact that something is wrong or the fact that nothing is wrong with our bodies we will call the factual aspect of health.

However, the reality of pathology or its absence is not the full story of health.

We are sentient or 'feeling' organisms. However, even more importantly, we both feel and understand. Sometimes this understanding can make us feel differently from what we would feel if we were objective about reality, like when we feel perfectly fine although something is amiss in our bodies or we feel bad even when everything is ok.

To understand this issue, consider a pet. It's amazing to realize that what we see as an injury may not impair Rex's basic functions and or even bother him. A veterinarian friend says that dogs have 3 legs and a spare – recognizing that amputation does not hold them back from doggy behavior and a lot of tail-wagging. Cats are another example. They may have badly diseased teeth (horribly commonplace) but seem to ignore the problem. We humans, however, understand what having diseased teeth means and we feel a threat the dog does not experience. This threat makes a dental infection carry much more impact (a psychic component to pain can dramatically enhance it!) because of our understanding. Health promotion and prevention agencies spend a great deal of time, effort and money trying to get us to understand that smoking, for instance, is doing damage to our bodies despite the pleasures of smoking. They are trying to make us understand – thereby affecting or recruiting the psychic component – the danger despite our feelings of pleasure and healthiness. So, one aspect of being healthy is our understanding of the threats to health and making them palpable to our consciousness. Humans feel more – and feel more correctly – healthy when they know more.

Our emotional state is also an aspect of our health. If we are depressed, we will not tend to take on challenging new problems or activate ourselves. On the other hand, if we are manic, we may attempt to do things that are injurious or even life-threatening. Our state of mind affects our health, even when this has no physical basis, and our health influences our state of mind.

Our understanding and our emotional state comprise what we will call the mind or mental aspect of health. It encompasses our thinking and feeling about our health. We will later encapsulate these in the word 'comfort.'

A second aspect of health is how health affects what we can do. An arthritic knee joint may impair our ability to walk. Similarly, an obstruction to our breathing, as in the case of chronic obstructive pulmonary disease (COPD), certainly impacts our ability to run in a marathon. We will call this the function aspect of health.

There is another aspect of health, is the possibility of hidden abnormalities. Some of these can affect the course of our lives, making us more vulnerable to certain threats or potentially shortening our lifespan. One example might be an inherited disorder that only exhibits its effects when we get older.

Finally, situations in which we are immersed, including the presence of those around us, influence how healthy we feel. Our relationships affect us. We may do more things better or few things well based on the community in which we find ourselves. Aspects, like the economic, social and physical surround, can be crucially important to how one experiences one's health and how likely we are to develop biologic abnormalities. We call this the environmental aspect of health.

Of course, the physical, environmental, function, innate and mental aspects of health strongly interact with each other.

Break it Down, Sure – but Remember that Health is Holistic

We can dissect our feelings of healthiness into these aspects and we can recognize the possibility of cognitive dissonance between our feelings of healthiness and our being disease-free. We, however, must remember the idea with which we started, that feeling healthy (or unhealthy, for that matter) is a holistic experience and it may not depend on actually being healthy.

When we are healthy, we say we feel good and we lack negative symptoms. For instance, we don't have a headache or a stuffed nose, a fever or a soft throat or a pain in one of our limbs. We also aren't depressed, terrified or fearful. We feel comfortable. We have the energy and the get-up-and-go to do things. We can carry out our daily duties. We feel reasonably happy, and we can think clearly and perceive the world around us in ways that enable us to make sense of it and to fit into our environment. However, this is all stated with the proviso that, if we have some sort of pathology, how we feel may not reflect how we physically are!

Clinicians evaluate our overall feelings of healthiness by asking us how we feel and what we can do. In more formal or research settings they may ask us to complete questionnaires related to overall feelings of well-being. However, one of their goals is to try to help us feel better regardless of our circumstance.

There are several dimensions of health, as summarized in FIGURE 1.8.1.

Comfort
Physical, mental, emotional, intellectual, vocational

Function
What one wants to do and can do

Longevity
A proxy for severity (the presence and extensiveness of disease in the body)

Context
Social, environmental, economic, nutrition

FIGURE 1.8.1: The Dimensions of health

THE PHYSICAL FACT ASPECT OF HEALTH – As we have stated, being healthy isn't just feeling healthy! In addition to the feeling, there is physical or biological fact.

We are healthy if we are reasonably fit and of reasonable weight, if no organism like a virus or bacterium has infected us, and if our cells and organs (including our brains and minds) are functioning properly and behaving as they should. We aren't truly healthy if we have latent problems like an undiagnosed cancer.

We might feel heathier than we are when we are in the early stages of many diseases. People with undiagnosed problems might feel well and be able to perform the activities of daily living but they are not healthy. When we consider the physical fact aspect of health versus the feeling aspect, we can see that there can be conflicts. We might smoke tobacco or drink too much alcohol, both of which change our organs and tissues and put us at risk of premature illness or death. It might also be that we absorb noxious substances from our environment. So, again, we can feel healthy and be healthy, or we can feel healthy but be unhealthy. We can actually be sick without knowing we are sick or without feeling sick.

THE FUNCTION ASPECT OF HEALTH – 'Function' corresponds to what we can do. People evaluate their own function by reflecting on what they can do (activities) versus what they want or need to do. For example, they might determine that they can successfully perform their desired activities of daily living, including eating and dressing themselves, interacting with friends, dealing with merchants in stores, running a marathon or walking around the block.

People also evaluate their function by considering how and how well their limbs and body systems work. They judge if they have full use of their arms and legs, and if their organs, like liver and kidneys work appropriately to eliminate the alcohol they drink. They ascertain if they can function sexually in ways they find satisfying. This self-assessment may be different for every one of us, some being satisfied with deft handling of the TV remote, while others demand of their bodies the ability to play the accordion while jogging up Currahee Mountain.[30]

Clinicians evaluate function by asking about and observing a person's ability to perform activities required of daily living. They also measure the function of organ systems through testing and they assess the performance of limbs and joints. For example, clinicians may ask if patients can climb stairs as a measure of overall function, and they may observe the function of various joints, determining, for example, if the patient's knees have full range of motion.

THE MENTAL ASPECT OF HEALTH INCLUDING COMFORT AND PAIN – Another aspect of health is our mental state, both our thinking and our feeling. This strongly interacts with and can be affected by – or we do not allow it to be affected by – the physical fact and function dimension. It is reality that, absent any physical problem, we can feel that things are not right. So, we need to differentiate between feelings that are a product of the mind – such as pain with no clear physiological cause, including the pain of sadness, fear, disappointment – versus an effect of our senses (the neural effect of a physiological event like itching or the pain of injury). Pain, for instance, can exist in the mind without there being any detectable physical cause of that pain. Some clinicians assert that mental pain can emulate physical/sensual pain. However, when someone complains of pain without a detectable abnormality to cause it, we can't determine if the pain originated in the mind or an undetected physical problem caused it. We now have three aspects of health that interact.

THE ENVIRONMENTAL ASPECT OF HEALTH – Environmental factors also determine our health and feelings of healthiness. We all know that people who have good living conditions and access to clean water and adequate nutrition have better health. In general, wealthier people have a longer life expectancy

30 https://en.wikipedia.org/wiki/Currahee. Accessed July 22, 2022.

than the less affluent. A person in inferior conditions and environment may not yet be sick, but that is not likely to last. This low end of the social spectrum is a fertile breeding ground for illness, disadvantaging its victims and making them more susceptible to illness. The social environment is an aspect of one's environmental situation and an aspect of health.

THE INNATE ASPECT OF HEALTH – We all live with our genetic inheritance and none of us is perfect in that regard. However, some are born with a flawed genome that sometimes means they may have body systems that are faulty as a consequence. Some are born without limbs or with organs that function poorly or that are in anatomically problematic locations. Others may have biochemical abnormalities or abnormal components of their blood. Until recently (with the advent of CRISP-CAS and like gene 'editors'), we could do little about this, other than perhaps avoiding ingesting certain nutrients or using drugs to stave off mortal consequence. Scientists have even discovered that an issue faced by a parent, like alcoholism, may affect how our genes, though normal, function in our bodies (epigenetic effects). We all have these innate factors that serve as the platform on which we live our lives. In terms of our health, we do the best we can with what we have received from our parents.

What does it Mean to be Healthy?

So, the answer to the question 'What does it mean to be healthy?' is:

1. We have nothing physically wrong with us (including imperceptible or difficult-to-diagnose medical problems). The physical fact aspect is positive.
2. We are able to do the things we need or want to do. The function aspect is positive.
3. The feelings derived from our senses or generated in our minds aren't disturbing us, we can think appropriately and have nothing mentally disturbing us (we aren't depressed, manic or inappropriately elated), and we are in a mental state that allows us to react appropriately to our situation and interact appropriately with others. The mental aspect is positive.
4. We live daily in an environment where continuing to remain healthy is much more likely than becoming sick. The environmental aspect is positive.
5. We can cope with our genetic limitations. The innate aspect is positive.

What does it Mean to be Sick?

We can deduce the meaning of being sick from the understanding we now have of what it means to be healthy. Being sick is the antithesis of being healthy as we have described it.

However, now it is clear that being sick means one, some, many or all of:

1. We do have something physically wrong with us, like an infection, an injury or a problem in our brain, like a tumor. The physical fact aspect is negative.
2. We either have an ache or pain, feel "out of sorts" or worse, or we eventually will because of the changes in our bodies.
3. We are unable to do certain activities of daily living because an organ system is not working properly, or our muscles and joints don't work the way we expect, or we have impaired sensation including touch, hearing, vision and balance. The function aspect is negative.
4. Our mental state is out of balance, causing delusions or hallucinations, baseless fear (including fear of being sick though we are not physically sick),

sadness or other negative feelings. The mental aspect is negative.

5. We live daily in conditions that make sickness more likely. The environmental aspect is negative.
6. We cannot go far enough to avoid, offset, ignore or correct for our genetic nature. The innate aspect is negative.

This becomes a little more complex when we consider that the fourth item may not be based on any physical or biological cause. We will discuss this thoroughly in the section on mental health when we discuss the mind and brain concept. We will argue that it is inappropriate to say that a person is 'sick' in many instances of mental dysfunction. Unless the brain itself is somehow damaged, disorganized or otherwise physically affected, saying that a person is 'sick' is pejorative related to mental health.

The conclusion of this is that not feeling well may or may not be an issue of being sick or not. Our brains have the ability to project feelings without reference to a physical or physiologic problem.

Our Mantra: The Dimensions of Health

How can we put all this together to arrive at a simple statement?

Throughout this book we have used "**comfort, function and lifespan**" as the dimensions of health. The 'function' part is easy to understand and corresponds exactly to our analysis above. 'Lifespan' is an addition to that analysis but a crucial one to each of us. It is the term 'comfort' that encompasses several different ideas.

Consider for a moment how people who are dying can declare being comfortable. What this means is that, although they face the end of life, they endure little or no pain, they accept the reality of death, fear is minimal and being alive is worth it. Similarly, people with spinal injuries who have lost the function of arms and legs can indicate being in a state of comfort. They likely have gone through a series of mental stages to accept the reality of impairments and have found adjustments, such as the use of mechanical devices or assistants or just acceptance.

Therefore, 'comfort' addresses a spectrum of states that go from what all of us would consider being appealing to very challenging states that some would find unacceptable, but many could work through them to achieve what we would call a copacetic or tolerable situation. These are mental adjustments to physical reality and apply to the physical fact aspect, the functional aspect and the environmental aspect of our health. The integrating and adjusting mechanism is the mind. The mind supports us in our efforts to achieve a healthy state (through decisions that help us become fit, for example) and helps us in adjusting when we face bodily problems such as inherited limitations, incurable diseases, injuries and origins in an economically depressed or environmentally compromised area. The mental aspect of health even gives us ways of managing mental problems, like depression, through steps we undertake to offset or correct our feelings on our own or with the help of others.

Comfort is the overriding state of good health that stands over all the challenges of our imperfect biology and mentation, making the very best of everything possible. In an important sense comfort overcomes physical reality, function, environmental situation and whatever the limits may be on our lifespan.

The World Health Organization Takes on Health

As we stated, the World Health Organization (WHO) defines health as "*a state of complete physical, mental and social well-being and not merely the absence of disease or infirmity*".[31] That is very much in keeping with what we have offered.

The WHO's definition of health is innovative because it recognizes not only physical health, but also emotional and social comfort. It recognizes that a person's social context and environment play important roles in overall well-being.

Unfortunately, if we think about it, the WHO definition does not identify anyone as actually being healthy! The definition is all-encompassing, but it is vague. Anyone bored, unmotivated, or tired and therefore uncomfortable, is not 'healthy' according to that definition. Achieving the condition of health connoted by the WHO definition is likely impossible, because no one is in a state of complete physical, mental and social well-being. Moreover, the WHO definition is not functional, because we cannot derive measures (metrics) of health based on that definition. Without metrics we cannot assess healthiness or of the effectiveness of healthcare interventions.

Descriptions that are more useful recognize the social and emotional components of well-being emphasized by the World Health Organization and include operational definitions[32] and measures of health. Later in this book and in Volume 2 we describe the measures professionals use to estimate physical and mental health.

31 https://www.publichealth.com.ng/world-health-organizationwho-definition-of-health/. Accessed July 12, 2022.

32 An operational definition is a definition that indicates the measures and operations necessary to describe the concept.

Chapter 9: Patient Engagement and Participation

KEYWORDS: Patient Participation, Patient Engagement, Informed Consent, Communication, Health Knowledge

ABSTRACT: Encounters between doctors and patients are most valuable when patients understand, negotiate with, and agree with a clinician's suggestions for care. Clinicians' roles include providing advice about medical conditions and providing emotional support so that the patient feels as comfortable as possible after each encounter. This chapter discusses what patients and clinicians can do together to make interactions most worthwhile.

Introduction

Good, bad or indifferent, we humans exist in a sea of relationships. We have friends, family, professional associations, dealings with authorities, enemies and even those we ignore. It is worthwhile to think about the relationship between a patient and the physician.

The type and quality of the relationship between the physician and patient dramatically affects the nature of the care process. Patients, in the past, sometimes felt they were visiting an oracle, who knew everything about Medicine and would fix whatever was wrong – if and only if patients did exactly as they were told. Perhaps because of this sometimes jointly held belief system, physicians could get away with being arrogant, authoritarian, aloof and dominant. Many weren't like that, though. Unfortunately, some patients were relegated to subservience, obeisance and obedience. But things happened to enable patients to participate actively in their own care.

Among the reasons that this mutual perception changed, were that patients began to realize that much of what was wrong with them could not be absolutely cured. Worse still, sometimes the oracle made mistakes and the patient got hurt. Quite a few patients became uncomfortable with just following orders. A major change occurred secondary to the existence of the Internet, which provided understandable medical information and made it very clear that, often, there were no easy fixes or cures. Over the last two decades, patients have often visited their care providers armed with information and well-thought-out questions based on this information. Gradually, physicians and patients have seen the possibility of a new kind of relationship, one based on mutual understanding and respect, open communication and intelligent discussion, negotiation and agreement.

The contents of this text will arm patients with a relatively comprehensive understanding of the nature of care, health, sickness, diagnosis, treatment and the issues associated with these. The ideas herein will help patients become knowledgeable and active participants in the care process. The relationship between physicians and patients is already changing. And it's moving in the right direction. What is here can accelerate that change and can prepare and empower patients and their clinicians, enabling them to carry out appropriate roles in the new patient-physician relationship.

It is worth asking why this is important.

Reasons to Change the Patient-Physician Relationship

There are a number of key reasons to alter how patients and physicians relate. They are the 'Four C's.'

The 4 C's
Compliance
Consent
Communication
Comfort

FIGURE 1.9.1: The 4 C's of the patient relationship

FIGURE 1.9.1 lists the 4 C's that encapsulate the main requirements of a good patient-physician relationship.

Compliance. Both experience and research have shown that, in the past, under the old physician-in-charge regime, physicians prescribed a course of treatment, but about 38% of patients didn't follow it – this is an enormous number, as about 48% of Americans receive a prescription every month.[33] The term physicians use for adhering to treatment advice is 'compliance' (you can see that is a loaded term: I command, and you comply). However, the fact is that quite a few patients do not comply with therapeutic regimens and that makes some encounters virtually worthless! As one example, it is common that a patient will stop taking an antibiotic, which is supposed to be taken for five days, after a day or three. One result of this – other than the patient's infection perhaps not being cured – is that we may see the emergence of antibiotic-resistant strains of bacteria. The bacteria that weren't completely killed off by the antibiotic while it was taken may have developed the ability to survive the application of that antibiotic (and possible similar ones) in the future. On the other hand, non-compliance is appropriate if an engaged patient understands the proposed intervention, like an antibiotic[34], is unnecessary or harmful. Blind compliance is also a mistake.

There are countless other examples. One piece of research[35] shows that just as many patients never even fill their prescriptions at the pharmacy (If you listen carefully, you can hear the time in the office, the money invested therein, the diagnosis and the treatment decision gurgling down the drain!) In other situations, patients abandon a treatment because they experience predictable (and potentially, if they had been properly prepared, manageable) side effects. Unfortunately, we currently lack the mandate, processes and systems to routinely track the fate of compliers and non-compliers.

We have learned that getting the patient's agreement – and this means a meaningful understanding and commitment – to the benefits and harms of the prescription is crucial. This depends on the patient grasping the issues with the medication, the need to acquire and take it and doing so for the entire recommended course and agreeing that the goals of treatment are compatible with the patients' values and personal objectives. This is not just so the prescribed medication deals with the immediate problem, but also to prevent other problems, like resistant bacteria or wasted healthcare dollars. So, we now recognize that a kind of negotiation needs to occur between the patient and the physician, and a pseudo-contract needs to be formed between them.

33 https://www.medscape.com/viewarticle/830616. Accessed August 24, 2022.

34 Pierre-Marie Roger, Eve Montera, Diane Lesselingue, Nathalie Troadec, Patrick Charlot, Agnès Simand, Agnès Rancezot, Olivier Pantaloni, Thomas Guichard, Véronique Dautezac, Cécile Landais, Frédéric Assi, Thierry Levent, Collaborators, Risk Factors for Unnecessary Antibiotic Therapy: A Major Role for Clinical Management, Clinical Infectious Diseases, Volume 69, Issue 3, 1 August 2019, Pages 466–472, https://doi.org/10.1093/cid/ciy921. Accessed August 24, 2022.

35 https://www.aafp.org/news/health-of-the-public/20140428nonadherencestudy.html. Accessed August 24, 2022.

This is so that the patient is properly treated and so that visiting the physician had a point.

Sometimes patients find out after the encounter, through friends or information on the Internet, that the recommended treatment was not appropriate in the circumstance. This may mean re-contacting the physician and discussing how to proceed. If honesty is part of the patient-physician contract, then non-compliance is a reasonable part of the discussion as well and there should be an opportunity for both the doctor and the patient to learn something new.

Consent. Another major subject, that of consent, is crucial to the care process. Consent is especially important if the patient is to undertake any regimen that could injure or potentially create transient discomfort, or perhaps even have some bad side effects. Consent means that the patient sees the point of the intervention and (really and actually) agrees with it and the chances of personal benefit or harm. Consent is a legal matter. The law requires physicians to get patient consent prior to the patient's participating in any intervention, let alone one that might potentially inflict harm.

Research has revealed the challenge associated with consent. An experiment was set up in which a surgeon – witnessed by another person – would explain breast surgery to a patient and (supposedly) get the patient's consent to any procedures. In the case of quite a few encounters, when the patients left the office and were asked about the consent they apparently gave, the patients denied that anything at all was explained to them! There can be good reasons for something like this happening. Sometimes, the sheer terror of the situation can cause people to appear to be listening, understanding and consenting, but they really aren't. Informed consent means the patient understands what is proposed and the likelihood of benefit and harm from a recommended treatment. Physicians should inform patients and patients should know where to find information about the potential benefits and harms of care.

Communication. Any visit to a clinician involves communication. This communication is in two directions. It is first from the patient to the physician explaining what's wrong. Then it occurs from the physician to the patient through questions the patient answers. Then it usually proceeds back and forth with the physician making suggestions or recommendations and the patient asking questions to get clarification, and so on. This communication is challenging! Not every patient is aware of human anatomy, physiology, pathology and treatment alternatives. Not every physician is fully aware of the patient's situation, including social environment, pain tolerance, understanding of the physician's recommendations, honesty, trust, and, very commonly, the patient's level of embarrassment… along with, sometimes, a bit of deception.

The care process is a communication process. To participate in communication, a common language is essential – and patients can have a problem with that when programmed during their upbringing with terms like bellybutton, peepee and the like. But communication is crucial! Patients must be, sort of like in court, able to tell the truth, the whole truth and nothing but the truth… or their best approximation to that and must be given time to do so. That will permit the physician to understand the patient's problems, situation and tolerance for advice. The physician, too, must participate in this communication process, because real communication is two-way; communication of any other kind is called nagging and ignoring. There needs to be real and shared understanding. To achieve that, there needs to be a kind of bilateral translation process and a communication protocol, so the patient can more clearly state problems and the physician can more plainly ask questions and express recommendations. That translator really needs to be interior to the two parties. We build consent and compliance on the basis of communication. Absent communication, there is no point to the engagement.

Comfort. Then there is comfort. That's a major reason the patient is there: to be comforted. We're sure that just about everyone, on seeing a doctor about a problem, felt somewhat better after the experience, even if no prescription was forthcoming. A key reason for patients being engaged in their care and participating in it is that a degree of comfort will result. This has been called the "laying on of the hands", meaning that just simple attention to patients has a positive effect on their comfort. Sometimes this can be augmented with an innocuous pill or an injection, both called placebos, which really are not specific to the problem at hand but that help the patient feel listened to and cared – something was done. The result is often an improvement perceived by the patient – and, despite the nature of it, a real medical effect can result. Isn't it also true that being able to take a hand in one's own care itself causes comfort? For example, one can exercise and feel good, because we've done something about our health. If we actually participate in what amounts to the ritual of the medical visit, we are more likely to reap comfort. This is one of the key effects patients seek in seeing a physician.

The Impact of the Four C's

These are the four C's, but let's reorder them: Comfort, Communication, Consent and Compliance. These four Cs explain what we can reap from becoming engaged and participating in our own care. We all will have problems, especially as we age or go through various aspects of life like growth, pregnancy and the wear and tear of just plain living. If we become engaged and participative in our care, we can quite dramatically improve our comfort with our lives. This will happen because we will be able to communicate what's wrong and understand what needs to be done. We will also be able to intelligently agree with and consent to what may be difficult interventions. And we will find ourselves more able to achieve compliance with what might be very worthwhile but challenging treatments.

These four Cs are really what this book is all about achieving, with our focus, of course, being on communication.

A Word that Describes You: What are You to Your Doctor?

When you read about healthcare processes, you will see different words applied to those who use services. In this book, we use the terms 'person' or 'patient'. However, some prefer the term 'client', while others prefer 'consumer' or 'customer'. What's the difference?

All of these words can apply to the receiver of medical services. Of course, we all deserve the label 'person.' We and others use that term to emphasize that the system is not dealing with an object, like a 'case'. The word 'case' is a common one used among physicians. Regretfully, this strongly depersonalizes the person with the problem, reducing people to objects. That is changing, however, as many physicians are careful to avoid saying: "I had an interesting case today". Rather, they use: 'I saw an interesting person or patient today". This is a meaningful difference because it emphasizes that those examined and treated are individual human beings, people, with feelings and concerns, not things or faceless medical conditions.

Some allied professionals, including psychologists and social workers, prefer the term 'client'. In this instance, they are trying to draw a comparison between those who use their services and those who use other kinds of services, such as stores, banks and garages. They all use the term 'client.' In considering this choice, recognize that 'clients' make a personal decision to use, and pay for, one of these services. The word 'client' indicates who chooses and controls the interaction with the service. With any of these business types of services, we have complete control when it comes to deciding which service provider will work for us. WE have options. We can choose which service we want and if we really need that service now or can put it off till next year. The is true of the term 'consumer,' but it is a more generic term that, unfortunately, smacks of the ingestion of a meal.

In the case of health care, getting help is not truly optional, the choices are fewer and the dependence on the provider is greater.

In Medicine and the healthcare system, the term 'patient' is most often used. There is a negative aspect of this term too, as it implies a kind of dominance of the provider, indicating a shift of control from the person to the service provider. To combat this, some have tried to use the terms 'client' or 'consumer' to indicate that the control must be and really is with the receiver of the service. We haven't, though, because of what those terms denote. Of course, when you are in an intensive care, festooned with tubes and facing complex interventions, you must be patient and accepting, and terms don't matter.

In this book, we use the term 'patient' as a kinder and more humane one than the terms 'client' or 'consumer'. In other words, we see the relationship as more intimate between the physician and the person than one's arm's-length relationship with a mechanic, retailer or banker. However, we can see the negative aspect of the word 'patient' relative to the concept we are promoting: the assumption of the mantle of the CEO of one's health care. The specific use of the word 'patient' is justifiable, though. The truth is that, in Medicine, the clinician and the receiver of care share a deeper connection than in these other cases. Patients trust and to some degree subject themselves to their clinicians. Furthermore, clinicians have a deeper fiduciary responsibility to the persons for whom they care. Care is not just a business activity; it is a deep and abiding concern about and relationship with those who present themselves with problems.

We just don't know of a better word to embody this relationship than the word 'patient' to express the subject of care.

Then There's the Word for the Interaction

Finally, there is a divergence in the terminology used for the engagement with the patient. Some prefer the term 'visit', while others prefer 'encounter'. What it really comes down to is the weight of emotional engagement with which we perceive these two words. We 'encounter' people on the bus or in line for a flight. When we 'visit' them, this involves more social involvement and a far more significant choice. Herein, we have used the word 'visit,' as it denotes something deeper than 'encounter.' For us the word 'encounter' sounded a bit too cold and we want to emphasize the intimacy of what occurs between a clinician and a patient.

Going too deeply into this would be making too much of simple words, perhaps. On the other hand, words are the atoms with which we compose our communications. The wrong words can convey the wrong meanings. It may be tricky to choose the right words, but we believe it is worth the effort.

Chapter 10: Understanding the Health System

KEYWORDS: The Health System, The Sickness System, Components of the Human Body, Components of the Health System, Complexity, Health Services Administration, Health Services Governance

ABSTRACT: The health system and the human body both comprise various interacting elements. Each element can function well or poorly on its own. Sometimes when one element of the human body or of the health system is dysfunctional, the other parts can adapt so that the complete system remains well-functioning. On the other hand, occasionally a change to improve one element disrupts the overall organizational balance and creates dysfunction. For example, in addressing sickness an antibiotic meant to kill a harmful organism may also harm the organisms in the gut that help digest food. Although the original infection may be cleared, new problems (such as diarrhea or an allergic reaction) create other problems. Similarly, in the health system, if people are moved from one department to help another one that is short-handed, the department losing workers might perform poorly and be unable to provide sufficient support thereby frustrating the organization's achieving its overall goals.

Introduction

Is there a health system or a sickness system?

Regrettably, the answer isn't obvious. We now understand the difference between health and sickness. Ideally, the 'health system' is the constellation of facilities and services we have evolved to help us remain healthy and to return us to health when we get sick. The part addressing 'helping us remain healthy' is, unfortunately, usually the virtual runt of the litter.

It is even worthwhile asking if any 'health system' is a 'system'! Looked at from the outside, the health system may, in fact, not look like a 'system', a term that connotes parts that work together as components of an integrated mechanism. Some say that calling it a 'system' is to apply that term too generously. It does not always function like a system. An industrial wag compared it to a helicopter, which some describe as a bunch of loose parts flying in close formation. There is truth in that! The reality is that the health system is large and multifaceted, internally competitive, jury-rigged to some extent, geographically distributed with gaps in communication, different from jurisdiction to jurisdiction and (this is a special word) 'complex'.

Complex systems are hard-to-understand entities where small changes may entail major or unpredictable consequences. The classical (and mythical) analogy links perturbations caused by butterfly's wings disturbing the air in the Amazon rain forest to the development of a hurricane over the Atlantic Ocean. Not really valid but you get the idea: tiny changes in the initial state of the system can have big effects on later states and the direction and magnitude of the change can vary capriciously. The health system may not appear to be a system because it is so incredibly complex. No matter, it is also not fully integrated or cohesive and, not infrequently, suffers from internal, if we can coin a pseudo-medical word, 'dysorganization', reminiscent of 'dysfunction'.

In health and health care, small changes may be followed by major unintended consequences in addition to the intended ones. To give a medical example, a doctor who prescribes a diuretic medication to someone with mild kidney failure might, unintentionally, have prescribed something the body cannot handle, with the consequence of total kidney failure and even death. An administrative instance would be where a health administrator closes one emergency department in a district to save money. This might, unintentionally, create a circumstance where other emergency departments become overloaded, wait-times become too long, and people die as a result. The aftermath might be higher costs.

Another and perhaps most important feature of complex systems is that they can adapt to change. They are organic, robust like we are. For example, when a person, a complex human system, receives more thyroid medication than needed, the pituitary gland adapts by reducing the amount of thyroid gland stimulating hormone it produces.

To help understand the health system, it is useful to think about the human being, human problems and disease, the need to find out the root causes of problems – called diagnosis – and provide treatment.

The Human Body

If we think about it a little, it is clear that the human body has characteristics similar to the health system. This is a clue to understanding the nature and structure of the health system. One could argue that the human being is not geographically distributed, or that it doesn't vary from jurisdiction to jurisdiction. But Public Health professionals will tell you we do! In reality, every human is different, and these differences often have geographical and even jurisdictional variation. For example, growing up in a poor neighborhood or in one contaminated with industrial chemicals can influence behavior and health.

As complex systems, all human bodies do not respond in the same way to identical stimuli. For example, someone who has been exposed to bacteria and viruses in the past will be more likely to have resistance when exposed again. This is one reason that some suggest that children who are exposed to dirt[36] might in the long run be healthier compared with those raised in a more sterile environment.

The human body is composed of an integrated set of organs and organ systems. Here are a few:

> The heart and blood vessels – they are called the 'cardiovascular' system, 'cardio' referring to the heart and 'vascular' referring to the blood vessels – the veins and arteries. This system distributes oxygen and nutrition to the body and transports waste products for disposal to the lungs and kidneys.

> The brain, spinal cord and other nerves – we call them the 'neurological' system. The brain and spinal cord combined is referred to as the 'encephalon'. We think, act and sense ourselves and our environment through with this system.

> The lungs and airways – we name them the 'pulmonary' system. This brings oxygen into the body and ships carbon dioxide out.

> The esophagus, stomach and intestines – are called the 'gastrointestinal' system, where 'gastro' refers to the stomach. This system enables us to ingest and digest nutrients and water and to eliminate solid waste products.

36 https://www.webmd.com/parenting/features/kids-and-dirt-germs#1. Accessed July 22, 2022.

- The genitals and urinary organs – we label these the 'genitourinary' system. These are both another component of the waste (liquid in this case) removal capability, as well as the means of pleasure and procreation.
- The ears, nose and throat – this is called the ENT system and is the domain of otolaryngologists ('oto' refers to the ear and 'laryng' to the larynx or throat. This is the entry point for air, food and water, as well as harboring key senses (taste, hearing, smell) and is responsible for the humidification of the air we breathe in.

The list goes on and on, but we'll stop there for now.

Medical and Surgical Practice

The fact is that every hospital and every area of medical specialization corresponds directly to the list of organs. For example, there are Cardiologists, Neurologists, Pulmonary and Gastrointestinal (GI) specialists, to name a few who deal with the areas in the list above. Almost always, hospitals have departments corresponding to the items in the list. A reasonably comprehensive list of common medical departments can be found in: https://www.nursesclass.com/2021/08/departments-in-a-hospital.html.

So, the components of the health system and the types of specialists that work in the health system are not mysterious. They are congruent with the components of the body. However, how components of the human body relate one to another is as mystifying as how the components of a healthcare system work together or collaborate to care for people. After all, it is the person as a whole, not the individual organs on their own, that is important.

Before we move on, we should note that those who offer clinical care usually perform one of two generic functions: diagnosis and treatment (often termed 'medical') care or surgical care. Many credentialed groups offer diagnosis and treatment, not only physicians. However, in most jurisdictions physicians are most often the professionals permitted to order tests or prescribe medication.

The first of these functions, diagnosis, involves figuring out what's wrong with the person. The second, treatment, involves offering recommendations to ameliorate the problem.

Medical care providers are usually able to provide corrective interventions that include counselling, giving advice, such as suggesting a dietary program, performing simple or complicated surgical procedures and prescribing drugs.

Surgical interventions can run from minor surgery, something done by virtually all physicians, right up to major heart (thoracic), abdominal (belly area), bones and joints and brain surgery. The areas of surgical practice exactly parallel those of general medical practice, although today there is often what is called 'hyper-specialization'. Examples of hyper-specialization are lung and heart transplantation surgery, where thoracic surgeons limit their practice to replacing patients' lungs or hearts, which are extremely challenging procedures. The comeuppance of all of this is that both medical and surgical departments exist that address extremely focal areas of the human body, such as children's cancer – Pediatric Oncology – which can combine both medical and surgical programs.

The key message of this is that the components of the health system parallel the components of the human body, but they usually divide into medical and surgical foci. Furthermore, pretty well every area of the human body has medical and/or surgical specialists who address its issues.

However, it is worth reiterating that humans are complex, and many people have illnesses that represent dysfunction in several body systems simultaneously (these are called 'co-morbidities'). Seniors, for example, might suffer from heart disease, lung disease, kidney disease, high blood pressure and diabetes. The treatment of each condition must recognize the influences of the other abnormalities. The treatment of and risk associated with an episode of illness are often different for people who have co-morbidities. This makes clear the need for an integrated approach to the patient, preferably with someone who knows the person serving as a coordinating figure, such as the family or general practitioner.

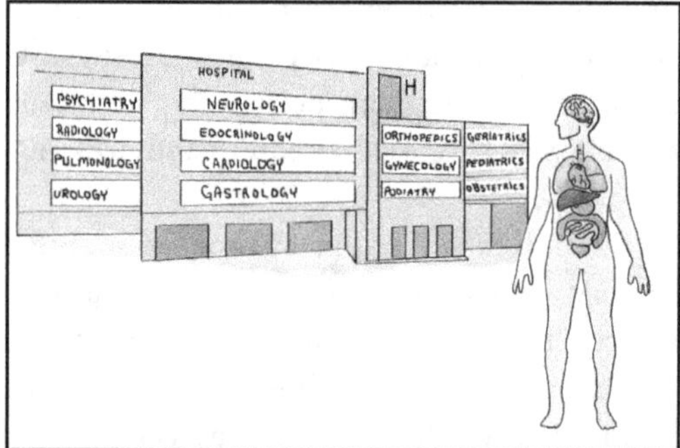

FIGURE 1.10.1: The health system reflects the nature of the body

The Health System Organizational Components

(See FIGURE 1.10.1)

Here we will tabulate the most important organizational components of the healthcare system, starting where patients usually start when they need its services. It is worth noting that the components reflect the nature of the human body and its need for care.

The Physician's Office

Most people enter the health system by visiting a physician, with or without preliminary interaction with a nurse practitioner – a more highly trained nurse who can manage many of the areas a physician can. Sometimes it will be through a clinician in an Emergency Department.

Physicians who see patients at this point in the care process are usually General Practitioners (GPs) or Family Practitioners (FPs), the latter having undertaken additional training. Emergency Departments are staffed by physicians with advanced training in emergency Medicine. Most of these medical practitioners can be found in a private medical office or in some kind of group practice or clinic. Lots of individual medical practices with one-person offices exist, but it is becoming more and more common for medical practitioners to band together in clinics.

Clinics

Clinics are health care's way of organizing multiple providers into working units.

There are many kinds of clinics. A group of general practitioners and/or surgeons may share an office facility, perhaps for financial reasons or so they can centralize and share support services. In another model, a variety of different medical specialists may do the same, so that patients see a common façade no matter what their problems are, and the clinicians share overhead including use of common waiting rooms. Maybe the best-known example of the latter is the Mayo Clinic. Another sophisticated example would be a clinic that provided a variety of surgical services. This is usually called a 'surgicenter.' Today, we have vascular surgical clinics, clinics that do hernia (a bulge of the intestine through the abdominal wall) repairs, ophthalmology clinics that do cataract-damaged eye lens replacements and so on.

These clinics may also have other kinds of practitioners, such as the nurse practitioners, physiotherapists, kinesiologists, psychologists, occupational therapists (OTs) and other types of, sometimes called 'allied professionals.' This allows the clinic to offer a wider range of services and also allows handling of patients by specially trained professionals. By the way, clinics have others on whom they depend, such as nurses, technologists, social workers, receptionists and even business professionals who handle the financial and logistical aspects of the clinic. So, a clinic that is large enough may be able to address virtually any problem that a patient faces. However, most individual practices and clinics focus on medical diagnosis, pharmaceutical treatment and minor surgical interventions.

Some clinics may have a mixture of general/family practitioners and specialists, like Cardiologists or GI (Gastrointestinal) specialists. This allows the easy and local referral of patients with especially complicated problems who require special advice or treatment. Family doctors and specialists all treat serious illnesses. Specialists, though, are more likely to treat people with illnesses that are unusual, uncommon and difficult to diagnose or require difficult or unusual treatment. In some jurisdictions, general practitioners or family doctors might not have access to the specialized hospital services required to treat certain illnesses.

With different varieties of clinicians in the same location, they can easily interrupt colleagues to get quick consults while the patient is still there. However, if patients need more comprehensive consultations, they normally must come back, as, in the busiest clinics, each of the practitioners will be engaged with other patients.

In clinics lacking needed experts on site, GPs will refer patients to external specialists to look into the patient's problem and intervene. This means either a telephone call or electronic communication with an expert located elsewhere or the patients' visiting a different site to see a specialist, rather than returning to the same clinic for follow up.

Again, there is a parallel between the way the health system organizes itself and the way in which people deal with, or should deal with, their health problems: in an organized and efficient way. Also, like with the human body, administratively intervening in one part of the health system can prompt change or dysfunction in other components. If an operating room is removed from service, this may affect virtually all specialist services, patient wait times can increase and patients may suffer or die before they are finally helped.

The Hospital

The most comprehensive and profound interventional component of the health system is the hospital. The hospital can provide services on an in-patient (i.e., in a bed) or outpatient (patients walk in for scheduled visits and leave the same day) basis.

In some communities, certain services, for example MRI or other diagnostic testing, are only available in a hospital building. In other communities, these services may also be available in clinics or at standalone or even mobile facilities. The choice of clinic or hospital location is dictated by (patients' or clinicians') economic or convenience factors.

An acute loss of function or significant discomfort can compel patients to go to an acute-care hospital, or a physician may send patients with chronic problems and an inability to care for themselves to a long-term care hospital or a continuing-care facility. Generally speaking, if patients require services unique to a hospital, then they must be admitted to the hospital. Usually, regions have one or more hospitals suited for dealing with the most complicated problems and these are often associated with universities. They are called 'tertiary hospitals', 'Academic Medical Centers' and 'university teaching hospitals' and serve another key function, the training of physicians and other health system personnel. In these organizations a variety of students and researchers participate in patient care, such as medical and nursing students, medical residents in specialist training programs, biomedical scientists and even administrative students, such as from MBA programs. They are the crème de la crème of our care systems offering broad-spectrum, hyper-specialized care for the most complex patients.

At the other end of the spectrum there are General Hospitals that address the more mundane medical problems. Specialty hospitals are uncommon, tending to focus on specific problems, like heart care or cancer care, but they are important. There are also institutions that focus strictly on mental health.

The Hospital Emergency Department

A person injured in a car crash may go directly to the hospital, typically being transported by an ambulance. In this case, the person enters the hospital through an Emergency Department (ED; other descriptors include 'Emerg' and 'ER' – Emergency Room – although it almost always is much more than a room!). The same would be the case if a physician at an office encounter found the patient to have an immediate, serious problem and sent the patient there.

The functions of an Emergency Department are several-fold.

The first function is 'triage' – the determination of the seriousness of the problem and the immediacy of the need for significant intervention. For example, if a patient is bleeding heavily (hemorrhaging) or unable to breathe well enough, this demands immediate attention. Patients less 'acute' will be in for a bit of a wait but will get their turn after others' more serious problems are addressed.

The second function of an ED is to stabilize the patient. As an example, it might be crucial to stop the bleeding or to establish an airway through which the patient can breathe.

The third major function of an Emergency Department is to either provide an immediate solution or to forward the patient to a specialty department within the hospital. If the patient remains unstable, this will mean transfer to the Intensive Care Unit (ICU) or to surgery. For example, if the bleeding cannot be stopped using pressure or a tourniquet or it is from a major blood vessel, the patient might be admitted to Vascular Surgery or to the ICU.

One can also enter a hospital the most usual way, through the Admitting Department directly. If a sick patient needs immediate treatment but it isn't as urgent, typically a physician in an office or clinic will send the patient to a hospital where that doctor has admitting privileges – meaning being authorized to send or care for patients there. Patients are admitted to one of the hospital departments, which could be a general ward or might be a specialty ward like a Cardiology, Psychiatry, a pediatric unit, or a Vascular Surgery unit. Most specialty departments have a number of beds in the hospital allocated to them based on the volume of patients they treat. Sometimes, care in the hospital is provided by physicians trained in Internal Medicine called 'hospitalists', who only serve within the hospital.

It is a goal of the health system to keep the originating general/family physicians in the picture, even though, in a sense, the patient has been swallowed up by the hospital. Unfortunately, that goal is not always achieved, and this can have deleterious consequences. Perhaps the most important impact is a communication breakdown between hospital physicians and primary care physicians, causing an increase in the rate of preventable harm. For example, when attending physicians (those caring for the patient in the hospital) don't know which drugs a patient is already receiving, the patient risks over-prescription and adverse drug reactions due to drug-drug interactions. Communication with the patient's GP or FP can prevent those.

Hospital Service Departments

In addition to Emergency, Admitting and the specialty medical and surgical departments, there is a service department infrastructure in all hospitals to support patient care. This set of services usually includes Diagnostic Imaging (X-Ray, CT, MRI, Ultrasound and other types of imaging examinations), a Clinical Chemistry Laboratory (for determining problems through blood, urine, or other body substance measurements), a Clinical Pathology department (to examine cells and tissues). It may also include sundry other services, such as a Pulmonary Function Laboratory (to determine lung function), a Neurology Laboratory (to study nerve conduction), a Blood Bank (for transfusions) and many other possibilities. This part of the infrastructure focuses itself on providing information to support diagnosis and treatment and reports back to the individual specialty departments.

The other obvious organizational component is that of surgery, which subsumes all the different types of surgical intervention, such as heart, vascular, neurological, gastrointestinal, etc., surgery. A patient is typically admitted to a medical ward, referred to a surgeon, who performs an intervention in the operating room (OR), the patient moves to a recovery room and then goes back to a medical ward, although sometimes specialty surgeons have their own wards.

The Resource Departments

Another infrastructural component of a hospital is Administration. Administration includes the senior executives such as the Chief Executive Officer, an array of vice presidents and departmental or divisional Directors, and a panoply of resource staff to support them. Every medical, surgical and infrastructure department typically has an administrator or manager from this group. One administrator is usually responsible for a number of departments and has an appropriate title.

When addressing Administration, it is important to note that there are two largely independent divisions with their own hierarchies in hospitals. One of these is the medical staff and the other is everyone else. Medical staff report to Division Chiefs who are physicians and these Chiefs, in turn, report to the Chief of Medicine or Chief of Medical Staff. It is easy to imagine that this represents an organizational challenge, as, in most hospitals, physicians are not employees of hospital administration. It has become common, however, that a Chief Medical Officer is a member of the institutional senior management team.

Finally, there is a group of other resource units to address matters like medical records management, human organization and hiring, purchasing and receiving and maintenance. Most commonly, these include the departments of Health Records Management, Human Resources (HR), Materials Management, Information Services (computers, hospital support software and electronic communications), Building and Maintenance, Finance, Quality Assurance, etc.

Administration is responsible for evaluating hospital performance (productivity, quality, efficiency, patient satisfaction) and making recommendations to improve the effectiveness and efficiency of care. Evaluating the costs of care for the benefits achieved is essential.

Ideally, administrations implement methods to track the health outcomes of patients cared for by the clinical departments. They also monitor costs and should try to link the financial and human costs to the health outcomes that follow. In many instances, that is merely a dream.

Types of Human Resources in Hospitals

Without going into a lot of detail, suffice it to say that, in addition to the physicians and surgeons who populate the various medical, surgical and service departments, there is a wide array of professionals that complement them.

Importantly, there are the nurses responsible for the day-to-day care of the patient. Perhaps it is worthwhile pointing out that some nurses are highly specialized, such as those who work in the Emergency Department or in the Intensive Care Unit to which very sick and often unstable patients are admitted until they can go on to a general ward. There are other kinds of nurses as well.

In addition to these professionals, there are Clinical Laboratory technologists and technicians who are responsible for handling, processing and examining specimens that come from patients. They subject those samples to analysis by electronic equipment that provides specific measurements. In fact, there are many specially trained technologists and technicians in most service departments. They can be found in Diagnostic Imaging, Pulmonary Function, in medical departments, like Cardiology (to perform electrocardiograms, do cardiac ultrasound examinations, and assist in special studies) and in most other departments.

Patients may also be seen by physiotherapists (also called kinesiologists) who help people regain as much function as possible. Occupational therapists help patients to recover skills for performing various cognitive (thinking) or motor (movement) tasks, such as reading, speaking, performing manual processes or walking.

We should also mention Health Information Management professionals, Health Informatics and eHealth professionals. The last two are computing and communications experts who evaluate, select and implement the information techniques and tools that clinicians and administrators use to assist hospital services and to evaluate and improve performance. These professionals are responsible for selecting, designing and implementing many kinds of care process support systems. The latter include medical records systems, systems to capture and aggregate data about care and to link care activities to subsequent health results, clinical prompting and diagnosis support systems, and systems that support the management and operation of almost every clinical department and service.

By no means does this exhaust the set of professionals dedicated to patient care. Nor is it all of the human infrastructure of the hospital. There are also staff responsible for patient transport, nutritionists, staff who serve meals, maintenance staff, administrative assistants, receptionists, cooks, staff who clean the facility and on and on.

This human fabric must function in harmony and with the degree of coordination that makes patient care high-quality, comforting, efficient and timely. Knowing the magnitude of this human component gives us an idea of why hospital care is so extremely expensive. Typically, hospital patient care costs in the thousands of dollars per patient bed per day. Care in the ICU and in Surgery is even more expensive.

Beyond the Hospital

The person originally seen by a family practitioner may be treated in a hospital and then return home, perhaps with various instructions and medications, and be followed up on by a GP or FP. Some patients, however, cannot simply be sent home. They may not be able to care for themselves and they may need further care.

A variety of institutional entities exist for continuing or further care. If badly injured, a person may need to be in an institution that can assist recovery over time or where, in the case of devastating injuries, life can only continue under continuous care. These institutions are often called Long-Term Care institutions. If the patient is badly injured but recovery is likely given assistance, he or she might be admitted to a rehabilitation hospital or center to receive ongoing physiotherapy and occupational therapy.

Rehabilitation centers aim to help the patient recover the maximal amount of function possible. For example, someone who has injuries that imply being wheelchair-bound for life might receive training in how to use the wheelchair to get around and to maneuver in difficult locations. These institutions are crucially important for the care of those wounded in military service.

Not every patient who leaves the hospital, however, may be able to recover. A patient with a devastating brain injury or cancer that has spread (metastasized) may need a place to receive care until death inevitably intervenes. This latter type of institution is usually referred to as a Hospice. Care in such a facility is called 'palliative care' and is intended to keep patients as comfortable as possible for as long as they live.

The Surround of the Health System

There are many entities that do not provide direct patient care but surround and support the healthcare system.

The largest of these is the government, which oversees health system regulation and, in some countries, also its management and finance. According to one's country, governing can exist at several levels: the country-wide (federal) level, the state or provincial level, and the region or city level. Government involves itself in matters like regulation, safety, quality assurance, performance assessment, funding and general oversight.

The Public Health Agency is a crucial player in the health system. Its role is the detection and identification of factors that influence the health of the wider population, such as detecting and dealing with newly appearing viruses or bacteria that can infect people or that people can spread from one to another (like HIV or Venereal – sexually-transmitted – Disease). In the United States, the Centers for Disease Control and Prevention performs this function.

There is also the Food and Drug Administration, Health Canada, or the equivalent in other jurisdictions. They are responsible for determining if food, ingested commercial products and drugs are safe or might cause sickness, like cancer, and are as effective as claimed.

Beyond this, there are organizations that provide health promotion (like fitness, not smoking and diet recommendations) and disease and sickness prevention services.

Let's not forget Dentistry for the care of the teeth and jaw, Optometry for eye care, Hearing Clinics for addressing hearing problems, Podiatry clinics for foot care, and many others.

We would be remiss not to mention the research institutions (academic and industrial) that interact with the health system, the pharmaceutical and device manufacturing companies, the care homes for the elderly, the insurance companies that provide funding, and much more beyond that. It is quite easy to see why health care is usually the largest cost element in a modern society.

Role of Government in Maintaining Health

As we mentioned, governments regulate and sometimes insure direct health services. However, the major role of government related to the health of communities and individuals are through government's influencing of the broader determinants of health. Where people live and the context of their lives has a major impact on overall health. Government policies influence education, the physical environment (e.g., clean water and air, housing, sewage management), overall and individual wealth and the availability of nutritious food. Although most government spending strongly affects the determinants of health, this influence is often not included in discussions of health systems.

The Big Picture

When a person is not feeling well or is in pain, visiting a doctor to get a prescription and/or some advice on lifestyle modification may be all that is necessary. If a person has a more serious problem, the first stop might be an emergency department or even admission to a hospital arranged by a doctor. In the hospital, the cause of the problem may be sought, and a definitive intervention undertaken, hopefully putting the person on the track to full wellness. Once the patient is well enough to be moved on, the person's destination might be back home or some sort of long-term care facility or hospice. Throughout the person's trajectory through the health system, professionals of many types will interact with the patient to diagnose what is wrong, to assess what to do next, to recommend some sort of intervention, to intervene and to help the person towards recovery or as much comfort as is possible as possible at the end of life.

The health system is a set of individually very sophisticated components that together provide the kind of adaptive complexity necessary to care for the complex human being.

It's time for at least a little bit on the ideas of complexity as it relates to the health system.

Chapter 11: Issues in Our Healthcare System

KEYWORDS: The Cost of Care, The Value of Care, Assessing Health System Performance, Assessing Individual Performance, Charlatans, End-of-Life Care

ABSTRACT: Individuals and institutions want to spend time and money on useful care. No one wants to spend money for useless or harmful healthcare activities. Evaluating care and knowing when it is useful or harmful is of vital importance. Unfortunately, charlatans—credentialed or otherwise—sometimes market snake oil – products that are not cost-worthy because they do more harm than good.

For Seniors, it is important to know when end-of-life care is likely to be helpful, wasteful, or harmful. Yet, it is important to avoid ageism and give both seniors and young people the care they need. We recognize that what is appropriate for a young person might not always be appropriate for an elder.

Introduction

It is perhaps no wonder that there are many issues associated with health care and the systems we have created to deal with it. In a certain sense, we will now do what a clinician does with a patient: we will observe, diagnose and suggest interventions.

The Cost of Health Care

Television, newspapers and think tanks routinely quote politicians and pundits about health care and health insurance. Presidents, Prime Ministers, Senators, Congressmen and assorted parliamentarians routinely consider health policy. Usually, proposed solutions involve more spending, not less, with little discussion about the expected health benefits or harms of each solution. The consequence is that Americans and Canadians seem comfortable to lavish money on health services. In Canada, at the time of writing, we spend about \$5,800 per person per year (11% of GDP) for health care, in the United States the amount is about \$8,900 per person per year (18% of GDP).[37] [38] Accounting methods do differ in the two countries; nonetheless, it is obvious that both spend more than pocket change for health care.

Headlines emphasize an emerging crisis in healthcare spending and proclaim that health care, as we know it, is unsustainable. Of course, no one really believes that 10, 20 or 50 years from now sick people will not be able to get expert health advice or find alternative ways to access answers to important health questions. However, excellent care might be unaffordable for some if

37 The World Bank Health Expenditure % GDP. https://data.worldbank.org/indicator/SH.XPD.CHEX.GD.ZS. Accessed Sept 8, 2023.

38 The World Bank Health Expenditure Per Person U.S. dollars. https://data.worldbank.org/indicator/SH.XPD.GHED.PC.CD. Accessed Sept 8, 2023.

costs continue to increase at the same rate... this is certainly true for many already.

The objective isn't only to make health care less expensive. A modest saving in health expenditures could free-up substantial funds to support education and economic development. The fact is that a significant portion of those expenditures is wasted, producing no benefit for the people or the payers (all of us). Individuals, communities and governments would surely prefer not to pay for health services that are harmful or wasteful. Better spending would not only potentially improve health care, but also enable the savings to be used to support other worthwhile services.

Determining the Effects of Health Care

Whether a person works in health care, manages health services or is a patient, there must be some way of knowing if care is effective. Linking health services to health results (outcomes) is necessary if we are to learn which activities are worthwhile. Therefore, it is important to identify which health-related activities lead to better health outcomes and which activities result in harm or no benefit. This means measuring the effects of health care by assessing and measuring health status before, during and after treatment (Section 4 discusses measures of health). Useful definitions of health must suggest the kinds of measurements that clinicians and assessors can use to link healthcare activities with health outcomes. This is called 'outcomes-based healthcare assessment.'

Everyone will eventually become sick and will likely seek health advice. Fortunately, clinicians assess and measure health to some extent at every visit and they usually make some formal or informal record of their findings. The quality and accuracy of these 'measurements' may be in question, but the locus of care is definitely a point of assessment. The key is to get good and valid measures of health and interventions routinely, to do so accurately, and to capture these measures in a form that can be analyzed.

The burden of recordkeeping is, regretfully, significant. Because of this, care providers debate about how much time they should spend doing recordkeeping versus the time they invest in clinical care. It has been a goal of Health Informatics professionals to provide clinicians with eHealth tools that afford efficient means of capturing accurate data at the point of care systematically, with minimal distraction from the primary task, caring for the patient. Health Informaticians have developed techniques that enable clinicians and researchers to capture quantitative information about health and changes in health associated with care. As of today, though, these techniques help, but themselves absorb significant time and cause much frustration.

Another issue is the breadth and depth of recordkeeping for which the clinician is directly responsible. Again, there is debate about the standards promulgated by medical regulatory agencies and what is reasonably possible and appropriate for immediate patient care. Elsewhere in this book, Dr. Campbell points out that recordkeeping can negatively impact psychiatric patient care.

The dream is that, eventually, many clinical activities can become self-documenting or verbally dictated to a recordkeeping device. An example might be an Internet-enabled clinical instrument that communicates data (like blood pressure) directly to a computer system. For our purposes here, we will simply note that linking clinical activities with health results is essential if we are to develop the clinical and administrative knowledge we need. Solving the practical problems of achieving this is a work-in-progress.

Today, many citizens only wish they had timely access to excellent health care. On the other hand, many wealthy people get quick access, but sometimes receive unnecessary services.[39] [40] [41] George Bush, the former President of the United States, a seemingly healthy, athletic 67-year-old at the time, had a routine checkup while President including a heart stress test. He felt well, and he functioned normally. During the exam, doctors found signs of the narrowing of his coronary arteries, which they interpreted as a hidden finding of disease, and decided to place a stent (an implant that holds the artery open). This is interesting, because research since then has shown that coronary artery stents do not confer any longevity benefit. They may relieve pain in those people who have exercise-induced chest pain. However, patients who are symptom-free do not appear to benefit. The medical literature suggests surgeons implant many stents that are of no benefit to patients unless they had symptoms. So, a stent may have done nothing for Mr. Bush. He was symptom-free before and symptom-free after the stent treatment. Research indicates that he is unlikely to live any longer with it than he would have without it, either. Unfortunately, some people who have surgery, whether or not it was necessary, can suffer because of unforeseen complications, like infections or clots to the brain. Unnecessary treatment can also be unsafe.

UNECESSARY CARDIAC STENTS - THE GEORGE BUSH EXAMPLE

The medical literature suggests surgeons implant many stents that are of no benefit.

George Bush, a seemingly healthy athletic 67-year-old, had a routine checkup including a stress test. In the course of the exam, doctors found signs of narrowing of the coronary arteries and decided to implant a stent (a stent is an implant that opens an artery).

He received a stent although our current medical literature suggests that athletic people who are not having symptoms do not benefit from cardiac stents. Sometimes these unnecessary procedures are not only inconvenient but also harmful.

In order to know when cardiac stents are useful, useless or wasteful, it is necessary to track the health state of people who received stents to learn the characteristics of people helped or harmed by treatment.

It is peculiar that, while some people receive unnecessary or harmful care, others suffer from rationing and excessive waits because they or their community believe they cannot afford worthwhile care.[42] [43] [44]

---

39 Larry Husten, Forbes August 6, 2013 Did George W. Bush Really Need a Stent? http://www.forbes.com/sites/larryhusten/2013/08/06/questions-about-president-george-w-bushs-stent/#13f8556c5569. Accessed July 22, 2022.

40 The George Bush stent controversy is pertinent. President Bush received a stent, even though the medical literature suggests he was unlikely to benefit. Cf. Initial Coronary Stent Implantation with Medical Therapy Vs Medical Therapy Alone for Stable Coronary Artery Disease Meta-analysis of Randomized Controlled Trials by Kathleen Stergiopoulos, MD, PhD; David L. Brown, MD published in JAMA Internal Medicine, Feb 27, 2012, V172#4, *Arch Intern Med.* 2012;172(4):312-319. doi:10.1001/archinternmed.2011.1484. http://archinte.jamanetwork.com/article.aspx?articleid=1108733. Accessed July 22, 2022.

41 Cardiovasc Revasc Med. 2013 Sep-Oct;14(5):251-2. doi: 10.1016/j.carrev.2013.08.008. To stent or not to stent: The President Bush stent controversy. Waksman R., PMID: 24034861 DOI: 10.1016/j.carrev.2013.08.008 https://www.ncbi.nlm.nih.gov/pubmed/24034861. Accessed July 22, 2022.

42 Key Facts About the Uninsured Population, The Henry J. Kaiser Family Foundation. http://kff.org/uninsured/fact-sheet/key-facts-about-the-uninsured-population/. Assessed August 25, 2022.

43 Stergiopoulos, K., Brown, L., Initial Coronary Stent Implantation with Medical Therapy vs. Medical Therapy Alone for Stable Coronary Artery Disease: Meta Analysis of Controlled Trials. Arch Intern Med. 2012;172(4):312-319. http://archinte.jamanetwork.com/article.aspx?articleid=1108733. Accessed July 22, 2022.

44 Waiting Your Turn: Wait Times for Health Care in Canada 2015. https://www.fraserinstitute.org/studies/waiting-your-turn-wait-times-for-health-care-in-canada-2015-report Accessed August 25, 2022. More recent reports are also available at the Fraser Institute Site.

Measuring Health (or Failing to Do So)

Science may have the answer in cases like President Bush's. Randomized, controlled clinical trials have investigated the effects of coronary artery stents on patients' symptoms and longevity. These trials have compared the outcomes of patients with and without the implantation of stents, both for patients with and without symptoms (such as heart pain – angina). A consequence of these trials is that we now believe that stents are minimally or not at all effective. This is the scientific way that experts have used to discover coronary stents' actual benefits and harms. Note that angina – usually causing chest or jaw pain sometimes starting in the arms or shoulders – is caused by an inadequate supply of oxygen to the heart, frequently because of narrowing or spasm of coronary arteries. Although it might seem logical that opening up a narrowed artery might improve blood flow, these results indicate that something else is causing the problem, such as failure further down in the circulation to the heart muscle (e.g., in the smaller vessels, the 'microvasculature'). In President Bush's case, he had no symptoms, so this questionably effective procedure was likely pointless.

Information about health outcomes (health after treatment compared to before) tells us if any procedure is worthwhile. When researchers collect information about the overall short- and long-term outcomes of many people, they can provide the information patients need to give informed consent. Before wagering that a treatment will help rather than harm us, patients need to know how many people who previously had the treatment did or didn't do well.

Anyone who has a clear idea of what health is and knows the expected effects of treatment is less likely to accept unnecessary and potentially harmful advice and services. This also applies to policy makers. Those who understand how health is measured and are aware of reported results are more likely to support worthwhile treatments rather than treatments that are dangerous or wasteful. The facts inform rational decision making.

Measurement is the essence of management, because without measurement it is not possible to know the effects of a treatment or any intervention, for that matter, or if a change will lead to better or worse results. Measurement itself, however, brings with it several issues, as illustrated in FIGURE 1.11.1.

KEY ISSUES IN MEASUREMENT

> *Reliability:*

- ***Repeat reliability**: test results or measurements agree when the test or measurement is repeated.*
- ***Inter-tester and intra-tester reliability**: results by different measurement or test performers agree; the results of a tester or measurer agree with own previous results.*

> *Validity:*

- ***Face validity:** the test or measurement appears to test or measure what it's supposed to test or measure.*
- ***Construct validity:** the extent to which a test or measure accurately assesses what it's supposed to test or measure.*

FIGURE 1.11.1: Key issues in measurement

There is a problem at the top, however. Most health organizations, governments and regulators, do not routinely monitor changes in health following care. Consequently, they do not know and cannot find out which recommended interventions are good, bad or indifferent. Moreover, most regulators do not monitor the impact of changed health policy on population health. For example, we might expect the American government could report on the effects of the increasing or reducing access to Obamacare. We might think that a new President would have this information before making other changes to health insurance. But no! That information is not available! Each decision maker must fly the healthcare airplane by the seat of the pants through the clouds of ignorance – there are no instruments to guide and help. They are flying VFR (visually) in situations, like storm clouds, that require IFR (instruments…data). Perhaps even worse, the 'instruments' the decision maker has are often flawed or malfunctioning and the decision maker does not know that. There have been many examples of an airplane pilot using a failed artificial horizon to fly right to the scene of a crash! No wonder there are so many administrators who end up at the scene of another healthcare 'accident'.

Each decision maker must fly the healthcare airplane by the seat of the pants through the clouds of ignorance – there are no instruments to guide and help. No wonder there are so many administrators who end up at the scene of another healthcare 'accident.'

Sadly, many of the controversies over health insurance relate only to costs rather than to measured health outcomes.[45] Without meaningful and useful measures of health, based on agreement regarding what health means (is it just that the patient survived or got home, not the patient's comfort or functioning?), it is impossible to validate the policy positions of proponents or opponents on any position. Nor is it possible to determine if communities achieve value for what they spend on health care. That value is achieving a given benefit.

One opportunity that would seem to be easy to take advantage of would be monitoring the influence of hospital care on health. Unfortunately, many hospital 'discharge reports' (formal documents that summarize the events of care) do not indicate if patients' health improved or worsened over a hospital stay. Seldom do hospitals formally assess health at admission, during a stay and at discharge. And they seldom follow up later to see how the patient is doing after discharge. Without that information about health outcomes, adjusting services is a shot in the dark.

In short, part of the problem in the management of health care and health services is that clinicians, regulators and policy makers:

Rarely measure or document the goals or purposes of care.

Rarely report the expected or achieved results of treatment.

Rarely can forecast how individual and community health will benefit from proposed changes in the administrative and regulatory frameworks for health care.

Rarely have quantitative or objective methods to measure or predict the effect of changes in health policy.

Rarely ask how many - and which - patients will have better health outcomes because of tests, treatments and changes in the delivery of health services.

We must be aware that every laboratory investigation and every treatment choice engenders not only the possibility of benefit but also the possibility of harm to our bodies or our wealth. Yet, few people ask about how they or their treatment might be affected by medical tests and treatments. Worse still, few health systems know if what they do makes a positive difference to their patients. It often comes down to "we've always done it this way" or "we feel that is the best way to proceed". Actual objective assessment is often AWOL (absent without leave).

45 About the Affordable Care Act US Department of Health and Human Services. http://www.hhs.gov/healthcare/facts-and-features/fact-sheets/aca-is-working/index.html. Accessed August 25, 2022.
The Affordable Care Act is Working from HHS.GOV. There are no measures of improvement or decrease in the health of people who are now covered. People who receive worthwhile care, otherwise not available, benefit. Those who receive unnecessary care may suffer from avoidable complications of treatment.

Consumers and Snake Oil

All of these ideas apply equally to consumers.

People watch TV and use the Internet. Exploiting these media, promoters bombard consumers with claims that this or that activity, food, drug, dietary supplement or a change in surroundings, weight or fitness will have a major influence on personal health. Unless we want to be whipsawed from one position to another or to be monetarily ripped off, we need to learn if these claims are valid. Evaluating claims requires some understanding of what we mean by health and the purposes of care and what we mean when we state that someone's health improved or became worse. The key is for each consumer to wonder if claims should be believed. If people are going to trust, then they would be wise to verify!

There are many examples of somewhat specious claims. Almost everyone has heard that drinking eight glasses of water per day is essential for health. I guess we should have wondered about this claim because a "glass" is not a metric or imperial measure of fluid, and a shot-glass might suffice (perhaps for some, it does!). It just ain't true! That claim is not based on actual evidence.

There are endless claims about a supplement for something: for your eyes, your brain, your intestines, no doubt even for your big toe. Of course, there is a cream to remove decades of wrinkles and there are shakes that will trim you down to a mere skeleton. We must question if these claims are valid. Almost uniformly, they are not. Yeah, that's true! Almost every vitamin and supplement that a huckster has claimed to be of value has been debunked in clinical trials – unless a person has a physiological deficiency. It is important to wonder about the ingredients and effects of any hyped product. Is there any possibility that those ingredients could actually be of help? Case in point, can a substance affect your brain if it is broken down by your gut? How? Is there a stomach-brain channel? Well, maybe after fasting for a day!

We can ask if there is any credible evidence that the supplement or nutrient has actually been of help. Without that evidence, we are all in the same position that we have cited for hospitals. We don't know if a product will be of any benefit whatsoever or if it might injure or compromise us in some way.

We must consider the measurables of health, discussed in the next chapter. These are the comfort, function and life expectancy we introduced back at the beginning. The question is: do any of the substances that peddlers promote to us improve our comfort, help us to be better able to function better or extend our lives? Very few have any of these effects and their objective impact seems to be the reduction of the contents of our wallets or pocketbooks.

Perhaps one or two brief stories will bring home some of the issues.

Some Clinical Scenarios

END OF LIFE CARE AND CLINICAL TRADEOFFS: SCENARIO-AGE DISCRIMINATION

Knowing the purposes of care helps understand why treatment choices are different at different ages. Usually, it is not only acceptable but also more appropriate to offer different treatment choices based on age and to emphasize the different purposes of care near the end of life.

Compare these two patients: Mary is a 92-year-old woman who feels well. She notices a neck lump and drives to her doctor's office. He investigates the lump and learns she has Hodgkin's Lymphoma (a cancer of the lymph system).

Michelle is a healthy, energetic, athletic, thoughtful 23-year-old full-time university student who holds a part time job with a major advertising agency. She also notices a lump in her neck. She visits the same doctor, who determines that she too has Hodgkin's Lymphoma.

The doctor discusses possible treatments and their up- and down-sides and recommends a different approach for each patient. Mary's family complains the doctor is 'ageist.'

The doctor discusses the purposes of care with Mary's relatives. Eventually they understand that the difference in treatment approach is appropriate, not based on ageism or on the differences in treatment success[46] *for young and old. Instead, good clinicians recommended treatment based on the knowledge of possible outcomes in each case. The danger for Mary is that the treatment would potentially shorten her life or make the time she had left very unpleasant.*

MAINTAINING FOCUS ON THE PURPOSE OF CARE

Fred is an athletic 54-year-old man, who has never shown signs of any disease. He sees his doctor because of an ankle sprain. By the end of the visit, he has a requisition for blood tests because his doctor believes in comprehensive care and screening for risk.

After two weeks, his ankle gets better by itself. His doctor tells him about his blood results and prescribes a cholesterol-lowering medication. Several weeks later, Fred feels fine except for some overall muscle aches, leg cramps and increased thirst and wonders why he received a cholesterol-lowering medication and if that might be what is causing his problems. Sure enough, he then reads that some of his new problems may be the result of the prescribed medication and that with or without cholesterol-lowering drugs his chances of a heart attack or a stroke were not altered. His suffering from cramps is in vain. In effect, his doctor actually prescribed unhelpful cramps!

46 Engert, A., Ballova, V., Haverkamp, H., et. Al. Hodgkin's Lymphoma in Elderly Patients: A Comprehensive Retrospective Analysis from the German Hodgkin's Study Group Journal of Clinical Oncology Aug 1, 2005:5052-5060; https://pubmed.ncbi.nlm.nih.gov/15955904/. Accessed Sept 8, 2023.

VOLUME 1

Section 3

THE NATURE OF DIAGNOSIS

FUNNY (SLIGHTLY EDITED) EXERPTS FROM MEDICAL RECORDS

Medical records are not known for good English, grammar or punctuation; they are often unreadable:

- *Patient has left her white blood cells at another hospital.*
- *Patient suffers chest pain when she lies on her left side for over a year.*
- *On the 2nd day the knee was better and on the 3rd day it disappeared.*
- *The patient has been depressed since she began seeing me in 2005.*
- *Discharge status: Alive but without my permission.*
- *Patient has 2 adolescent children but no other abnormalities.*
- *Ms. Charles slipped and apparently her legs went in separate directions in early December.*
- *Patient was seen by Dr. Smith who said we should sit on the abdomen and I agree.*
- *The patient has no previous history of suicides.*
- *She is numb from her toes down.*
- *She stated she had been constipated for most of her life until she got a divorce.*
- *Both breasts are equal and reactive to light and accommodation.*
- *Examination of his genitalia revealed that Mr. Jones is circus-sized and had an orchidectomy. (An 'orchiectomy' is a surgical procedure to remove testicles, while 'orchidectomy' would mean to remove an orchid!)*
- *Patient was found in bed with her power mower.*
- *She says she is cold, though not shaking; but her husband reports she was hot in bed last night.*

A Story: The Wages of an Incomplete Differential Diagnosis

Many people have experienced the consequences of delayed and mistaken diagnoses or faced problems that are ignored when a clinician uses the medical description of the problem – 'epistaxis' is just a medical word for nosebleed that doesn't explain its cause – as if it were a diagnosis. Patients' vigilance and their participation in their care often can avoid the harms that result from diagnostic delay or error.

Ross Douthat, writing in the New York Times[47], provided a moving tale of his experiences about the causes and consequences of delayed diagnosis. Sadly, many have had his experience. For him, though, participation and insistence led to more rapid (but nevertheless delayed) diagnosis. This is a lesson for everyone.

Mr. Douthat, a successful opinion columnist for the New York Times and a rare user of medical services, and his pregnant wife were expecting their third child and bought a house in rural Connecticut. Subsequently he complained of insomnia, "blazing pain," a stabbing pain in his teeth and head, and vibratory sensations throughout his body. He also had dizziness and disorientation and felt that his body was "slightly disassociated" from itself.

Many doctors claimed, "there was too much going on in his life" and attributed the problem to "stress". They neglected to explain why his stress presented as the problems he described, nor why he did not have similar experiences in previous, more stressful periods in his life.

He eventually persuaded one doctor to treat him for Lyme disease. Unfortunately, he experienced a rare, and short-lived complication from the antibiotic – the Jarish Herxheimer reaction, with flares of symptoms sometimes associated with the death of the bacteria in his body. Sadly, that doctor, though an infectious disease expert, was unfamiliar with this reaction and said: "we just don't know". Mr. Douthat persisted, and eventually doctors gave him an appropriate antibiotic, at the proper dose and for sufficient time. Despite this, he developed the chronic symptoms of Lyme disease (arthritis, joint pain, headaches, to name a few). His book "The Deep Places: A Memoir of Illness and Discovery"[48] is an excellent, moving and informative description of his medical adventures, the importance of participating in your own care, and why doctors must consider all possibilities before jumping to a diagnostic conclusion. Mr. Douthat shows that with persistence and an interest in researching a problem, ordinary people can find pertinent information related to the diagnosis and treatment of complex, sometimes difficult-to-diagnose, problems.

---

47 https://www.nytimes.com/2021/10/23/opinion/lyme-disease-chronic-illness.html. Accessed Sept 13, 2024.

48 The Deep Places: A Memoir of Illness and Discovery, Ross Douthat, Convergent Press, New York, Oct. 26, 2021. https://www.amazon.com/Deep-Places-Memoir-Illness-Discovery/dp/0593237366. Accessed Sept 13, 2023.

Chapter 12: Introduction to Etiology

KEYWORDS: Diagnosis, Nature of Diagnosis, Causes of Illness, Patient Wagers, Doctor's Thinking, Misdiagnosis

ABSTRACT: Medical diagnoses are efforts to understand the origin of a medical problem. When a patient identifies having a problem, doctors think of some of the possible reasons for the problem – a diagnosis. Detecting the cause of an individual problem is sometimes difficult because most problems can have many plausible causes. Most doctors can't easily remember the rare causes of some problems. Consequently, these problems may go unrecognized for many years. It is important for patients to understand how doctors can compile lists of reasons for a problem and then focus their attention on excluding certain problems and confirming a particular problem as the cause.

Introduction

We have touched on the nature of the patient's interaction with the physician and provided a basic overview of the health system. Now we will address what diagnosis is all about and what it enables. It is crucial for informing what physicians do and the effects they have. One must understand the nature and limits of diagnosis to fully appreciate medical care. Furthermore, for patients to become engaged in their care, they must become amateur diagnosticians and be able to participate intelligently and actively in the diagnostic process. This is because diagnosis is how we reach an understanding of the cause of medical problems and of possible treatments.

The Nature of Diagnosis

Mysteries intrigue us. They are puzzles about something happening, but we do not know what caused it. In fiction, the story reveals a crime of some kind, the discovery of the aftermath, and then the efforts of a brilliant detective to figure out who or what caused the incident.

What a physician does in diagnosis is similar. Solving some crimes is simple because of lots of compelling evidence and possibly witnesses or videos from surveillance cameras. Other crimes are difficult to solve and require help from many people and the use of sometimes lengthy and sophisticated forensic investigations. In the same way, in Medicine, some disorders are easy to recognize and not at all puzzling. Other disorders may be difficult to understand and interpret. Finding out their cause may require the help of decision support tools and other medical professionals.

Causes of crimes can be immediate or remote in place and time. A shooter is an immediate cause of death for a murder where a firearm is used. We recognize that reducing access to guns would help us to avoid many firearm deaths, as access to a gun is a necessary condition for every shooting death. However, eliminating guns is not sufficient to prevent murders. We need to eliminate or prevent the action of the immediate cause, murderers.

Think about a mystery involving a person killed crossing the street. The first issue is determining what happened and then, what caused it. Let's assume the person was hit by a car at dusk. Getting hit by the car is the immediate cause of death. The next issue might be finding out who was driving the car and under what conditions. The cause of the pedestrian's death may seem obvious, but the situation could be deeper than it appears. Suppose, for example, the driver was inebriated or that the driver had a grudge against the pedestrian. It might also be that poor visibility played a role in what occurred, in which case better street lighting would reduce the chance of another similar accident. If we decide that the person with a grudge was the cause, then this is crucially important – it wasn't an accident. Sure, the immediate cause was the impact of the car but, in fact, the car was used as a weapon and the real cause of the pedestrian's death is the action of the driver. It's now a murder, not an accident!

So, there are general types or kinds of causes. One example of a kind of cause is an 'accident' – unintentional circumstances, including pure chance; weather and poor visibility caused it. Another kind of cause is 'murder' – the driver weaponized the vehicle, and there are many grades of murder. Then there is 'unsafe driving' – inebriated driving, as we mentioned, as well as other unsafe driving behaviors. An 'etiology' – a type of cause – in the lists below is analogous to one of these kinds of causes of the pedestrian's death.

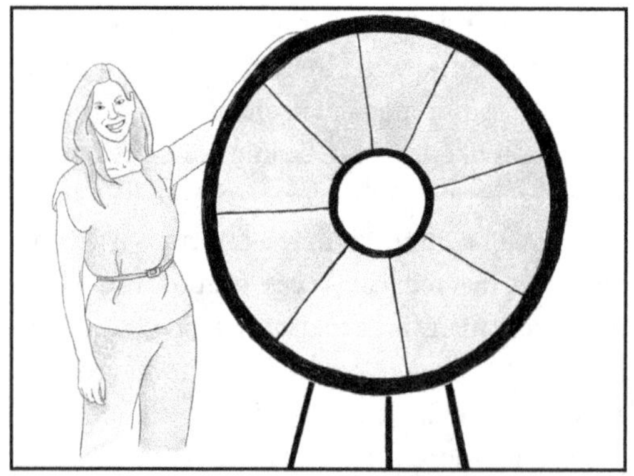

FIGURE 1.12.1: Choosing a treatment is a wager

Patients' Wagers

In health care there are lots of mysteries, specifically related to the causes of patients' problems. The challenge physicians face is to identify what is wrong, figure out the cause and to give it a meaningful name (a valid diagnostic term, a 'diagnosis') that can guide treatment to correct or ameliorate the problems. Instead of the police concluding that it was murder, not an accident, the physician concludes that the cause of the patient's problems is a bacterial infection, not a viral one.

However, accepting a diagnostic conclusion represents a wager on the patient's part that the explanation offered is correct and that the solutions (treatments) proposed will be acceptable, helpful and not harmful. FIGURE 1.12.1 emphasises the wager the patient makes. We are faced with taking our chances.

Unfortunately, physicians are confronted by challenges like those the police encounter: tests to confirm or disprove any diagnosis and there will always be an associated error rate. The police may do breath-alcohol tests, interrogate witnesses and maybe access the driver's cell phone to see if distraction was a factor. However, each of these will be associated with uncertainties. None will be perfectly accurate, complete or unbiased. Physicians may order many investigations, as well. Their results are not always correct or accurate, either. Confidence increases, however, when many types of evidence all point in the same direction.

Related to the results of tests, another analogy from our common experience may be helpful. Everyone is familiar with screening at airports. The goal of that screening is to identify people who are dangerous, while subjecting everyone else to as little inconvenience as possible. Sometimes, a safe person is misidentified as a danger (a false alarm or false positive test result). At other times a dangerous person might be identified as safe (a false negative test result). Screening experts try to develop systems and procedures that result in as few misidentifications as possible.

The personal characteristics of those screened are also important. An 85-year-old grandparent is less likely to be a dangerous terrorist compared with a seemingly athletic 25-year-old. Similarly, in a prison, tests that suggest someone is not harmful are more likely to be wrong compared with the same tests performed in a monastery. This realization about the importance of the characteristics of populations has important medical analogs. A pap smear showing that a virginal 18-year-old has cervical (the outlet of the uterus or womb) cancer is more likely to be wrong compared with the same result in a 35-year-old prostitute. Young virgins rarely have cervical cancer (often caused by a sexually transmitted virus); it is far more common in older prostitutes. The 'prevalence' (frequency of the condition in the population) has a major influence on whether or not a test is likely to produce a helpful result.

Correct interpretations of the cause of a problem, what we call 'diagnoses', are important because they may lead to treatment possibilities. Incorrect diagnoses often can result in incorrect treatments or unnecessary risk. When patients accept treatments, they are betting that the diagnoses and the treatments proposed are the right ones for them. They hope the treatments suggested by the diagnosis will be more likely to help than harm and that the treatment will hasten recovery.

The Physician's Thinking

Back to airplanes. Physicians and pilots are similar. Both have an intuitive approach to problem-solving based on pattern recognition for dealing with many, especially urgent or time-constrained, problems. However, both also use – often in parallel with their intuitive approach – a systematic approach to help ensure they consider both common and rare possibilities for some problems. Flying itself becomes intuitive (called 'flying by the seat of your pants'), but any deviations from normal flight or unusual behaviors of the aircraft or instruments demand a systematic response. Pilots and physicians must be vigilant to see an unusual symptom or discover a sign (like an observation or test result) that does not fit with an innocent or common diagnosis. Then it becomes necessary to engage in a systematic thought process to figure out what is going on. For airline pilots, it's the lives of the 'souls' behind them; for physicians, it's the lives of the persons in front of them.

Whenever patients complain about a problem, the doctor listens carefully to them, examines them and begins creating a more-or-less complete mental list of the possible causes of what is bothering the patient. This is called a 'differential diagnosis.' The words connote that it is a list of possible diagnoses – possible causes of a problem – that doctors need to differentiate from one another and choose the one most likely. For any problem, the differential diagnosis will include a list of very common diseases, as well as a long list of obscure conditions. Few clinicians can recall all the possible causes of problems, as our example, fatigue, with more than the 2000+ causes, illustrates. Consequently, whenever clinicians have difficulty identifying the reason for a problem, it becomes important to consult a checklist or seek human or computerized help to get information about possible diagnoses and how to distinguish among them.

Some doctors use the lists of possible problem-causes that they carry in their own minds, and make little effort to consult comprehensive lists, like those in books or online. The strategy is time-efficient and is usually effective for patients who present with common, well-known problems. However, physicians cannot always recall all the possibilities and can fail to reach the right conclusion when patients have unusual problems, failed to mention some symptoms or have a condition the doctor has not learned about.

Other doctors (and, sometimes, their patients), when stumped or just as a verification step, use subscription and free computerized decision support tools[49] to help them exhaustively identify all the possible causes of a problem and the tests necessary to help confirm or reject each possible diagnosis. This latter strategy is most useful and sometimes necessary when a patient has an uncommon condition or presents with a common condition in an unusual way.

Finding the Medical Culprit

Going a little deeper, a person seeing a physician usually has some concerns or discomfort, will likely exhibit certain symptoms, and the results of the examination and tests might suggest what is amiss. The physician puts all this together to develop hypotheses about the cause of these problems. For example, the physician may determine that the cause of pain and weakness is a neoplasm ('new formation' – abnormal tissue growth) and will state that the diagnosis is 'cancer'. That may not be the end of it, however, as the person might live in an environment besotted with chemicals and that have caused the cancer (i.e., the chemicals are 'carcinogenic', cancer-causing). Based on this, we can see that there may be a chain of causes and getting to understand each link of the chain may be crucial. It may not be good enough to treat the cancer if exposure to carcinogens continues. The diagnosis, cancer, which is the immediate reason for the patient's problems, is the result of prolonged environmental exposure to carcinogenic toxins. A step deeper might be that the person is poor and uneducated and that necessitates working in that environment.

Considering this example, we will define the initiating cause as the 'primary cause' or first cause. In this case, the exposure to carcinogenic compounds caused the cancer; it's the primary cause (although, the World Health Organization might state that poverty was really the primary cause). The secondary cause of the patient's condition is the cancer itself and the effects that cancer has on bodily systems. The truth is that the medical literature and its vocabulary are a bit confusing when it comes to this thinking.

Physicians use the term 'etiology' (the study of causation or origination) to describe the cause of a disease (actually, the kind of cause). The word 'etiology' comes from the Greek and means 'giving a reason for'. Merriam-Webster defines etiology as the branch of medical science "concerned with the causes or origins of disease" and also as "the cause of an abnormal condition". Sometimes it is difficult to relate the secondary cause of a condition to the primary cause. It's akin to figuring out if the driver of the car in our example had a grudge, was impaired or was faultless because the pedestrian stepped out onto the road suddenly or a manufacturing error caused brake failure.

From time to time, circumstances compel doctors to treat diseases without putting a lot of effort into learning what caused the disease. One reason is that the patient is in serious discomfort and the doctor is convinced of the reason for the patient's suffering, based on the probabilities of a person getting certain diseases. Another reason is that sometimes major effort is not necessary as the physician can simply use pattern recognition to recognize that a constellation of problems reflects a specific illness. The risk is that the clinician might harm the patient by treating for the wrong diagnosis/problem. On the other hand, being

49 For example, Isabel https://www.isabelhealthcare.com/. Accessed Sept 8, 2023. or Diagnosis Pro https://jamanetwork.com/journals/jama/article-abstract/413942 Accessed Sept 8, 2023 - DiagnosisPro is the ultimate medical and differential diagnosis tool (informer.com). Accessed July 19, 2022. or BMJ Best Practice https://bestpractice.bmj.com/info/subscribe/ (requires a subscription). Accessed Sept 8, 2023.

meticulous can be harmful by engendering delays in diagnosis and intervention. A quandary indeed!

Sometimes it takes information from many patients to deduce the real cause of a problem. It is only when many people in a neighborhood develop similar symptoms that clinicians and researchers see a pattern that indicates a possibly unexpected cause. Doctors faced with one instance of thyroid cancer or food poisoning are unlikely to search for a specific or primary cause. However, if many people present with similar problems, clinicians and epidemiologists will search for environmental causes (like radiation) for the thyroid cancer, or food contamination (e.g., food poisoning caused by E. Coli).

From this material you can see the confusion. Suppose a doctor is seeing a patient and it soon becomes clear that liver cancer is causing the observed symptoms. However, it may be that the person has been abusing an intoxicant (e.g., alcohol) for many years. That intoxicant abuse, in fact, was the primary cause of the cancer. Of course, one could again continue this chain of reasoning and make a claim that there was a 'more-primary' cause, perhaps the socioeconomic environment of the patient, which the World Health Organization codifies as a cause of disease. For our purposes, however we will stick with alcohol as the primary cause, even though we know that alcohol is neither a necessary nor sufficient condition for the development of liver cancer. Some people who are heavy drinkers never get liver cancer even though they might severely damage their livers. Others who drink hardly at all might get liver cancer from a viral infection (e.g., Hepatitis C) or an unknown reason.

The lists of etiologies provide an overarching indication of the kinds or types of causes of disease. When clinicians are having difficulty making a diagnosis, they will, as we indicated, run through a more or less complete checklist of possible etiologies to make sure they have considered the all the possible causes for a problem.

The next section cites a quite detailed appendix that can be left till later. The general ideas are important, however.

Lists of Etiologies, Causes, Diagnoses

Physicians consider etiologies or types of causes of the problems of their patients and then reflect on specific causes. Disorders of almost any bodily system can be responsible for most medical problems. For example, many diagnoses, each associated with a different bodily system, might explain fatigue or muscle soreness or even a sore throat. In the early stages of most illnesses, people usually present with non-specific complaints, for example, tiredness, weight loss or muscle discomfort. This means that many possible diagnoses may apply. Sometimes, fatigue represents a normal response to life's circumstances – overwork, poor diet, lack of exercise, insufficient sleep. At other times, fatigue signifies a significant, easily-treatable malady – like hypothyroid (low levels of thyroid hormone from that organ). At other times fatigue is an early warning of important problems (for example, some cancers) where early diagnosis and treatment substantially improve the chances of a good outcome.

Clinicians and patients benefit when they apply a systematic approach that considers all of the possible kinds of causes of problems. However, the lists are challenging to recall, so people develop mnemonics as an aide-memoir. One useful mnemonic uses the word 'vitamins,' where the letters stand for each vitamin. A, B, C, D, E and K are vitamins, and the mnemonic is VITAMINSABCDEK[50] (See Appendix X[51]). Each letter stands for an etiology. People use this mnemonic to help them remember many of the kinds of causes of illness.

Remember that each kind of or general cause can have many specific causes. Consequently, many groups have developed differential diagnosis handbooks that anyone can use to help consider all the conditions that influence each body system. This document includes thousands of conditions and is beyond the scope of this book. Mnemonics are endemic in Medicine. Maybe the 'M' in Medicine stands for **M**nemonics!

The letters in the mnemonic VITAMINSABCDEK listed in Appendix X remind us of most of the types of preventable and non-preventable conditions that cause medical problems. The list encompasses most of the reasons for illnesses, given the current state of knowledge.

Knowing how diagnoses are made and the categories of diagnosis will help everyone, physician or not, develop hypotheses and an understanding of what is contributing to or causing an illness. With that they should be able to identify the diagnostic term that describes the cause. Understanding the nuances of diagnosis is crucial to the understanding and diagnosing of the illnesses that afflict people.

We are fortunate, however, that a small number of conditions cause much of the illness and suffering that plague people. Physicians and often patients are usually able to easily recognize and diagnose these more usual problems.

For example, according to the Centers for Disease Control, about 74% of all deaths result from 10, usually easy-to-diagnose causes.[52] The leading causes of death, in order of frequency, are:

1. Heart Disease.
2. Cancer.
3. Unintentional Injuries.
4. Chronic Lower Respiratory Disease (often smoking related).
5. Stroke.
6. Alzheimer disease.
7. Diabetes.
8. Influenza and Pneumonia.
9. Kidney Disease.
10. Suicide.

It is worth noting the 10 leading causes of death shown in FIGURE 1.12.2.

50 Zabidi A Zabidi-Hussinm, Practical way of creating differential diagnoses through an expanded *VITAMINSABCDEK* mnemonic Adv Med Educ Pract. 2016; 7: 247–248. Published online 2016 Apr 22. https://www.ncbi.nlm.nih.gov/pmc/articles/PMC4853007/. Accessed July 19, 2022.

51 Zabidi A Zabidi-Hussinm, Practical way of creating differential diagnoses through an expanded *VITAMINSABCDEK* mnemonic Adv Med Educ Pract. 2016; 7: 247–248. Published online 2016 Apr 22. https://www.ncbi.nlm.nih.gov/pmc/articles/PMC4853007/. Accessed July 19, 2022.

52 Centers for Disease Control and Prevention, NCHS Data Brief No. 328, November 2018. https://www.cdc.gov/nchs/products/databriefs/db328.htm#Summary. Accessed July 19, 2022.

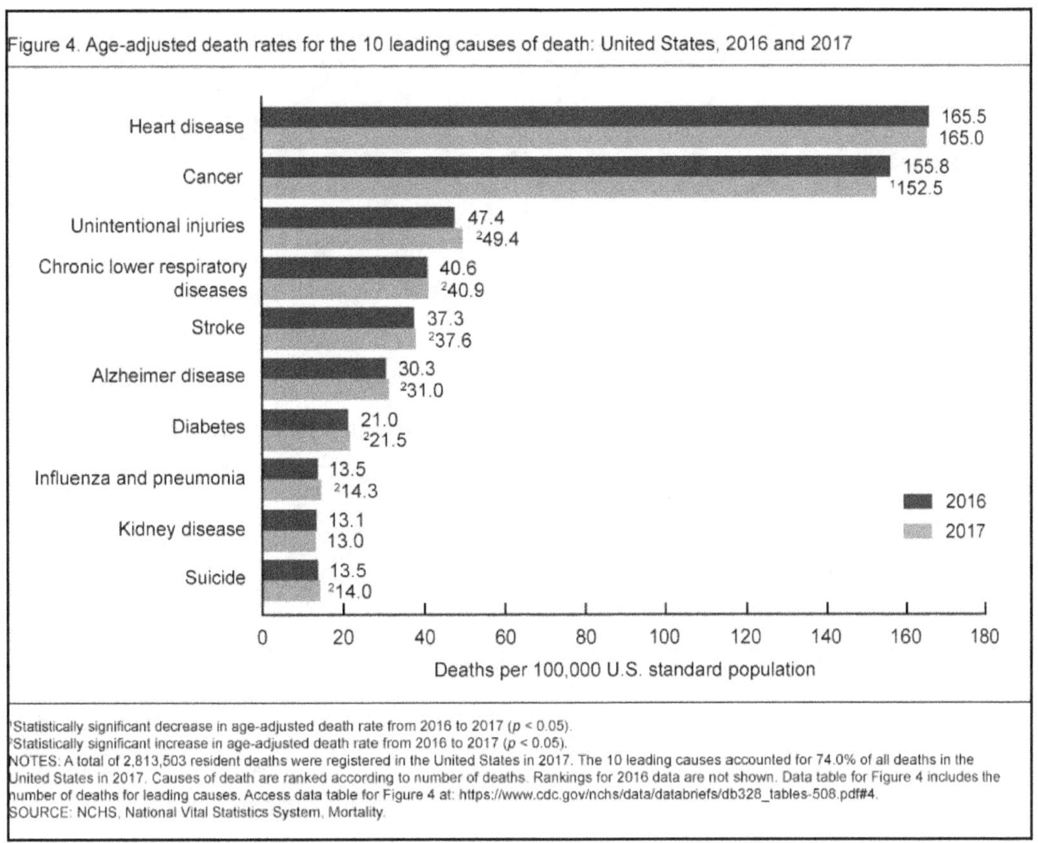

FIGURE 1.12.2: Mortality causes in US 2017-2017[53]

53 Sherry L. Murphy, Jiaquan Xu, Kenneth D, Kochanek, Elizabeth Arias. Mortality in the United States, 2017. https://pubmed.ncbi.nlm.nih.gov/36598387/. Accessed Sept 13, 2023.

Chapter 13: Understanding Diagnosis

KEYWORDS: Diagnosis, Flowchart of the Diagnostic Process, Strategies for Diagnosis, Watchful Waiting, False Alarms, Therapeutic Trial

ABSTRACT: Some problems are easy to diagnose, and some problems appear to involve self limited disease. An upper respiratory infection or cold is usually caused by a virus and clears up on its own. Sometimes, however, the cause is less benign. However, investigations aren't without risk, so occasionally doctors will try either tincture of time – waiting to see if the problem gets better – or a therapeutic trial – suggesting a medication to see if the problem resolves.

I'm tired all the time! Is something wrong with me?

Medical books are loaded with descriptions of the many (over 3,000) possible causes (diagnoses) of fatigue and of various other aches, pains and causes of death. But who needs medical books? Today, that same information is available to anyone with a library card or an Internet connection.

Diagnoses Can Often be Made Using Information Available to Everyone

Readers can search for lists of clinical decision support systems. One excellent example of these is called 'Prodigy', which can be found at http://prodigy.clarity.co.uk/home (Accessed July 19, 2022). The reputable British National Health Service supports it at no cost to people in the U.K. Another site, eHealthme.com,[54] provides useful information about drugs and their benefits and harms. Through resources like these, we can get at least an idea of what is wrong with us, our families or friends. They empower us and help us to determine when we need expert assistance.

E-HealthMe also enables people to ask other website users about their experiences and their solutions to problems.[55] Much as clinicians find decision support tools to be helpful;[56] readers and patients with access to online tools not hidden behind paywalls will find them helpful too.

Of course, to understand how to confirm or disprove a diagnosis, it is important to know something about how to interpret various test results and what they imply. Another section of this book deals with the predictive value of laboratory investigations: how often test results are correct or misleading and what you need to know about the prevalence of disease in a community to interpret tests correctly. It

54 http://www.ehealthme.com/. Accessed July 19, 2022.

55 http://www.ehealthme.com/. E-Health Me web site. Accessed July 19, 2022.

56 Alya Porat_Brendan Delaney and Olga Kostopoulou: The Impact of Diagnostic Decision Support System on the Consultation. BMC Medical Informatics and Decision Making BMC series – open201717:79. https://pubmed.ncbi.nlm.nih.gov/28576145/. Accessed July 19, 2022.

can get be confusing or overwhelming, though, and that is why we need physicians.

Making the Diagnosis

We all see ourselves as unique and having esoteric and complex problems, but is that true and is that the physician's experience?

Reality is that 'common things are common', an adage learned by every medical student. It states that the diseases many people have will, of course, be the diseases physicians commonly see. We also say that, if it looks like a duck and quacks like a duck, it is a duck (and not a flat-footed albino raven simulating mimicking a duck). Sometimes, however, other distant rare birds might look and sound like ducks.

It is heartening to realize that doctors and knowledgeable people can diagnose most problems without relying on elaborate physical examinations or sophisticated laboratory investigations. Studies show that over 75% of diagnoses are made based on a patient's reported history alone, another 12% require the information from a physical examination, and only about 10% require information from laboratory or other investigations.[57]

This is the good news: most of the time, a diagnosis can be made simply from information the patient tells the clinician or based on visual or auditory clues (called 'signs') that anyone can notice. Many computerized tools do help doctors and can help patients develop the lists of possible diagnoses and indicate what is necessary to confirm or disprove each diagnosis. Most people have problems caused by innocuous or at least not life-threatening problems. The lengthy lists of possibilities should not be scary despite including many serious, harmful and dangerous – but fortunately rare – causes.

What people see and sense about themselves will help them as well as their doctors reach an appropriate diagnosis and solution. Laboratory test results can reduce any residual uncertainty and help confirm that conclusion.

It is worth emphasizing again that readily available information is adequate to diagnose about 90% of diagnosable medical conditions.[58] Sophisticated tests, that only physicians can order, are not necessary to solve most medical problems.

Why Doctors Diagnose

Whenever people have problems – that is they are uncomfortable, have limitations of activity or are worried about survival – doctors try to interpret the problem in a way that explains it – defines its cause – and points to a solution.

People suffer unnecessarily when clinicians miss or take too long to diagnose an important problem. Delayed diagnosis of important problems, like certain cancers, leads not only to prolonged short-term suffering but also to worse long-term outcomes. People who understand the basics of diagnosis can assist their doctors in not missing or delaying a diagnosis.

A physician's life would be simpler if each of our problems had only a few possible explanations or possible treatments, but most abnormal signs (what we see), or symptoms (what we feel), or abnormal lab results (what we objectively measure or visualize) have many possible causes and, usually, several acceptable treatments.

We already mentioned fatigue, a very common complaint. Fatigue may be caused by mundane problems, sleep deprivation for one, but also by significant problems, among them hormonal abnormalities and cancer. In fact, no one can remember all of the over

57 (Peterson MC, Holbrook JH, Hales D, Smith NL, Staker LV: Contributions of the history, physical examination, and laboratory investigation in making medical diagnoses. West J Med 1992 Feb; 156:163-165). http://www.ncbi.nlm.nih.gov/pmc/articles/PMC1003190/pdf/westjmed00090-0053.pdf. Accessed July 19, 2022.

58 (Peterson MC, Holbrook JH, Hales D, Smith NL, Staker LV: Contributions of the history, physical examination, and laboratory investigation in making medical diagnoses. West J Med 1992 Feb; 156:163-165) http://www.ncbi.nlm.nih.gov/pmc/articles/PMC1003190/pdf/westjmed00090-0053.pdf. Accessed July 19, 2022.

3,000 possible reasons for feeling fatigued. Sometimes even the most astute clinician is more efficient in diagnosing if patients help or the doctor uses checklists of all the possible diagnoses and the examinations and tests required to confirm each.

On the other hand, people may also suffer and sometimes die from the consequences of too many investigations. Most medical tests produce helpful results. Unfortunately, tests also carry risks of their own. There must be a balance. A dangerous risk is the rare complication of a bowel puncture during a colonoscopy. False alarms are also harmful. A false positive mammogram[59] (breast imaging) result, indicating breast cancer that isn't there, can prompt an unnecessary breast biopsy (tissue removal) that leads to an infection, not to mention scaring the patient. A false positive result from testing the biopsied tissue, indicating the tissue is abnormal when it isn't, can then lead patients to not have further, necessary, investigations.

Two Strategies for Diagnosing

Doctors try to use efficient strategies to arrive at an explanation of a problem. Worthwhile strategies will recognize the possibility of serious threats to the patient, without exposing patients to the unnecessary risks that come with invasive or excessive investigation. We deal with strategies later, but we will mention two here: 'watchful waiting' (or 'tincture of time') and 'therapeutic trials' of safe medications. (We deal with these in more detail later, but we will touch on them here.) Tincture of time means waiting to see if the problem resolves spontaneously. Therapeutic trials involve prescribing medication to see if the problem resolves with the use of a benign medication.

Most doctors normally assume, correctly, that one of the common causes of a condition is, in fact, the actual cause of patients' problems. For the sake of the patient, however, doctors must also routinely consider rare but serious problems, because the consequences of delayed diagnosis can be disastrous. The physician's differential diagnosis might have just 2 possibilities, but there must always be a third virtual one: "Can it be anything else?"

For example, suppose a patient had a sudden onset of a cough. A cough is normally a sign of either a self-limited viral infection or easily treated bacterial bronchitis (inflammation of the breathing tubes caused by bacteria). Less common and potentially more serious causes, though, include whooping-cough, drug-induced (e.g., ACE inhibitor – a heart medication) cough, lung cancer, a rare fungal infection of the lung, or a systemic illness.[60] The latter ones would potentially threaten the patient's life.

Diagnosis is fraught with opportunities to be caught flat-footed or to over-react. Careful consideration of all the relevant facts and possibilities of causes is necessary. The breadth and depth of the diagnostician as well as attitude and experience all play roles in making good decisions. The patient's eyes, ears and brains and willingness to speak up can also play key roles in concert with the physician.

Forming a diagnosis sometimes requires a quite complex decision-making process. We have illustrated a simplified one in FIGURE 1.13.1 to show the kinds of steps involved.

---

59 Mammogram is an x-ray examination of the breast, often used for screening and sometimes to investigate a known breast lump or breast discomfort.

60 Rare systemic illnesses that might present as cough include sarcoidosis (and lupus erythematosus). Kefang Lai, Jiaman Tang, Wenzhi Zhan, Hu Li, Fang Yi, Li Long, Jianmeng Zhou, Xiaomei Chen, Lianrong Huang, Zhangyu Sun, Ziyu Jiang, Yuehan Chen, Hankun Lu, Wei Luo, Ruchong Chen, Nanshan Zhong. The spectrum, clinical features and diagnosis of chronic cough due to rare causes. Journal of Thoracic Disease, Vol 13, No 4 (April 2021). https://www.ncbi.nlm.nih.gov/pmc/articles/PMC8107567/. Accessed July 19, 2022.

Patient Complains of Sore Throat (a symptom).

Physician's Findings: inflamed throat tissue, mild fever. [Quandary: is cause a virus or bacterium.]

If no or minimal fever: suggest analgesic and tell patient to call or return in a few days if doesn't get better. If high fever or other concerns, swab throat so lab can determine organism. Treat as above and prescribe an antibiotic but suggest using it only if symptoms worsen.

If result from lab indicates a potentially problematic bacterium, contact patient and suggest take antibiotic or prescribe a different one based on the type of bacterium. Suggest a return visit if no improvement.

FIGURE 1.13.1: A simplified view of a decision process

Chapter 14: Reflections on the Diagnostic Process

KEYWORDS: Elusive Diagnosis, Explaining Health Problems, Strategies to Make a Diagnosis, The Differential Diagnosis, Uncertainty

ABSTRACT: The differential diagnosis is a list of possible causes for a problem. Reaching a proper diagnosis requires a systematic approach. Sometimes, diagnoses are elusive, and it is important that clinicians let patients know when they are unsure of the cause of the problem. Nevertheless, despite uncertainty, clinicians often feel the need to offer comforting solutions, including relieving pain and restoring function. This might involve giving treatments that influence the biology that might be contributing to the problem, even though the biology is unsure. Fortunately, the response to treatment provides additional information that can be used to make a definitive diagnosis.

I still don't know what's wrong with me and neither does my doctor!

What if the Diagnosis is Elusive?

Those are not joyous words! We worry until we know what's going on. We have a sense that no news may be good news but that may not be the case. Not hearing from the doctor after testing might mean the test results were normal or unimportant, or it could mean that someone mishandled or lost them. Getting test results that do not reveal a solution to the patient's problem could mean that further investigations are necessary to find out what is really causing it.

Delayed and mistaken diagnoses are leading causes of preventable death, disability and discomfort.[61] Estimates are that, for as many as 15% of patients, the diagnosis is incorrect.[62] Clearly, there is need for improvement! Fortunately, though, patients, health services administrators, informaticians and others can work together to increase the likelihood of correct and prompt diagnosis. In addition, many sources can assist diagnosis and suggest potential treatments of just about any problem. The World Wide Web is fertile ground for nurturing engaged and knowledgeable patients.

If people understand how physicians make a diagnosis, they can better participate in their care and improve the accuracy of diagnosis. This is important, as it has become increasingly difficult to find a full-service personal family physician. However, even if we have a family

61 Improving Diagnosis in Health Care, Erin P. Balogh, Bryan T. Miller, and John R. Ball, Editors; Committee on Diagnostic Error in Health Care; Board on Health Care Services; Institute of Medicine; The National Academies of Sciences, Engineering, and Medicine, ISBN: 978-0-309-37769-0. DOI: 10.17226/21794 2015. http://www.nationalacademies.org/hmd/reports/2015/improving-diagnosis-in-healthcare/improving-diagnosis. Accessed August 25, 2022.

62 Graber ML The incidence of diagnostic error in medicine. BMJ Qual Saf 2013;22: ii21-ii27. https://qualitysafety.bmj.com/content/22/Suppl_2/ii21. Accessed August 25, 2022.

doctor, it often takes too long to discover what is wrong and what to do in the case of vague, uncommon or rare patient problems, some of which have serious implications.

Explaining Health Problems

Whenever people have a problem, like feeling uncomfortable, having limitations on their activity, or being afraid of dying, doctors try to find an explanation that does more than merely describe the problem. It should also reveal its cause and point the way to treatment that can potentially improve the patient's comfort, function and life span.

As we have mentioned, most abnormal symptoms, signs or abnormal lab results have many possible causes. Information about diagnosis and treatment is readily available in user-friendly form. Those who understand where to go can search the Web and can help increase the speed and accuracy of their diagnoses. Being knowledgeable means knowing which questions to ask, seeing the importance of giving their doctors complete information, and being able to interpret and supplement what their physicians say.

Strategies to Make a Diagnosis

To understand how physicians solve problems, we need to go more deeply into the nature and process of diagnosis. In this this chapter we describe how doctors make diagnoses to find both the common and rare causes of problems. Everyone can use these very same methods.

Doctors might, off the top of their heads, stimulated by a patient's symptoms and signs, remember more of the possible causes of problems because of their training. Readily available information may, in fact, enable anybody to determine the causes of 80-90% of diagnosable medical conditions.[63]

Sometimes, however, it is necessary to go further than observation. In that situation, clinicians may order tests to confirm a diagnosis that the clinician made based on just symptoms or signs. The results of tests allow physicians to discover, clarify, explore or exclude diagnoses. Some causes of problems just are not apparent from the patient's descriptions of symptoms, from the physical exam or even from all of these together with the patient's family and personal history. Being sure sometimes requires more.

When doctors see patients, they mentally consider the possible reasons for the patients' problems. Naturally, they think of the common, more likely conditions first. Most patients have conditions that are common. But not all do. This means that most of the time, doctors who only consider the most common conditions will come to the correct diagnosis. Note, however, that it is possible that they might come to an incorrect conclusion the very time that it is important to be right. If so, the patient can suffer.

Consider the following. Many patients with Hodgkin's disease, an important blood cancer, suffer from delayed diagnosis because the clinician interprets an enlarged lymph node (the lymph nodes are components of the body's immune system) in the neck as consistent with the more usual cause, a common viral infection. The lymph nodes enlarge while trying to fight the infection. Depending on the tolerance of the patient and the suspiciousness of the physician, the diagnosis of Hodgkin's disease might be delayed for a short time – one or two months – or a long time, possibly years. If diagnosis is delayed too long, this can mortally endanger the patient.

The problem is that the initial presenting symptoms for Hodgkin's disease are usually non-specific and not particularly alarming. These include fatigue, an enlarged lymph node

63 Hampton J R, Harrison M J, Mitchell J R, Prichard J S, Seymour C. Relative contributions of history-taking, physical examination, and laboratory investigation to diagnosis and management of medical outpatients. Br Med J 1975; 2 :486. http://www.bmj.com/content/bmj/2/5969/486.full.pdf. Accessed July 19, 2022.

or recurrent infections. Often the fatigue and enlarged lymph nodes seem innocuous.

The challenge, of course, is to reduce the time it takes to arrive at a definitive diagnosis for Hodgkin's and other important diseases, without inflicting unnecessary testing on the patient. It would not be right to expose the larger proportion of people, who have non-threatening, benign and self-limited problems, too expensive and potentially harmful testing. Or at least not as the first move. As a rule, it is best practice to undertake aggressive investigations if a problem persists for longer than a couple of months without a definitive diagnosis. Sometimes, though, even short delays are unacceptable because some even briefly delayed diagnoses can have serious consequences. Of course, if the problem significantly interferes with the patient's comfort and function, more immediate and aggressive investigation is a must.

More on the Differential Diagnosis

Remember what we said about the 'differential diagnosis' (or just 'differential'). It is the set of all medical causes that might be responsible for a patient's problem. Most problems have many possible causes. This means that their differentials could include hundreds of possibilities, but only a few of them are common causes.

A comprehensive differential for any medical problem, let alone for all medical problems, will only be found online or on a computing device – it is simply beyond most human cognition and memory to have that volume of complicated information 'in mind.'

We have mentioned elsewhere of the thousands of causes that might be responsible for fatigue. Luckily, many fewer causes account for most cases of fatigue. Recognizing the number of possible causes, it is not surprising that it takes a long time to make a correct diagnosis for some of the rarer conditions. Nor is it astonishing that, when they have not concluded a definite cause, clinicians might still try a variety of interventions (like an antibiotic or Tylenol for an unexplained fever) to attempt to provide symptomatic relief or just to be safe.

It is usual that, at least initially, most physicians consider far fewer possibilities than would appear in an all-inclusive differential. They appropriately consider at first only the most common reasons for a problem. Even though a computer-generated differential diagnosis can list hundreds of possible diagnostic candidates, the probability of most of them being valid is vanishingly small. To deal with that, some diagnosis-support systems (e.g., DXplain[64]) provide the user with a probability that each possible cause is the correct one. They, in addition, indicate how to eliminate certain diagnoses from further consideration, as well as how to confirm a diagnosis. Eliminating and confirming diagnoses usually entails ordering specific tests and determining if the results are positive or negative.

The game of diagnosis has quite simple rules, one of which is to focus on a likely diagnosis and to eliminate the next most likely possibility.

Sometimes, doctors give up and report they cannot think of a reason for a problem even though they have only considered common causes and have not consulted the complete list of all possible causes. The chapters that follow discuss common diagnoses and indicate the most common causes for those diseases, as well as 'red flags' that demand timely, aggressive, investigation.

As we have written, accepting a diagnosis or explanation of a problem is a wager that the explanation is correct. To estimate the chance that a diagnosis is wrong, clinicians must have information about how frequently conditions occur in the community (their prevalence), and how often the tests they use give false alarms (their 'specificity') or false reassurance

64 Massachusetts General ICS, DXplain. http://www.mghlcs.org/projects/dxplain. Accessed July 14, 2022.

(their 'sensitivity'). The chapter on testing later in the book discusses these scientific concepts in more detail.

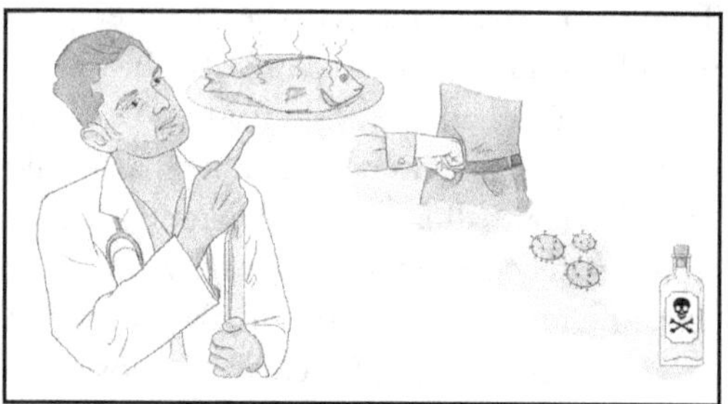

FIGURE 1.14.1: Considering possible causes – the differential diagnosis

Reflections on Differential Diagnosis

The use of Differential Diagnosis is not by any means limited to Medicine and the physician's office. Other users of the concept may not call it that, but they use the same process. A differential is essentially a list of possible causes of a problem, as we have illustrated in FIGURE 1.14.1

If one watches airplane accident documentaries, crash investigators (e.g., from the NTSB or Transport Canada) develop a list of possible explanations for crashes and then consider them one at a time until only the right explanation remains. They use passengers or witnesses to discern 'symptoms,' like what they felt, heard or saw, such as that the plane was shaking, making unusual noises or doing weird maneuvers before it crashed. The investigators view accident remains, look at videos and review 'black box' and cockpit voice records to get objective 'signs' of a problem with the plane or the pilots. They subject metal and mechanisms to 'testing', including chemical, microscopic and other imaging studies. As they are gathering all this, they develop a formal or informal list of possibilities: a differential. As they examine all the things observed and measured, they add new possibilities to the list or remove others. At the end, usually one or a very few causes emerge as the explanation(s) for the accident: the investigators' 'diagnosis'. Their determinations completed, they make a set of recommendations that serve as their treatment... in this case, sanctions or steps to prevent the next crash.

The same type of process is used by engineers to figure out why a bridge collapsed, or by a mechanic to determine why your automobile went flaky. Mechanics and engineers start with a simple mental list and might eventually consult manuals or other literature to find obscure causes for a problem. Perhaps the most general case of a differential can be found in one of the Thinking Tools defined by Edward De Bono.[65] He presented his 'Consider All Factors' (CAF) tool to help people generate a comprehensive list of all the causes of an administrative problem, for example. He delineated other tools to help consider each as an explanation for the problem.

The differential diagnosis process is a powerful thinking technique limited in its power only by one's memory (or other information resources available) and the time, attention and discipline one devotes to listing and considering possibilities. It should now be easy to see why not considering all factors might harm patients. If a visit is rushed, the gathering of information is truncated or the mind is not put to the analytical challenge, it becomes less likely that the clinician will reach a definitive diagnosis. That is why those steps are crucial; without any one of them, the differential diagnosis process might not arrive at the desired destination. Then the patient will be untreated or mistreated.

Furthermore, having the patient think along with the physician provides a kind of co-pilot, another brain, another set of eyes, ensuring

65 https://www.biggerplate.com/mindmaps/85PUiPeS/edward-de-bono-thinking-tools-caf-consider-all-factors. Accessed July 19, 2022. This reference shows a mind map tool for Consider All Factors.

that the diagnostic process proceeds as well as is humanly possible.

Hearing "I Don't Know"

Suppose a patient went to the medical office and complained about being tired all the time. The doctor examined the person and ordered tests. A week later, the patient returned to the office and the doctor performed another examination. After answering more questions and leaving with an order for more tests, the patient left still feeling tired. A week later, back at the office, the doctor stated a very scary thing: "I don't know what is wrong!" After a bit of additional discussion, the doctor suggested that the next step might be additional tests. Another possibility is that both the patient and the doctor might realize that people with normal test results usually recover without intervention – there might not be anything medical awry. Therefore, the patient might agree that it would be most appropriate to wait at least a few weeks to see if anything changed. Are doctors really allowed to say: "I don't know"?

Reality is that physicians sometimes realize that they simply do not know what is going on. It may be that the patient has a very esoteric illness that will take some time, sophisticated testing and effort to discover. Right now, though, which disease is causing the patient's problem is not known. Among many possibilities, it may be that there is no medical cause and the patient just needs more rest, better nutrition, counselling or some aerobic exercise. Until the doctor investigates all the possibilities, or the suggested nonmedical interventions help the patient, the correct answer may very well be: "I don't know" and both the physician and patient must tolerate the ambiguity. This does not mean giving up, however, and further investigation might have to follow. Uncertainty permeates human matters.

Everybody Must Be Honest about Knowing

For professionals of any kind, the words 'I don't know' may seem like a copout. But they are not! In a certain sense those words are a commitment to trying to solve a problem, not avoid it. Perhaps they should be followed with the word 'yet' to recognize this, but the words are honest. They should impel committed people to look further, perhaps beyond their present state of knowledge and into unknown territory.

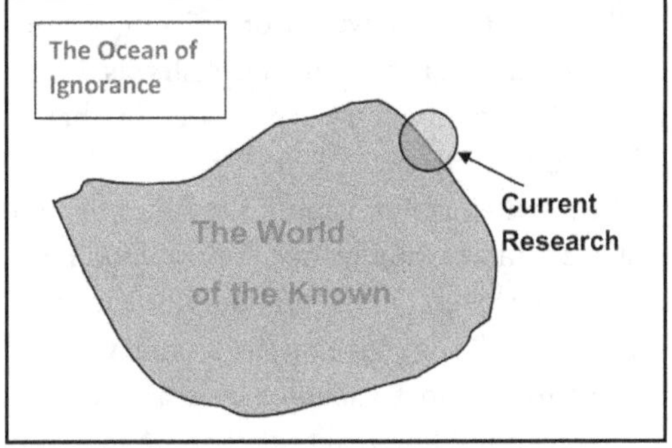

FIGURE 1.14.2: Science reveals a lot, but there's a lot we still seek – hence research

One can think about what we 'know' as the 'island of our knowledge' we inhabit. We illustrate this in FIGURE 1.14.1. To arrive at a judgment, we search that island, which embodies the things we know, for solutions and we hopefully find answers. But every island is of finite size. No one knows everything about anything, let alone everything about everything. Even more concerning, we often know things incompletely or imperfectly. In other words, we think we know something but, on trying to apply that knowledge, it proves to be inadequate or possibly even wrong. The situation is worse when we get off the island of what we know and into the 'ocean of ignorance' containing things we don't know or about which we know just a little. There we are in dangerous waters because what we know about out there may be even more spotty, incomplete or incorrect. This is especially true of those of us who are Jacks or Jills of all (or many) trades.

Perhaps you remember the famous statement by Donald Rumsfeld when he talked about 'knowns'.[66] He described the 'known knowns', these being the things we deeply understand. Then there are the 'known unknowns', where we are aware of them but completely or largely ignorant of their nature or their details. Finally, there are the 'unknown unknowns', about which we do not even know we are ignorant. One might add to these the 'unknowables', at least given the current limitations of science. We cannot understand those as there is no frameworks or existing frameworks are inadequate to accomplish this. Note, Rumsfeld's commentary is preceded by that of J. Luff and H. Ingram in 1955.[67] [68]

Rumsfeld's analysis applies to all of us, not just the military intelligence community. How often have we discovered that our knowledge is incomplete? Today, given a little time, we may be able to fill those vacuoles by searching the Web. The humbling reality is that we may not know enough to know that retrieved information might be incomplete, biased, confused or incorrect. Elsewhere in this compendium, we address the problems of searching for medical information.

There is also what is called the Dunning-Kruger Effect[69], where we know a little bit about something but really just have a naïve or inflated view of our expertise.

Admitting Being on an Island

The interesting thing is that knowing when to say, and being able to say, the words 'I don't know' takes a critical examination of our knowledge. Further, it requires quite a bit of security be honest about what we know and to reveal that we are not perfect. For all of us human beings there will always be a question we cannot answer, cannot answer correctly or cannot answer in a way that isn't confused or confusing to others. Very knowledgeable clinicians, endowed with excellent thinking skills, will, from time to time, speak the words 'I don't know'. People who hear those words should be grateful that they are in the hands of someone secure and honest enough to utter them. Together with that clinician they can be assured that their journeys to finding the causes of their problems will be as fruitful an expedition as is humanly possible.

66 https://en.wikipedia.org/wiki/There_are_known_knowns. Accessed July 19, 2022.

67 https://www.habitsforwellbeing.com/johari-window-we-dont-know-what-we-dont-know/. Accessed July 19, 2022.

68 http://www.convivendo.net/wp-content/uploads/2009/05/johari-window-articolo-originale.pdf. Accessed July 19, 2022.

69 Mahmood, K. (2016). Do people overestimate their information literacy skills? A systematic review of empirical evidence on the dunning-kruger effect. Communications in Information Literacy, 10(2), 199-213. (9) (PDF) Do People Overestimate Their Information Literacy Skills? A Systematic Review of Empirical Evidence on the Dunning-Kruger Effect (researchgate.net). https://files.eric.ed.gov/fulltext/EJ1125451.pdf. Accessed Sept 13, 2023.

Chapter 15: ——— Strategies for Diagnosing

KEYWORDS: Strategies for Diagnosing, Tactics for Diagnosing, Physical Examination, Tincture Of Time, Confirming A Diagnosis, Testing, Common Problems.

ABSTRACT: This chapter outlines the strategies and tactics that clinicians and anyone might use to systematically find the reason for a patient's problem. These include developing a differential diagnosis of possible causes, and deciding which investigations, including physical examinations and lab tests might be helpful in confirming the cause. These systematic steps recognize that it might be preferable to start with benign tests for less common causes, rather than invasive, possibly harmful tests for a more likely condition.

It's one thing to figure out what's caused a kitchen appliance or a TV to fail, and even that can be challenging. Trying to determine the cause of a medical problem is a bit harder. In fact, those who fix appliances or other equipment use a systematic approach: a strategy. They proceed in a structured way do some things first, like examining the device, measuring electrical parameters, plugging it in and checking all the switches, then they repair the motor, for example, or debug the electronics.

Physicians have strategies, too, that are intended to be time-efficient and effective. If not, they could not fix problems (like a patient in respiratory distress or chest pain) before it was too late, not to mention dealing with a waiting-room full of people. Without worthwhile and efficient strategies, doctors would be more likely to miss important signals, make mistakes, take too long to solve a problem or 'solve' the wrong problem. We sometimes forget that physicians need sufficient time to care for the sheer numbers of people who need their help.

STRATEGIES AND TACTICS

For our purposes in this book, we use the following structure:

*A **GOAL** is the ultimate end point we want to achieve. In Medicine this is to improve patient health.*

*A **STRATEGY** is our overall approach to achieving our goal. This might involve the use of a structured approach for moving from interviewing, observation, measurement, testing, confirmation, coming to a definitive diagnosis and using an evidence-based intervention. We can call this strategy the 'Clinical Decision Paradigm.'*

*An **OBJECTIVE** is an essential waypoint in the process, for example making a diagnosis or choosing a treatment. We would have the objective of achieving each of the steps above: getting as much as possible from the interview, observation and measurement, etc.*

*A **TACTIC** is an approach to achieving each objective,*

The goal and the overall strategy of medical care should be clear from the anecdote. Let's consider some of the objectives and the tactics used to achieve them.

Diagnostic Tactic: Obtain a Thorough and Complete History

Physicians interview their patients and ask many questions about what is bothering them. They ask what is causing discomfort; what the discomfort is like; when it started; how often and when it happens; what other problems exist and if other family members or neighbors have similar problems. This is called 'taking a history.' A comprehensive history is often – at least 70% of the time – enough to reach a reasonable understanding of the possible causes of a problem. While listening to the patient's recitation, the physician begins forming a set of hypotheses about what is going on to cause the patient's problems. Questions may also probe for points the patient might have ignored or not recognize or was embarrassed to mention.

Diagnostic Tactic: Complete an Appropriate Physical Examination

Next, the physician will usually do a physical examination, even if reasonably sure of the diagnosis. This examination, guided by the possibilities evoked in the physician's mind during listening to the history, will provide additional information to support this or that diagnosis. The physician will do things like listening to chest sounds; looking in the patient's mouth, eyes and ears; examining the skin; checking out nerve reflexes and asking if this or that hurts. Relating to the specific problems the patient reported, the exam may focus on certain areas.

The physical examination can help confirm the physician's initial suspicions about a cause, but it can also stimulate considering alternate or additional possibilities. The physician is using every sense to home in on what is wrong even if the patient is unaware of a problem. The history and physical exam are harmless and yet can yield great returns... setting the stage for proper intervention. One purpose can be to validate a hypothesis regarding a cause. Another is to eliminate other possibilities. Often, the history and physical exam together can clinch the diagnosis, especially if the physician examines all relevant body systems and is careful to try to evoke any signs that would invalidate alternate causes. Sometimes, though, it can take more effort and time to arrive at the definitive diagnosis. It is worth it, though. Intervention to manage or correct the patient's problems depends on getting the diagnosis right.

Diagnostic Tactic: Think About and Consider What was Heard or Seen

Although thinking (such as forming or considering hypotheses) is embedded in all the steps above, the physician needs to think more about what is happening. Is the patient being honest and comprehensive? Does the story hold together? Are there other or confounding factors? What else should I look for and ask about? What do I think is going on? What can I ask about that would validate or invalidate what I think? What is the full set of possibilities that explain the patient's problems? How can I confirm or eliminate possibilities? How shall I tell the patient what I think and what might the reaction be?

There is an antique picture of the famous physician, Dr. William Osler, standing by a patient's bed contemplating what he has seen and heard and then thinking about what the cause might be (FIGURE 1.15.1). Every physician must do this. Failure to fully comprehend the situation and, rather, to just order tests, will delay care, endanger the patient and likely cost the patient and the system wasted time and money.

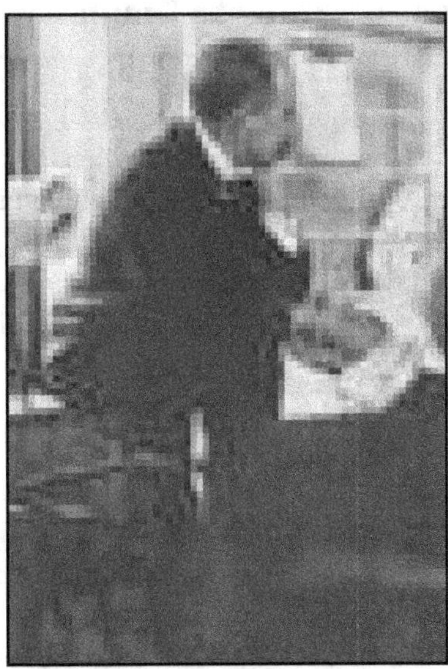

FIGURE 1.15.1: Osler considering the possibilities

- ✓ Obtain a Thorough and Complete History
- ✓ Complete an Appropriate Physical Examination
- ✓ Think About and Consider What was Heard or Seen
- ✓ Allow Self-Healing to occur - the Tincture of Time
- ✓ Get Confirmation through Testing - Imaging and Body Fluid Chemistry
- ✓ Try a Therapeutic Trial
- ✓ Close the Loop and Undertake Definitive Intervention
- ✓ Critically evaluate the outcome

FIGURE 1.15.2: Major diagnostic tactics

Diagnostic Tactic: Allow Self-Healing to Occur – the Tincture of Time

FIGURE 1.15.2 is an outline of the key diagnostic tactics most physicians use.

Sometimes, problems are transient and resolve on their own. Remember that 'Tincture of Time' means not rushing to judgment, but rather waiting to see if the problem does resolve spontaneously. Many problems, including fatigue, muscle aches, joint pain, upper respiratory symptoms (runny nose, cough, simple sore throat and some fevers) resolve in a few days without any intervention. If clinicians do not see any red flags (warning semaphores – see Chapter 14 and this one) indicating the need for earlier intervention, they are comfortable asking the patient to wait to see if the problem resolves without medical intervention. The good news for most of us is that many problems do.

Diagnostic Tactic: Get Confirmation through Testing – Imaging and Body Fluid Chemistry

When the history and physical examination together do not lead to a conclusive diagnosis, clinicians will order laboratory tests, imaging (x-ray, ultrasound, CT, MRI and microscopic) and measurements of electrical activity in various organs. Examples of the latter include an electroencephalogram – EEG – that measures brain activity and an electrocardiogram – ECG or EKG – that measures heart activity. These can provide objective indication of the function of various key organs, like the kidneys, liver, nerves and heart, which are not discernable in the physical examination.

Diagnostic Tactic: Try a Therapeutic Trial

If the cause of the patient's problems is not obvious, the physician might try what we called a 'Therapeutic Trial'. This means trying an intervention to see if it helps. In a therapeutic trial (note: this is not the same as a 'clinical trial', a research technique, which we discuss later) the doctor might prescribe a medication believed to treat an assumed diagnosis – but one not yet confirmed – of the patient's problems. The most common therapeutic trial is prescribing antibiotics for the fever and cough associated with flu-like symptoms. The doctor acts as if the patient has a bacterial infection, which is all antibiotics can cure – they have no effect on viruses that are the common causes of these symptoms. If the problem resolves, the doctor assumes the antibiotic cured the problem and may never do the testing that would show that the antibiotic contributed to a cure and that the problem simply resolved by itself. This isn't ideal, but sometimes it demonstrates an 'abundance of caution'. In doing this, the doctor has not acted with a clear and definite understanding of the cause (the definitive diagnosis) of the patient's problem.

Diagnostic Tactic: Close the Loop and Undertake Definitive Intervention

Once the physician receives the results of tests (and patients should get a copy!), it should be possible to form a definitive diagnosis. Ideally, the physician had arranged a return visit date and can discuss the results with the patient and suggest the definitive intervention. Sometimes it may not be necessary to have this return visit, or the doctor might tell the patient to expect a message if the results indicate one is needed. The problem in this latter case is that test results may never arrive at the office or someone may misplace them internally. Closing the loop in one or other way is crucial and can be assured if patients receive test results directly and call the physician if they aren't called. There may be instances in which directly receiving test results is inappropriate, though. This may be a matter for discussion between the patient and the physician.

Overall Strategy to Diagnosing a Problem

Medical strategies, if they are good ones, are systematic and depend on numbers, like the frequency of problems in the community or the likelihood that a treatment will help. Truly effective systematic efforts to solve a medical problem often have their basis in statistical analysis. Physicians use statistical information to estimate the probability of a patient's having a given condition and to identify the frequency of the benefits versus harms of investigation and treatment. So, there is a degree of science. However, many decisions are a product of the Art of Medicine.

Some diagnostic choices are artful, because clear-cut information about the chances that a patient has a specific diagnosis or about the effects of investigation and treatment is not readily available. Reflecting on our colonoscopy example, the chance of bowel perforation from a colonoscopy differs by region because of variations in the skills of doctors doing the investigation and differences in the status and resilience of patients. It may be difficult to find out for the patient's region.

Often doctors use pattern recognition to quickly diagnose a problem. They may use this to diagnose asthma in a wheezing patient who has had prior episodes of asthma. Often, doctors using pattern recognition arrive at the correct diagnosis. Sometimes, however, the failure to follow the Clinical Decision Paradigm can have disastrous consequences. For example, doctors might incorrectly conclude that a young, breast-feeding woman with a breast abscess (a collection of pus) has mastitis (inflammation of the breast) related to breast feeding and not caused by breast cancer, just because breast cancer is rare in young, breast-feeding women.

Doctors use a strategy to diagnose problems to avoid harm from delayed, missed or incorrect diagnoses.

When doctors implement a systematic diagnostic process, they consider what is unique about the patient. Are there familial or genetic issues? What risks has the person been exposed to? Was there travel to an exotic location? Does the patient work in an industry that uses toxic chemicals? Has there been contact with someone who has a communicable disease? Each answer makes one or other interpretation of cause more or less likely. If the person has never been to a malaria-infested area, it is very unlikely that a fever is caused by malaria.

WHY PATIENTS SEE DOCTORS

What is unique about the patient – the person's 'risk factors' and the patient's personal beliefs and preferences – have important influences on the appropriateness of different diagnostic and therapeutic approaches.

Participating as an active member of the team looking after one's health helps to ensure that the recommended diagnostic and treatment approaches will be acceptable to the patient. Providing as much information as possible, including describing relevant situations or other factors may help the physician to determine what is causing the reported distress. This will make the clinician's job easier and hasten the selection of an appropriate intervention compatible with the patient's desires.

It turns out that a relatively small number of problems represent a large proportion of visits to family doctors. The Center for Disease Control and Prevention listed the following most common reasons for patients to visit as family doctor:[70] These lists change over time as citizen demographics change and as diseases become more or less prevalent.

1. Cough.
2. Symptoms referable to sore throat.
3. High blood pressure.
4. Knee symptoms.
5. Fever.
6. Skin Rash.
7. Abdominal pain.
8. Back symptoms.
9. Visual problems.
10. Earaches.

The commercial information company, IQVIA, looks at this a bit differently. IQVIA produces a list that focuses on the diagnoses or conditions doctors eventually assigned to patients. This list includes 'Check-up' and 'Unknown cause' as reasons for a visit, indicating that doctors recognize that not all problems find a clear solution or interpretation.[71]

The diagnoses or causes of the problem addressed in the visit, as listed by IQVIA, only become known after investigations are underway. The IQVIA list is:

1. Hypertension.
2. Diabetes.
3. Check-up.
4. Depression.
5. Anxiety.
6. Acute respiratory Infection.
7. Normal pregnancy.
8. Hyperlipidemia.
9. Esophagitis.
10. Unknown cause.

When coders (professionals who assign formal terms to index the content of medical records) consider the reason for a visit to a doctor, they will usually list the name of the disease, i.e., diabetes, the doctor found as the cause of the patient's problem, which was excessive thirst. That is the reason the patient went to the doctor. This explains the difference

70 Hing, E,, Uddin, S. Visits to Primary Care United States 2008. https://www.researchgate.net/publication/47678129_Visits_to_primary_care_delivery_sites_United_States_2008. Accessed Sept 8, 2023.

71 https://www.iqvia.com/-/media/iqvia/pdfs/canada-location-site/top-10-reasons-en-2016.pdf?la=en&hash=5E609230DF0B8E119D1CB276A5665E629276093D&_=1517508473394. Accessed August 25, 2022.

between the two lists and why the University of Ottawa list is more helpful for those who wish to determine if a problem is not likely to be one that demands immediate physician attention or where a delay is unlikely to be harmful.

Patients usually visit a doctor because of a problem (their symptoms) they need addressed. Hence, researchers at the University of Ottawa developed another list of the 10 most common symptoms leading patients to visit a family physician.[72] The Ottawa list is very similar to the CDC's and includes (from most common to least common symptoms of the ten) the items below. In addition, the Ottawa list indicates the red flags that should prompt patients to seek more immediate advice. The next chapters discuss each problem including its common causes.

1. Cough.
2. Fatigue.
3. Low Back Pain.
4. Fever.
5. Dyspnea (shortness of breath).
6. Generalized abdominal pain.
7. Headache.
8. Vertigo/Dizziness.
9. Chest pain.
10. Edema (swelling of arms or legs).

The Treatment Patients Receive

We have mentioned that some problems disappear spontaneously without medical intervention. Others clear after treatments meant to reduce discomfort and increase function, even though no one really knew what the underlying problem was nor has the intervention actually treated it. Often no one can explain the patient's signs (objective observables) and symptoms (subjective sensations) in a satisfying way. However, they resolve spontaneously without anyone discovering the real cause.

Almost everyone has had a cough or stomach pain that resolved without treatment and without learning the cause. Sometimes, people elect to take remedies that may reduce discomfort and improve function despite not knowing what's wrong. Over the counter (OTC) cough and cold remedies and non-steroidal anti-inflammatory drugs (NSAIDS) such as Aspirin (acetylsalicylic acid) and Motrin (ibuprofen) are examples of remedies that people take without knowing the exact cause of their discomfort. People often feel better after and it is often impossible to know if the agent hastened recovery, or if the problem would have resolved on its own.

Some conditions present (show themselves) in obscure ways and take a long time to explain. Solving these important problems requires a systematic approach, including the development of the list (a differential diagnosis list) of both common and obscure causes of the problem. Because many problems have many possible causes, when a doctor says: "I've checked for everything and can't find anything", it is wise to ask for the list of diagnoses considered.

Patients' Common Problems

Listening to patients is an important skill for physicians. Seven of the ten most common problems[73] are 'symptoms' – the rest do have some objective signs, in addition to being symptoms – issues that patients complain about because they experience discomfort from them. As you can see in the lists above,

72 The whole series is available from Canadian Family Physician The following is an example of what is available Top 10 differential diagnoses in family medicine: Chest pain | The College of Family Physicians of Canada (cfp.ca). Accessed July 19, 2022. David Ponka, Michael Kirlew. Top 10 differential diagnoses in family medicine: Chest pain. Canadian Family Physician Dec 2007, 53 (12) 2146. https://www.cfp.ca/content/53/12/2146. Accessed July 19, 2022.

73 Most common problems from the Ponka, University of Ottawa list.

the most common symptoms reported are fatigue, low back pain, dyspnea (shortness of breath), centralized abdominal pain, headache, vertigo/dizziness and chest pain. The ones that physicians can observe directly (i.e., they have objective findings) are cough, fever and edema (swelling of body parts).

Understanding these common problems, their causes or explanations and their treatments goes a long way to understanding a goodly portion of the work of doctors. This is why we will discuss, in the next chapters, common problems, possible explanations and red flags (warning signs) that should prompt for further investigation or treatment. Knowing about these issues will ensure that more people get satisfactory and satisfying care. There are many sources for formation to solve each of these problems.

Medical students often hear the adages "common things are common" and "when you hear galloping sounds in the West don't think of zebras." It is true that common things are common, but uncommon causes are not necessarily rare. There are several thousand rare diseases. What we call 'rare' is a movable feast. Accepted definitions usually classify a disease as rare if it afflicts fewer than one in two thousand people. On the other hand, the European Organization for Rare Diseases estimates that approximately 7% of the European population is afflicted with a rare disease.[74] Using this estimate, for every 100 members of the community, 7 will have an uncommon affliction. The average doctor has between 1,000 and 2,000 patients in her practice. Based on the European data, we would expect that about 70 of the average doctor's patients would have an uncommon affliction. When doctors give up before exploring rare explanations for a problem, they can be sure that at least some patients will suffer unnecessarily. This indicates that, in every practice, some people will have diseases that are not easily recognized or interpreted. The reluctance of some clinicians to explore rare conditions makes it even more important that all members of healthcare teams, including patients, develop an understanding of how to reach a diagnosis.

Because of the large number of possible causes of problems, it becomes important that the healthcare community and patients themselves develop systematic approaches to identifying the likely and not so likely causes of any problem. They should also develop methods to sort through these causes and to determine which of the many is most likely to be valid.

When clinicians think about an overall strategy for diagnosis, they must know what steps to take to find a diagnosis, the information they need about the patient, where to find it, information about possible causes for a problem and where to find those causes.

74 Rare Diseases: Understanding This Public Health Priority. European Organisation for Rare Diseases (EURORDIS). https://www.eurordis.org/IMG/pdf/princeps_document-EN.pdf. November 2005. Accessed Aug 1, 2022.

Chapter 16: ——— Risks in Diagnosis

KEYWORDS: Medical Errors, False Positive Test Results, Unnecessary Alarm, False Negative Test Results, Inappropriate Reassurance, Over-Testing, Other Diagnostic Issues

ABSTRACT: Usually clinicians make an accurate and helpful diagnosis. Sometimes, though, they tell patients they have the condition they don't have, a so-called 'false positive.' Other physicians may tell patients they are healthy when the test results provide incorrect and harmful reassurance. Patients and clinicians must be aware of how and why these errors occur.

Reasons for Error in Diagnosis—

News flash: Doctors Aren't Perfect! They are human, they make mistakes and, oh yes, they can't do miracles!

Physicians, like all of us, can make many kinds of mistakes, even though they might be smart, highly trained, experienced and of good will. The causes of mistakes physicians make are familiar: physicians can be distracted or upset by something in their own lives (why won't my car start?), or just plain tired. They can forget. They can be biased ("I never liked George's article about Aspirin"). They can be ignorant or lazy ("I haven't had any time to read a journal on the topic" or "I have not found pertinent material"). They are indeed humans!

The National Academies of Medicine in the U. S. devoted an entire 472-page report[75] to issues of diagnosis and how to reduce diagnostic error.

Physicians and patients should be aware of three important kinds of mistakes that expose patients to the risk of erroneous diagnosis. Elsewhere in this book, we explain the kinds and nature of biases, the natural human predispositions that afflict our minds and ensure that we are never perfect. For now, we will discuss mistakes.

The first mistake, **ignoring possibilities**, happens when clinicians do not reach a diagnosis because they have not deliberated on all the possibilities and have not considered and tested for the complete set of both common and rare possible causes. If this is the case, patients will continue to suffer or will receive only symptomatic treatment, while doctors could have identified the actual cause of their problems and could have treated them appropriately.

We have pointed out that clinicians simply cannot remember every possible cause of every problem. Neither could any of us. The list is thousands long! That's why reminder systems that assist clinicians and patients in considering all possibilities are essential.

Serious rare conditions behave like military snipers. They hide in the bushes and in places where people least expect to detect them. Sometimes they even blend in and look like common causes. Without a thorough and attentive search, doctors may not detect rare conditions or they take a long time to

75 National Academies of Sciences, Engineering, and Medicine. 2015. Improving diagnosis in health care. Washington, DC: The National Academies Press. https://www.nap.edu/catalog/21794/improving-diagnosis-in-health-care. Accessed July 19, 2022.

find them.[76] In the meantime, patients suffer unnecessarily or develop avoidable complications. Patients can help their clinicians by doing their homework and researching further information and possible causes of problems that doctors have not yet explained. There are many stories of people who have invested years in libraries and online in order to find out what was wrong with a newborn or young child[77].

The second mistake patients face is receiving a **false positive diagnosis**. That happens when clinicians, after examining and testing, diagnose a condition different from the one actually afflicting the patient and recommend treatments that are at best pointless and possibly harmful.

MISTAKEN PANCREATIC CANCER – A FALSE POSITIVE

The 62-year-old mother of a health professional visited her family doctor who told her that she was 20- to 30-pounds overweight. So, she went on a diet. She lost 20 pounds and returned a year later. For some reason, the doctor was concerned about the magnitude of her weight loss and ordered abdominal investigations. An ultrasound suggested she had pancreatic cancer. Her doctor referred her to a surgeon, who performed an aggressive surgery (Whipple's procedure), removing her pancreas and other tissue from her abdominal cavity. A week after the surgery, she complained of blood in her urine. Her family doctor attributed the bleeding to a bladder infection. Ten days later she died from a complicated clotting disorder (disseminated intravascular coagulopathy) related to the surgery.

Subsequently, the pathology report on the tissues removed during her initial surgery did not find any signs of cancer. Her death was totally avoidable and was a consequence of a false positive diagnosis of pancreatic cancer. Unfortunately, neither the family doctor nor the surgeon bothered to confirm the diagnosis of pancreatic cancer suggested by the ultrasound. Instead, they undertook very aggressive corrective surgery for a non-existent problem. Sad!

The third risk is receiving a **false negative diagnosis**. This happens when the physician tests for many conditions, including the one that is causing the affliction, but the test results come back negative (indicating no disease). That result indicates the patient is disease-free when the patient actually has a disease.

Another cause of error is **bad testing choices or poor handling of results**, which provide the doctor and the patient with false reassurance:

1. When the doctor ordered the wrong test for the condition.
2. When the doctor ordered a test that is not sufficiently sensitive to detect the disease (more on that in the chapter on testing).
3. When the doctor misreads or misunderstands a result.
4. When the laboratory made an error. That does happen!
5. When the one patient's report gets mixed up with another's. This can happen when there is confusion regarding names, a computer error or miscommunication.
6. When the report is misplaced, misfiled or lost.

A PHYSICIAN PAST HIS BEST-BY DATE

Many years ago, when DC was awaiting admission to the university, he received a form requesting he have a medical exam and be tested for Tuberculosis (TB). He was in an area where there was still a lot of TB, so that may have made some sense – it didn't seem that way at the time. There was a very elderly physician located near campus who did these exams. DC passed the physical and sputum was sent to a lab for testing. The form came back saying 'negative' to TB. However, the wording caused the physician to read it differently. He wanted to indicate in his report that he

76 Engel PA, Gabal S, Broback M, Boice N. Physician and patient perceptions regarding physician training in rare diseases: the need for stronger educational initiatives for physicians, J Rare Dis. 2013;1(2):1-15. https://ojrd.biomedcentral.com/articles/10.1186/s13023-019-1285-0. Accessed August 22, 2022.

77 http://care4rare.ca/patient-stories-1/. Accessed August 25, 2022.

was positive that the DC did not have TB by putting the word "positive" in his report. It took quite a bit of argument to get him to write "negative"! Needless to say, it is likely that he was past his Best-By date, and memory has it that he was permanently 'recalled' a few months later. Speaking up can prevent harm, and that is at least as true when dealing with younger physicians as it is for older ones!

There are many possible errors related to the testing and reporting process.

Loss of the report can be a serious issue. Sometimes test results are lost either on the way to the doctor (even in the case of digital communications, such as in the office or when the lab sends the report to the wrong email address or fax machine). Also, the doctor might have tested for the condition, but the test result was mishandled, and the diagnosis is at least delayed. Personal communication of results can, too, be problematic. When a doctor does not call a patient to report a result, it does not necessarily mean that the result was normal or unimportant; no news may not be good news. Consequently, patients benefit if they get a copy of a report and make certain that the doctor has thoughtfully reviewed the results of their laboratory investigations.

NO NEWS IS BAD NEWS

Most people think that computers are pretty hot stuff and that they never make mistakes. Would that were true! Sometimes information can be modified or destroyed by software and other times it can be lost inside the machine and nobody knows it's there. A large radiology practice used computers to assist in dictating, storing, communicating and printing reports. One day, a curious staff person looked at the list of reports and discovered that there were approximately 1,000 in what's called the 'printer queue'. She could not figure out what was going on, but on examining the contents of the queue, realized that none of those reports had been printed or sent out. This turned out to be a very serious problem as many weeks of patient reports were trapped in the computer and the physicians who ordered the radiological examinations had not received their results. One can realize the serious impact of this by understanding that physicians often await reports before contacting their patients. It turned out that many patients had not been contacted and therefore had not been properly followed up. Although the practice informed the company that sold the system of the software problem, a year or two later the same thing occurred again in a different practice.

Just a Taste of False Positives and Negatives

We previously mentioned another example, screening at airports. The goal is to detect people who are dangerous, while not inconveniencing everyone else. Sometimes, however, a safe person is identified as a danger (a false alarm or false positive result). At other times, a dangerous person might be identified as safe (a false negative result).

Another issue that influences the likelihood that a diagnosis is correct is the presence of the problem in the population at hand (its 'prevalence' – the frequency of the condition in the population tested). As we indicated previously. an investigation of gang members that suggested a member is not harmful is more likely to be wrong compared with a similar investigation performed on monks or nuns. The frequency of a condition in a population affects the chances that a positive or negative test result provides accurate guidance.

Similarly, a pap smear (an abbreviation of 'Papanicolaou Smear' – a test to detect cancerous cells from the female cervix, the opening to the uterus), as we mentioned, is far more likely to be correctly positive among prostitutes than young virgins. Prevalence has a major influence on whether a test result is more or less likely to be an accurate reflection of the patient's condition. Willie Sutton, the famous bank robber was reputedly asked why he robbed banks. He is said to have answered: "Because that's where the money is!" Thereafter this was called 'Sutton's Law.' The 'money', so to speak, is mostly found where there is more money.

Because the prevalence of cervical cancer becomes greater with age, there is wide agreement that routine pap smears should not be started until age 25.[78]

A FEW ADDITIONAL WORDS FOR CLARITY.

A test for a specific disease that correctly or incorrectly reports that a patient has the disease is called a 'positive test result' or just 'positive'. If the patient actually has the disease, this is a 'true positive test result'. On the other hand, a test for a specific disease that correctly or incorrectly reports that a patient does not have the disease is called a 'negative test result' or just 'negative'. If the patient actually does not have the disease, this is a 'true negative test result'. They are 'false positives' or 'false negatives' if the result is incorrect.

There is a lot more on this in the chapter on testing.

People who create tests for diseases try to develop ones that report as few false negatives and as few false positives as possible. In other words, they want the test to provide the correct results: that the patient does or does not have the disease. However, they rarely succeed in producing perfect tests. The chapter on testing provides an analysis of the technical qualities of tests and how to interpret them. The simple truth is that almost no test is perfect. And tests that aren't perfect will inflict patients with false positives and false negatives. Testing is fraught!

This lack of perfection is hard on patients. The errors in testing cause anxiety if a patient gets a positive test result when the person does not have the disease. It also isn't good to get an incorrectly reassuring negative test result when the patient actually <u>does</u> have the disease. Either can cause a delayed diagnosis or the patient may be mistreated or untreated.

NOT SO FAST!

DC once had the chance to work with a brilliant, young Pediatrician who specialized in child cancers (Pediatric Oncology) and worked in an ICU. During discussions, DC naively suggested that getting positive test results as quickly as possible from the lab should be a priority. He was set straight by the pediatrician, who emphatically said words to the effect: "No! I need to know most urgently if a test result is negative, because that means that my hypothesis about what was going on (and to confirm which I ordered the test) was wrong and I need to straightaway reconsider it and figure out what is, in fact, going on. A life may hang in the balance!"

Doctors are likely to think of more common conditions and find them sooner. What's more, positive test results for common conditions (because they are more prevalent!) are more likely to be an accurate reflection of the person's condition compared with a positive test result for a rare condition.

AMERICANS PANICKED: ANECDOTE

Americans panicked when headlines reported that a Liberian man with a high fever and severe pain died from Ebola (a deadly virus that causes widespread internal bleeding and is usually isolated to certain African countries) after having been released from a Texas emergency department[79]. Ebola had not been considered as a possible diagnosis because it was a rarity in Texas and because the clinicians had not noticed that the patient had come from a high-risk area (Africa). If clinicians had tested for Ebola, they would likely have detected it. On the other hand, if they had tested for Ebola on millions of North Americans who use emergency services, they would have wasted virtually all that testing and millions of dollars... although they might have gotten a few false positives and upset even more people! Nothing is perfect! However, it was unreasonable to not test for Ebola on the very small number of patients who had

78 New Canadian Task Force guideline: Start Pap tests at age 25, not 18 The Canadian Task Force on Preventive Health Care 2013. https://canadiantaskforce.ca/guidelines/published-guidelines/cervical-cancer/. Accessed August 22, 2022.

79 Ebola patient sent home despite fever records show, by Manny Fernandez and Kevin Sack, New York Times, October 10, 2014. https://www.nytimes.com/2014/10/11/us/thomas-duncan-had-a-fever-of-103-er-records-show.html. Accessed July 14, 2022.

travelled in a high-risk area and whose symptoms were compatible with Ebola.

The headline in the anecdote above reflected a common problem, though. Patients, their relatives and sometimes their communities suffer when diagnosis and treatment are delayed or are incorrect. This can lead to inappropriate or delayed treatment and, sometimes, to avoidable disability, discomfort and death. These ensue when doctors fail to consider all possible diagnoses and therefore do not order appropriate blood tests or imaging studies (see the 'Scopes' examples below) to examine organs. Unfortunately, as the National Academies of Medicine report emphasized, delayed and mistaken diagnoses occur far too frequently.

EXAMPLE 'SCOPES'

Doctors often use instruments, called 'scopes' for short, to directly visualize internal parts of the body. Examples include:

- *Looking into the eye with an 'ophthalmoscope', which enables the doctor to see blood vessels, the retina and the optic nerve. An ophthalmoscopic examination provides direct evidence of damage to or deterioration of blood vessels or the retina or evidence of pressure around the brain.*
- *Using a 'bronchoscope', which enables the doctor to directly visualize lung tissue to find evidence of lung diseases or lung cancer.*
- *Introducing a 'gastroscope', which enables the doctor to examine the esophagus (the swallowing tube) and stomach.*
- *Inserting a 'colonoscope', which is passed through the rectum and enables the doctor to visualize and biopsy the lower bowel.*

The National Academies book 'Improving Diagnosis in Health Care'[80] suggests patients can prompt doctors to consider all possibilities by asking: "What could be causing my problem? What else could it be? When will I get my test results and how should I follow up?"

Consequences of Over-Testing—

People suffer and sometimes die from the consequences of inappropriate investigations or too many, not just too few.

Medical tests usually produce helpful results. Unfortunately, most tests also carry risks of their own. An example we have mentioned is when a bowel is punctured during a colonoscopy, when a false alarm led to an unnecessary test. Unnecessary and potentially harmful treatment might also follow. Remember, a false alarm occurs when a test result is positive, but the person does not have the illness. Another example is an infection[81] consequent to an unnecessary breast biopsy prompted by a false positive mammogram[82] (breast x-ray) result.

As testing procedures improve, it will become easier for doctors to order additional tests to confirm or disprove a diagnosis without invading the body. This can be good – the body is not injured – or it can be bad, as it is easier to over-order and give less consideration to the value the test result. The crucial change we need is developing better non-invasive tests that produce correct results more often. Scientists and commercial organizations[83] are developing tests that search for objective disease biomarkers using the air patients exhale, for example. One example is a breath test for H. Pylori which infects the stomach and can

80 National Academies Press, Improving Diagnosis in Health Care, Balogh, E.P., Miller, B.T., Ball, J.R., ed., Committee on Diagnostic Error in Health Care, The National Academies of Science, Engineering and Medicine, 2015. https://www.nap.edu/catalog/21794/improving-diagnosis-in-health-care. Accessed July 19, 2022.

81 Ray, J.E., Gardner, Suzanne, M., Cushing, R.D., Determinants of surgical site infection after breast biopsy, American Journal of Infection Control 33(2):126-9 · March 2005 https://www.ncbi.nlm.nih.gov/pubmed/15761414. Accessed July 19, 2022.

82 Mammogram is an x-ray examination of the breast, often used for screening and sometimes to investigate a known breast lump or breast discomfort.

83 https://www.owlstonemedical.com/. Owlstone Medical is developing methods to do breath analysis to detect biomarkers for a variety of diseases. Accessed July 19, 2022.

cause ulcers or cancer. Though the testing procedures themselves may become less harmful, any residual false positives they produce will continue to be harmful. This is because people will likely endure follow-on investigations or treatments they do not need. Don't forget, also, that tests cost money, and some are quite expensive.

There are other consequences of over-testing. People who have been falsely reassured by test results may subsequently be less likely to seek appropriate help, even if they develop new or worsening symptoms. They believe the test result and feel they are in the clear, despite the occurrence of disturbing symptoms.[84] The falsely reassured individual, told that chest pain was innocuous, might not seek advice when the pain becomes debilitating or other symptoms of cancer or heart disease reveal themselves.

Doctors try to use efficient approaches to explain a problem. They recognize the possibility of serious threats, but proceed in small steps (simple things, like careful examination and questioning) that minimize exposing patients to the unnecessary risks and worry that come with invasive or excessive investigation. Harmless approaches like 'watchful waiting' or 'tincture of time' allow the physician to see how things progress and maybe undertake a therapeutic trial of a safe medication.

Remember, no test is perfect! Tests, like the humans who develop and use them, are not flawless!

---

84 Renzi C, Whitaker KL, Wardle J Over-reassurance and under-support after a 'false alarm': a systematic review of the impact on subsequent cancer symptom attribution and help seeking BMJ Open 2015;5: e007002. doi: 10.1136/bmjopen-2014-007002. http://bmjopen.bmj.com/content/5/2/e007002. Accessed July 19, 2022.

Chapter 17: Diagnosis[85] Urgency and Rarity

KEYWORDS: Common Diagnoses, Rare Diagnoses, Urgent Diagnoses, Less Urgent Diagnoses, Diagnostic Harm Reduction

ABSTRACT: Rapid diagnosis of some medical conditions is important because the consequence of a delayed diagnosis can be fatal. Other medical conditions may be self-limited or progress slowly. For self-limited and slowly progressing problems delayed diagnosis is less important.

Introduction

To understand diagnosis more fully, it is useful to parse the causes for illness into several overlapping groups:

> Illnesses with common and uncommon causes.

> Important and unimportant illnesses.

> Urgent and non-urgent illnesses.

Common and Uncommon (Rare) Causes of a Condition

Diagnoses can be grouped as common or rare. For example, self-limited viral infections and post-viral tiredness are common causes of fatigue. Addison's disease, on the other hand, is a rare (but important) cause of fatigue. People with Addison's disease commonly experience a lengthy delay in diagnosis because the problem is not near the top of most doctors' lists of possible causes of fatigue. Often people are given the explanation 'depression' to account for the problem and this (inappropriate or non-useful) 'diagnosis' persists until a clinician does specific tests for the hormones that are deficient in Addison's disease. Suddenly it becomes clear that it only looks like psychiatric depression; rather, it is a diseased organ causing a symptom that can masquerade as a mental problem.

Important and Less-Important Causes of a Condition

Another way we can group diagnoses is by their importance. Ebola virus is a serious but very rare, at least outside Africa, viral cause of fever, weakness and fatigue. Despite rarity in the developed world, a missed diagnosis is important, not only for the patient but also for those people the patient contacts (it is highly transmissible via contact with infected bodily fluids), whom they might also infect.

Ordinarily, a simple viral upper respiratory infection is less important because, while being contagious, the disease is self-limited for most people. The word 'important' really refers to the magnitude of the disease's effects or impacts on the patient and others, whether minimal, minor, major or mortal.

A child with a fever and mild headache usually has a simple viral infection. However,

85 A later chapter indicates how doctors confirm or disprove diagnoses, including the use signs, symptoms, tests and therapeutic trials.

a small number have meningococcal meningitis (a bacterium-caused inflammation of the tissues that encase the brain and spinal column, called the 'encephalon') – a condition that could progress rapidly and is usually fatal.

AN IMPORTANT PROBLEM UNRECOGNIZED – MENINGITIS

In DZ's own practice, an emergency department physician saw an infant in the ER. DZ was unavailable because he was tied up with an obstetrics case. The emergency doctor judged that the infant's symptoms were those of a simple viral infection and sent the child home. Subsequently, the child became progressively worse and the mother, who had been reassured by the first diagnosis, did not return for several hours. The child was moribund and died shortly after returning to the emergency department.

Timing in a case like this might be everything. If the mother had been less concerned, and the first visit had taken place later in the course of the illness, the ER doctor would probably have seen more dire symptoms and would probably have recognized the severity of the condition. In their earliest stages, even the most serious and progressive diseases can mimic benign conditions.

Serious, important conditions might initially look like more common, minor and unimportant conditions.

Clinicians cannot aggressively investigate all seemingly minor problems as if they are serious because aggressive investigation can not only entail discomfort and inconvenience, but also, they increase the risk of harmful false alarms. We might state it thusly: if you are seriously ill, it is better that you look seriously ill! The diagnosis always starts with the patient's symptoms. It is not possible to have Superman's x-ray vision and gaze into the body. Unfortunately, there is no Star Trek 'Tricorder' either! The illness is seen by the diagnostician "as through a glass, darkly", interpreted in the context of the looks, behaviors, reactions and statements of the patient.

Malignant melanoma, a skin cancer, is important because it can spread and have deadly consequences. Early detection is crucial and can be lifesaving. On the other hand, a 'pigmented seborrheic keratosis' (which sounds awful but is an innocuous colored mole) is less important because it normally is a cosmetic problem with no influence on other body systems. Although malignant melanoma is rare and seborrheic keratosis is common, clinicians often biopsy (remove a piece of tissue for lab examination) skin lesions to reassure themselves and the patient that the lesion is unimportant. This means that many skin lesions are biopsied "unnecessarily" because they are not of any importance. But we can't know that until the tissue is examined microscopically. Luckily, only a very few people suffer because they develop infections at the biopsy site.

Today, 'dermatoscopy' (the use of a skin-microscope usually with a camera attached) allows dermatologists (doctors specializing in skin diseases) or other physicians to visualize a lesion to determine if it is benign (won't spread) or malignant (cancer that may spread). With microscopic visualization, dermatologists reduced the biopsy rate substantially because the visual clues are usually enough to determine that a lesion is benign and therefore that a biopsy is not necessary. Aggressive investigation with a dermatoscope is not harmful because the test is not invasive. Today, this device can even be used remotely over the Internet.

Urgent and Less Urgent Diagnoses

Another grouping is of serious possible causes that demand urgent attention. In these cases, delays in diagnosis could lead to serious harm. Some forms of meningitis, for example, cause very rapid deterioration and death, as is clear from the anecdote.

Generally, the most common causes, the ones doctors are most likely to remember and consider, are the least serious. Uncommon conditions are often more urgent to address, as their victims are likely to suffer from delays in diagnosis. A good example is headache caused by meningitis. Early detection of meningococcal meningitis is crucial, as it is serious and demands urgent attention. Delays in its diagnosis are, far too often, associated with fatal outcomes.

Delay in diagnosing psoriatic arthritis (a disease of the skin and joints) also leads to harm. Patients whose diagnosis is delayed suffer from increased erosion of joints and poorer overall health. While prompt diagnosis[86] benefits many, in the words of Larry the Cable Guy, it is important to "Git Er Done!"

Patients themselves also can contribute to delays in diagnosis. Women are more likely to have poor outcomes following a heart attack[87] because they are more likely than men to delay seeking hospital attention. This is often because their symptoms, like pain from their heart problem, are different from men (being sometimes right sided or presenting as jaw pain). Sometimes, men are also stoic, holding out in getting help until it's too late.

As we mentioned before, Family Medicine researchers from the University of Ottawa report that fatigue is the second most common symptom leading people to see a family doctor. Most cases of fatigue are temporary, benign, and self-limited. Fatigue frequently results from a poor diet and lack of exercise, sleep deprivation or minor viral illnesses. Unfortunately, fatigue is also an early symptom of serious and sometimes fatal conditions, including serious infectious diseases and cancers. So, fatigue can cut either way.

Because some serious and urgent problems are uncommon, the doctor might not think of a serious possible cause and may not search for factors that prove or disprove the diagnosis. No news, well, is no news!

Harking back to fatigue, the dilemma for doctors is deciding when and how to investigate and for what to test. There are just so many possible causes. Most people do agree that unexplained fatigue lasting more than three weeks deserves urgent attention. However, one group of reputable investigators suggests (incorrectly, in DZ's opinion[88]) that it is appropriate, in many situations, to wait as long as six months before starting in-depth investigations.[89] A long wait means that some people with serious and urgent problems will suffer because of a delayed diagnosis.

The tables below illustrate the categories of diagnoses. Clearly, it is most appropriate to order inexpensive and non-invasive investigations (at least initially) to try to make prompt diagnoses for common and uncommon, serious and less serious conditions.

It is also necessary to do the proper investigations, whether or not they are expensive or potentially dangerous, in order to avoid the consequences of delayed diagnosis for a serious and urgent condition.

Investigative caution relates not only to the possible diagnoses but also to the possible harms of testing. See FIGURE 1.17.1.

---

86 Haroon M, Gallagher P, FitzGerald O. Diagnostic delay of more than 6 months contributes to poor radiographic and functional outcome in psoriatic arthritis Annals of the Rheumatic Diseases 2015; 74:1045-1050. https://ard.bmj.com/content/74/6/1045. Accessed July 19, 2022.

87 Bugiardini R, Ricci B, Cenko E, et al. Delayed Care and Mortality Among Women and Men with Myocardial Infarction. Journal of the American Heart Association: Cardiovascular and Cerebrovascular Disease. 2017;6(8): e005968. doi:10.1161/JAHA.117.005968. https://www.ncbi.nlm.nih.gov/pmc/articles/PMC5586439/. Accessed July 19 2022.

88 Zitner, D., Caution advised when testing for causes of fatigue, Canadian family physician May 1999 45:872-3. https://www.ncbi.nlm.nih.gov/pmc/articles/PMC2328310/. Accessed August 22, 2022.

89 Godwin, M., Delva, D., Miller, et.al., investigating fatigue of less than six months' duration Canadian Family Physician, Vol 45, Feb 1999, pg. 373. https://www.ncbi.nlm.nih.gov/pmc/articles/PMC2328284/. Accessed August 22, 2022.

	SERIOUS - POTENTIAL DANGERS	NOT SERIOUS
URGENT	Requires immediate aggressive investigation and treatment.	Unimportant diagnosis-self-limited, few consequences for delay.
NOT URGENT	Cancers where a short delay does not increase harms, or knee problems where delayed diagnosis does not affect eventual outcome.	Self-limited, coughs, colds.
There are urgent and not urgent presenting complaints and some of each of these are serious or not serious.		

FIGURE 1.17.1: Severity groupings

Chapter 18: The Levels of Evidence

KEYWORDS: Knowledge, Evidence, Anecdotal Information, Case Studies, Systematic Reviews, Expert Opinion, Randomized Controlled Trials, Cohort Studies.

ABSTRACT: Clinicians and patients develop beliefs about what tests and treatments are likely to be helpful or harmful based on various types of information. Some beliefs are based on stories told by other doctors or patients, in other words, anecdotes. Other beliefs are based on stronger evidence. This chapter reviews the types of evidence and the strength of conclusions that lead to clinical beliefs and consequently interventions.

Levels of Evidence

How many of us have been whipsawed from one medical belief to another based on articles in the press? Take Vitamin E to enhance healing! Take Vitamin B3 to prevent heart disease! (Spoiler Alert: studies have not proven that these vitamins actually have those effects!). Consciously or unconsciously we surely wonder how many people have to take the treatment for someone to benefit? And how many people will be harmed? What are the kinds of evidence that help answer these questions?

Remember reading that we should all be drinking eight glasses of water a day? That was published in probably thousands of newspapers and on thousands of websites as if it were the gosh-darn absolute truth! Some may have wondered what the quantity called a 'glass' was. Was it a large glass, small glass, martini glass or shot glass? That should have raised suspicions. Luckily for us, someone eventually did the hard digging to find out the source of this recommendation in the research literature. There was none![90 91 92] Furthermore, it turns out that thirst may be the best indicator for how much water we need. In addition, its form might be as tea or coffee or plain old faucet water. This is an important example, as it illustrates the challenge we all have in coming to rational and firm beliefs about how to care for ourselves.

What is Evidence?

It is crucial to understand what evidence is. Many years ago, DC asked a well-known lawyer and former judge that question: what is evidence?[93] The answer he gave was an important lesson. He explained that evidence is just about anything. Consider a person murdering

90 Guppy Michelle P B, Mickan Sharon M, Mar Chris B Del. "Drink plenty of fluids": a systematic review of evidence for this recommendation in acute respiratory infections BMJ 2004; 328 :499. https://pubmed.ncbi.nlm.nih.gov/14988184/. Accessed Sept 8, 2023.

91 McCartney Margaret. Waterlogged? BMJ July 12 2011; 343: d4280. https://www.bmj.com/content/343/bmj.d4280. Accessed July 19, 2022.

92 Science News, Advice to drink eight glasses of water a day "nonsense" argues doctor, July 13, 2011. https://www.sciencedaily.com/releases/2011/07/110712190822.htm. Accessed Sept 8, 2023.

93 Dominic Covvey, Personal Communication: Justice Horace Krever. 1979.

another person. If there exists a person who was told by another person who the murderer was, that is evidence…very weak evidence, but evidence, often called circumstantial evidence. If there was a witness to the actual murder or maybe even a photo, that is evidence – much, much stronger evidence, but evidence. If there were 10 witnesses, each being a trained observer, who recorded a video with sound, then that is really good evidence. However, lawyers would be unable to defend alleged murderers, if even this were the final word.

What is evidence that a medical treatment works?

Perhaps the lowest level of evidence of the effectiveness of a drug is where a physician gives it to a bunch of patients and believes that it worked. However, there are problems with this minimal level of evidence, usually called 'anecdotal evidence.' Not all the patients who received the treatment might have actually been sick or sick from the same disease. Perhaps some just felt bad, and given time, they would have felt better. Perhaps the physician was overly hopeful or biased in favor of the effectiveness of the treatment and mistakenly perceived that the patients improved when they really didn't. The actual treatment here might have been the 'tincture of time' and the medicine applied might have made no difference at all.

One can potentially improve on anecdotal evidence by upping the numbers and maybe ensuring that the patients are in fact sick. For example, a physician might look at a group of 100 patients who have certain signs and symptoms, apply a certain treatment, and then observe if the treatment worked or did not. That sounds like much better evidence, and kind of is, but again there are problems. For example, it may be that not all 100 patients had the same kind of sickness, despite their symptoms and signs. It might also be that the physician, hoping for a good result, felt that certain patients had gotten better, but they had not. Or the physician might have had a bias that the medication was going to work, and that bias resulted in either including less-ill patients or assessing that they were less ill after the treatment. Or there might be other reasons, like luck. This type of study is often called the 'case study.' It is better evidence, but we don't have proof that the treatment <u>caused</u> a genuine improvement. There is perhaps a degree of association but not actual causality.

Of course, if lots of physicians looked at lots of patients in lots of case studies, that makes somewhat better evidence, but not much. The reason is that the same conditions apply! In none of these studies can we assure ourselves that the level and type of illness were the same for all patients, and that the result of treatment wasn't just a red herring or somewhat biased. This is a fair accusation, particularly if the person doing a study has some interest in the outcome, such as selling a product or getting recognition in the literature. Another issue is that studies can be 'cherry-picked', by selecting only ones that produced the hoped-for results. The sum of a lot of weak or questionable studies does not equal a good study!

Good Evidence

The way that Medicine dramatically improves the quality of evidence is by having what are called 'clinical trials.'

A clinical trial is a relatively simple concept that is extraordinarily difficult (and usually expensive) to carry out in real practice. The general idea, though, is that we take steps to avoid some of the problems with anecdotal evidence and the results of case studies. The way to do this is to carefully define the types of patients included in the study and to significantly increase our assuredness that their type and level of sickness are similar. Think of this as a kind of standardization of patients.

Let's assume we have a population of patients with a disorder, for example, high serum cholesterol (a kind of fat in the blood). Suppose that we measure their cholesterol levels using objective and standard methods. Let's also make sure that the population of patients has an appropriate mix of factors that might affect their outcomes (like different body weights, genders, ages, smoking histories, etc.). We then randomly divide this population into two or more groups, applying a medication (e.g., a 'statin', which lowers blood cholesterol) of one type to one of the groups, or a statin of another type (or a sugar pill) to another group. Then we let the clock run and periodically we measure the serum cholesterol of the members of both groups, we tabulate the number of patients having heart or blood vessel problems in both groups, record the number that died in each group, and so on. A study like this typically takes tens of thousands of subjects and several decades. However, the outcome will have a certain probability of telling us if a statin produces more benefit than harm or if one statin is better than another or no intervention at all.

There is, though, a fly in the experimental ointment. We must realize that even in the case of a well-designed and executed clinical trial, a different group of patients even with the same screening criteria (that determine who is in the trial population) will have differences. Furthermore, the various assessments done have only a finite level of accuracy and can be wrong. It might also be that some patients snuck off and took another medication or altered their diets or started or stopped smoking. The next time we did a trial like this even on tens of thousands of patients over decades, the outcome of the trial could be, and often is, different – sometimes significantly so. So, even a clinical trial is not perfect evidence. We do have more of an indication that the medications caused the effects that we observed, so we do get a modicum of cause and effect. But the result is often not certain because the differences between the outcomes of the trial groups are often not enormous, to say the least.

Alas, the fact is that we cannot achieve perfection! However, we can do better! The most advanced level of evidence we can get in this mortal coil is called a 'systematic review' or a 'meta-analysis' – an analysis above (meta) the corpus of clinical trials. There are many researchers and organizations that perform this type of study (such as Cochrane Collaboration: https://canada.cochrane.org/cochrane-canada and the Health Information Research Unit (HIRU) at McMaster University: https://hiru.mcmaster.ca/hiru/, as well as NICE in the UK: https://www.nice.org.uk/). What's done in a systematic review is to take all the clinical trials that have been published – and that can be a problem as trial failures are often not published – then to eliminate any trials that were imperfect (yes, another judgment that can cause problems). Then we look at the remaining studies overall, comparing or even combining their statistics. So, the very best evidence we have on this planet in this era, our 10 witnesses to an assault all with video cameras and sound, is the systematic review.

The formal definitions of the levels of evidence used in the categorization of research findings are listed in FIGURE 1.18.1.

1a:	Result of systematic review of randomized controlled trials.
1b:	*Result of individual randomized controlled trial.*
2a:	*Result of systematic review of cohort studies.*
2b:	*Result of individual cohort study.*
2c:	*Result of "outcomes research".*
3a:	*Result of systematic review of case-control studies.*
3b:	*Result of individual case-control study.*
4:	*Results of Case series.*
5:	Expert opinion.
Oxford Centre for Evidence-based Medicine Levels of Evidence[94]	

FIGURE 1.18.1: Levels of evidence

94 OCEBM Levels of Evidence Working Group*. "The Oxford Levels of Evidence 2". Oxford Centre for Evidence-Based Medicine. https://www.cebm.ox.ac.uk/resources/levels-of-evidence/ocebm-levels-of-evidence. Accessed August 10, 2022.

The Problem with Tracking the Medical News

It is amazing how quickly the results of clinical trials appear in the press or on the evening news. However, as we have seen, these trials don't give us the necessary level of evidence. Even worse, sometimes results that just happen during the trial, but not the subject of actual testing, are promulgated. This latter point is illustrated by considering the investigation of church fires. Suppose that every church that burned down had a red door. Someone might conclude that red doors caused church fires – an incidental finding. The BBQ News broadcasts: "New study reveals that painting church doors red causes fires!" You can get the point.

The comeuppance could be, in an area like nutrition, that after patients watched the nightly news a year ago they switched to a high-fat diet. However, after the morning news today they switched to a low-fat diet. They got whipsawed!

The lesson from all of this is that treatment decisions must be based on the highest level of evidence possible, preferably systematic reviews or meta-analyses. But even these are not perfect evidence and other later analyses might change the recommendations. They are just the best that we can do at the moment.

So, What Do We Do?

We need to recognize that, just like the judge and jury, lower levels of evidence might be all we have, so we must rely on the results of one or a few clinical trials or even on anecdotal experience. The art of Medicine is often based on this anecdotal evidence…experiences of a physicians in their practices. It may work; it may not work. If it works, good for that patient. If it doesn't work, that's the way the cookie crumbles. Doctors do the best that they can with their human minds, human perception, the available 'facts,' their human biases, the effects of human emotions and their experiences as human beings. Not we, nor the world, nor our science are perfect. But we try our best.

Most encouraging is that after drugs have been approved, many treatments are subjected to post-marketing surveillance. Unlike clinical trials, or even meta-analysis, post-marketing surveillance occurs when people track the fate of almost everyone who takes a drug to learn if overall the drug takers are healthier or worse off for having taken it.

The thalidomide tragedy is one example where better post-marketing surveillance might have reduced the time it took to learn that pregnant women who used thalidomide were more likely to have babies born with limb deformities or missing limbs.

Life and health depend on our knowledge and how certain it is!

Some interesting reading:

https://journals.physiology.org/doi/full/10.1152/ajpregu.00365.2002. Accessed Sept 13, 2023. (Debunking excess water drinking.)

Chapter 19: Introduction to Health Informatics

KEYWORDS: Health Informatics, Health Informaticians, Collection and Use of Health Information

ABSTRACT: Health informaticians must understand Computer Science, Information Science, Health and Health Care, and Social Science especially as it applies to care. They use this knowledge to design and develop more effective approaches, as well as systems, processes and information management and analysis tools to support clinical activities, health-related research and administration.

Before revealing the details of the roles and functions of this group of professionals, it is worth noting that some of them call themselves 'Health Informaticists,' 'Biomedical Informaticians', or 'Biomedical and Health informaticists/Informaticians'. As a bit of humor, some reject the term 'Informaticist', because it can be misspelled 'Informaticyst', which sounds like a bit of pathology to those of the medical persuasion! Quite a few years ago, there was a near endless debate about the proper designation for people in the field and the decision was that any one of the three terms mentioned here was appropriate.

We have used the term health informatician throughout.

Health Informatician Roles

There are many roles and functions of health informaticians. For one education presentation, we produced a listing of almost 500 different areas of specialization of these professionals based on a survey we did. This list was too vast to be of practical use, so we boiled it down to 11 general areas of practice:

- Health Information Content, Vocabulary, Semantics, Structure and Management.
- Translational Bioinformatics (the extension of genetics into health information).
- Intelligent Health Systems (Artificial Intelligence – AI – and Machine Learning).
- User Interfaces, Human-Computer Interaction, Usability and Human Factors.
- Health Communications, Telehealth, Information Usability and Health Education.
- Digital Imaging, Image Processing and Image Management (addressing x-ray, ultrasound, MRI, CT, Clinical Pathology Imaging, and so on).
- Mathematical Computing and Algorithms in Health.
- Human Aspects of Health Informatics, Effects on Work, Workflow, Roles and Ethics.

> The Health Technology Infrastructure (Computers, Software, Peripheral Devices and Networks).
> Competencies, Curricula and Education in Health Informatics.
> The Informatics of Clinical, Laboratory and Health Systems Research.

Readers might find it useful to have a concise definition of Health Informatics, so this is included as FIGURE 1.19.1.

HI is the discipline that, firstly, aspires to comprehensively understand, in all their aspects, health and the health system, healthcare processes, and the roles, functions and needs of care providers, patients and other stakeholders.

HI then conceptualizes, develops, applies and evaluates concepts, theories, structured methods, and information tools to address the need to evolve as well-monitored, efficient and effective a health system as possible that satisfies the needs of all stakeholders.

FIGURE 1.19.1: Definition of health informatics (HI)

Health Informatician Knowledge and Skills

Health informaticians necessarily have a wide spectrum of knowledge and often several areas of specific focus (Example: physicians who are Health Informaticians and who work in medical imaging and decision support systems). They are called Clinical Informaticians and contribute to clinical care, health services administration, health services research and patient and clinician education. Many are also health professionals, like physicians and nurses.

Health informaticians make important contributions to clinical care by conceptualizing, designing, developing and implementing methods and systems to capture and store the data clinicians collect and use for ongoing clinical care, research and health system performance assessment. They also develop clinical reminder and prompting tools meant to help clinicians consider diagnostic and therapeutic possibilities and attend to laboratory and other results and findings.

Health informaticians make important contributions to health services administration, as they develop methods and systems that use data from clinical encounters to estimate the efficiency, cost and value of various health system services.

Health informaticians also contribute to clinical research, as they develop and implement systems linking healthcare activities and the health results of those activities.

In addition, health informaticians support patient and provider education by educating, producing information to support care, and reminding doctors and patients about important issues in clinical care.

Perhaps at the top of the heap are health informaticians who do research. However, many in the field, sometimes in addition to doing research, work in practical areas that are of potentially great support to the practice of Medicine and the operation of the healthcare system. The latter groups are often called 'Applied Health Informaticians' (and sometimes designated 'eHealth Professionals').

The Work of Health Informaticians

The nature of the work performed by these professionals is interesting. First of all, they observe, study and measure just about any aspect of health care. As examples, they investigate how patients provide and receive information, how clinicians must capture and store information and how they diagnose, why and how they decide about and provide treatment and how care processes work. Their objective is to understand health care in the deepest and most complete sense, noting its problems, inefficiencies, mistakes, results, and so on. Once they have this kind of in-depth understanding, they apply their knowledge of a variety of fields like those mentioned above to improve the care process and both care providers' and patients' experience with it. In other words, they devote themselves to improving the efficiency and effectiveness of health care.

Health informaticians come to this field with a variety of types of knowledge. Some are experts in Computer Science or Information Science, language (Linguistics), vocabularies, the social sciences, Economics, and dozens of other fields. There is even a well-known Health Informatician who has a Ph.D. in History, and others have advanced degrees in Psychology, Anthropology and the STEM (Science, Technology, Engineering and Medicine) disciplines. What they all have in common is the observing, studying, measuring and analyzing of healthcare patients, providers and care processes. They are primarily observers and 'comprehenders.' Then, according to the specific disciplines they bring to the party, they apply these so that we have a better healthcare system and a better experience with it.

To get a more detailed view of Health Informatics, it is worth looking at a compendium of professional competencies.[95] Health Informatics (the name of the science itself) is among the most variegated and interesting fields of endeavor.

Health informaticians, and anyone else working in health care, benefit if they understand the fundamental ideas in and the nature of Medicine and the healthcare system.

Another Motivation for this Book

One of the motivations for this book has been DZ's years of teaching in a program dedicated to Health Informatics at Dalhousie University in Halifax, Nova Scotia. He has taught students a deep appreciation of the nature of Medicine, medical practice and its impacts. To his surprise, students who understand the important ideas are able to find worthwhile answers to meaningful clinical questions.

It became clear that it was possible to teach the fundamental nature of Medicine and medical practice to students who did not have backgrounds in Medicine. Furthermore, without the kind of knowledge embodied here, these students would have been significantly impaired related to understanding of health care. It turned out that an even more general audience could advantage itself with the content herein. So, in reading this book, you are also getting the gist of an advanced course fundamental to the development of effective health informaticians. Health Informatics might even be an area of endeavor that could interest you. It certainly is fascinating and satisfying even to those of us who have been involved in it for over 50 years.

95 Pointing the Way Competencies And Curricula In Health Informatics Saved 2 3 22 3 27 01: Dominic Covvey, David Zitner, Robert Burnstein and many collaborators: Free Download, Borrow, and Streaming: Internet Archive; https://archive.org/details/pointingthe-way-competencies-and-curricula-in-health-informatics-saved-2-3-22-3-27-01. Accessed Sept 8, 2023.

Chapter 20: Biases – Human Nature's Spin

KEYWORDS: Biases, Cognitive Bias, Mistaken Thinking, Overconfidence, Framing

ABSTRACT: Why people make thinking errors has been well-studied. This chapter describes several types of thinking errors that everyone should be conscious of and try to avoid. These errors occur not only in health care but in other areas of our lives as well.

"I'm not biased, I've been around for a long time and have heard all of that before! Some of the ideas you expressed were good, but I didn't like the way you said them!" These are statements expressing different types of bias. Being biased, though, is not always obvious, and avoiding or minimizing the effects of bias is quite challenging.

People also show bias when they select the information they use to make choices because they just do or don't like it. People likewise limit their choices by saying "I can't consider that possibility" when they could. To overcome potential bias by a doctor, a patient may ask the doctor to consider a very rare diagnosis as a possible explanation for a set of problems.

Cognitive Biases

Bias is a popular topic. A Google web search produces over 360 million possibilities. It turns out that we each harbor many biases and it is often surprising to discover them in ourselves. One might even say that bias is a universal human characteristic.

Wikipedia lists over 180 'Cognitive Biases', also called 'Cognitive Errors'. It divides these up into: (1) decision-making, belief and behavioral biases, (2) social biases and (3) memory errors and biases. It lists almost 120 biases in the first category and a total of about 70 across the others. We can define 'cognitive biases' as "systematic pattern

s of deviation from [the] norm or rationality in judgment..."[96] In other words, cognitive biases are factors that influence our thinking and our conclusions. They turn out to be powerful forces that are subtly interwoven into the fabric of our minds, affecting all the thinking we do. If any of us, especially clinicians and researchers, face the challenge of making what we call 'objective decisions' and 'objective recommendations', we must recognize the effect of biases.

COGNITIVE BIASES

A few years ago, Vimla Patel, a star in the Health Informatics community, sent out an email regarding a video her students had produced about cognitive biases. When we searched for it recently, we were unable to find the original video, as it was not available at the cited location. We were able to find either that one or another at: https://www.youtube.com/watch?v=3RsbmjNLQkc. We highly recommend listening to this, as it is a memorable way of learning about biases.

96 https://en.wikipedia.org/wiki/List_of_cognitive_. Accessed August 31, 2022.

Of course, DC, with tongue-in-cheek, wrote back to Vimla, (you only will understand this after watching the video): "Very interesting, but I heard it before, knew it before I heard it and considered the video pedantic. I particularly didn't like the strumming and initially thought it was just another YouTube teen video. I was unable to listen to the entire thing because it ran against my grain, and it isn't nearly as good as videos I've done. What they sang was really ultra-right drivel. At least if my memory serves me correctly... when I saw it before, I felt the same way." That is DC's early contribution to the understanding of cognitive biases.

Some Crucial Biases

In an excellent article in the Journal of the Royal College of Physicians in Edinburgh, O'Sullivan and Schofield list 10 cognitive biases that affect clinical medicine.[97] We will address each of these briefly:

Availability Bias: This is what we do when we base our thinking and conclusions on easily available material. It is especially likely to occur if we recently read something and can remember it, unlike material we read perhaps years ago and may have forgotten or poorly recall.

Base Rate Neglect Bias: When a clinician is with a specific patient, there is a tendency to ignore information based on conditions known to exist in the overall population. The physician ignores the prevalence in the population and feels that this patient is somehow special. We see this often in forensic investigations, where investigators ignore the likelihood that a person-of-interest committed a crime, despite statistics that say it's more likely to be a person like the one at hand. For example, there is a horrible likelihood that, despite the person's attractiveness and apparent sincerity, if he or she is a family member, guilt is more likely.

Confirmation Bias: All humans jump to conclusions. Each of us quickly forms conclusions based on what we first see. As further evidence of what actually happened becomes available, we remain somewhat resistant to abandoning our initial conclusions. We see each piece of evidence as confirming what we thought. This is a fundamental problem in diagnosis. The first step of diagnosis must be to get data and put it together into useful information and <u>only</u> then to begin forming conclusions. It is extraordinarily dangerous to be driven by initial perceptions and thoughts. This can cut either way, as we can see a patient who looks well but is sick, or we can see a patient who looks sick but may have an innocuous condition. Physicians form first impressions on seeing a patient but there are traps in that.

Conjunction Rule Bias: In this case, multiple pieces of information can stand against a single crucial piece of information. It could be that a constellation of quite minor symptoms leads to an innocuous diagnosis, distracting from the possibility of a serious illness. It seems that we are more likely to take strength in numbers, rather than in the quality or importance of the information.

Overconfidence Bias: Sometimes physicians become simply too sure of themselves and believe, possibly even based on their sophisticated credentials, that they are great diagnosticians and can use intuitive judgement to reach conclusions about diagnosis and treatment. They may have huge confidence but be totally wrong. It seems that humans lack or are impaired related to self-critical thinking. The ultimate solution to overconfidence is harboring a degree of humility and always wondering about how we think.

Representativeness Bias: This may also be called the Aggregation Bias. In this instance, we decide on something because we note it is like other things we have seen or learned about. Similarly, we may assume that what is true for a group must be true for an individual or part of the group. It may be, for example, that we grew up in a violent neighborhood and the people

97 Cognitive bias in clinical medicine, ED O'Sullivan, SJ Schofield, J R Coll Physicians Edinb 2018, pp. 225-232;. https://pubmed.ncbi.nlm.nih.gov/30191910/. Accessed August 22, 2022.

who were violent had certain characteristics. If we see a person with those characteristics, we begin forming a conclusion that this person is just like the others who looked like that. Racial biases have at least one leg in this domain. In Medicine, the physician may think that a patient has been smoking (it turns out he just came in from a smoke-filled vehicle) and judges the patient to be a liar because of the denial regarding smoking. This could even lead the physician to withhold certain care because of the assumed behavior or the perception of prevarication.

Search Satisfying Bias: This is also called 'Premature Closure'. This is where we stop looking for information, once we think we have the answer. What we have not done is consider other possible answers, even when they can be better ones. It is usual for people who access the Internet to have a few favorite information resources, which may be reasonably accurate in one area but weak or misleading in another. For instance, there has been a long-term effort to establish a process for certifying sites for health-related information, but this has been an elusive goal. The same can be true about consulting any information source, such as another person. The person consulted may be expert in one area, let's say motor mechanics, but terribly deficient in another, such as the treatment of an infection.

Diagnostic Momentum Bias: Once a medical process is underway, it can be quite difficult to stop. There are several anecdotes in this book that illustrate this problem. Even when contrary information becomes available, there is a tendency to proceed along the original track. This isn't just in Medicine, either. There are many people in prison because the justice system began a process to convict them based on certain information and the investigators looked only for information to confirm their conclusion; they might even have withheld information that pointed to another perpetrator. However, despite contrary information (such as DNA analysis) becoming known, the process sped along right up to incarceration or execution.

Framing Effect Bias: It can be a lot of fun presenting information to people in an apparently scientific and professional way, but where the 'information' is nonsense. Some of us awful parents have done this with our children and thoroughly enjoyed their credence. In "You're a Good Man Charlie Brown," Charlie often explains things to Linus or Lucy, like how trees grow. The mode and quality of presentation can make things believable. Ads on TV exploit this fact. This means that a fraudster acting as a physician can relatively easily fool people by sounding and looking authoritative, assertive, confident and physician-like. It is also not unusual for people to present a meaningless measure, like a p-value (a measure of statistical confidence), that sounds cogent but isn't. The only thing that stands between a physician being convinced by well-presented but incorrect research results or a pharmaceutical rep's sales pitch is critical thinking. Those bombarded with assertive and well-spun claims must ask entertain scepticism, ask probing questions and do personal research. The same is true for a patient whom a physician is trying to convince about something, but who is dead wrong. It isn't nice to have been talked into being wrongly dead!

In pharmaceutical marketing one example of framing effect bias occurs when a pharmaceutical representative provides information about the presumed mechanism of action of a drug without substantial information about how many benefit or are harmed. For example, in the 1970's drugs were marketed as effective in reducing strokes because they dilated the arteries supplying blood to the brain. Unfortunately, the drugs also dilated the blood vessels in other parts of the body. Consequently, the brain got less, rather then more blood than before.[98]

98 Today's Drugs, British Medical Journal, June 19, 1971. https://academic.oup.com/bjs/article-abstract/59/4/329/6191620?redirectedFrom=fulltext. Accessed Sept 8, 2023.

Commission Bias: On being challenged, we all want to do something, just anything, sometimes. This has trapped many spouses. Let's say your partner cries out with frustration. Often the response is to immediately try to find solutions or to do something. Sometimes, just empathetic listening may be the only intervention the partner desired. A doctor needs to fight against commission bias when facing a crying child and a frustrated parent. It could be that waiting a day and applying over-the-counter pain relievers would be the best answer. However, the parent might not perceive that as responsive action. There may be the pressure to do something 'real,' like prescribe an antibiotic. The same can be true related to people who are dying. Family members may demand that the physician do something to stop this, but the truth may be dying is inevitable and intervention would only distress the patient.

It is worth noting that there is also **Omission Bias**, which is the tendency to inaction or to not consider other possibilities.

Many Other Biases

Another bias we frequently encounter is the **Gambler's Fallacy Bias**. This is when the person assumes that something that happens more frequently than is typical, will happen less frequently later – or the opposite. Gamblers often assume that, if a number comes up 3 times in a row, it won't come up a 4th time, or, if they lose several times in a row, then they are bound to win next throw, spin or hand.

Every one of these biases has many aliases. In another analysis, the Canadian Medical Protective Association (CMPA), which provides malpractice insurance to Canadian physicians and must pay up if they mess up, calls "Diagnostic Momentum Bias" the "Bandwagon Effect". You can see the similarity. As an insurance agency, the CMPA focuses on the set of biases related to the behaviors of physicians who have been sued or threatened with such. So, the CMPA's selection of biases is biased!

The CMPA uses the term '**Anchoring Bias**' to describe focusing on one piece of information or a particular diagnosis and not making adjustments when there is evidence for others. Another bias it addresses is called '**Premature Closure**', where a physician does not rethink an initial diagnosis and does not seek further information. This overlaps with the Anchoring Bias.

Yet another that also overlaps somewhat is called '**Search Satisfaction**,' where, after finding one thing, the doctor does not look for anything further. For example, a radiologist may immediately see the image of a tumor in a patient's right lung and not notice that the image of the heart shows it has a problem.

In this book we have mentioned a number of times what the CMPA calls '**Zebra Retreat**' bias, where the physician ignores a rare diagnosis just because it's uncommon. The aforementioned '**Bandwagon Effect**' is a good example to illustrate that, the more people that think something is right, the more the diagnostician should question it. Finally, the '**Attribution Error**' bias cited by the CMPA is very similar to what we call above, the "Representativeness Bias".

So Many Biases; So Little Time

In reviewing the literature on cognitive biases, something like depression descends on one. We exist in a thicket of biases like the viruses that surround us. A better metaphor might be travelling through a desert with quicksand every few yards. Even reading through the long list of biases requires significant effort and a fair amount of time. The problem of eliminating or moderating the impacts of these biases is an even greater challenge. The truth is that they are embedded in our brains, as they represent quick ways to form conclusions and make decisions. They are cognitive heuristics, or rules of thumb, that reduce the time associated with thinking things through. Unfortunately, these mental-efficiency tools are extraordinarily dangerous and can have harmful consequences when applied to real people in real situations.

Scientific Thinking – Attempting to Address Cognitive Biases/Errors

Everybody faces a significant challenge in attempting to recognize their biases and do something about them. In his excellent series of 4 articles, Justin Morgenstern suggests some ways of at least reducing the magnitude of the effects of bias.[99] He suggests that our real objective is to keep our rational minds active and thinking about what we often do intuitively – and intuition is necessary! He suggests asking oneself five questions in each situation, e.g., when dealing with a patient: (1) Which traps might I be falling into? (2) What else can the problem be? (3) Is there anything about the patient's symptoms, signs and the results of tests that does not fit with my hypothesis about what is wrong? (4) Could it be that there is more than a single problem? (5) Is this a situation where I must be more systematic and take the time to figure out what's going on?

We should remember that science is based on disconfirming theories, finding evidence that conflicts with them. This is because it is often impossible to prove or even to completely confirm a theory or totally reject it. Therefore, the scientist is left with attempting to strengthen the cogency of the theory by trying to show that the theory does not hold overall or in certain situations, by finding counterexamples, for instance. This scientific thought process would be the action of the rational mind: thinking about the thinking one is doing, and/or the conclusions reached and trying to find something that proves it is not so. What about the patient isn't explained by my diagnosis? If the physician finds something that does not fit, then the diagnosis is flawed, incomplete just wrong.

To assist this kind of thinking, one of the major computer-based diagnosis decision support systems, DXplain, provides prompts that suggest tests one can do or signs one can elicit that would obviate a given diagnosis. The idea of some of the other interventions suggested by Morgenstern is to reduce bias by recognizing that the mind can be distracted or clouded with issues and overloaded. Practices are often busy environments and just taking a pause to give enough time for thinking can make the difference. This approach has worked in the operating room, where, before surgery starts, the head nurse calls a 'pause for safety' to make sure that the team is dealing with the right patient, the correct surgery is planned, the surgeon has selected the correct limb for surgery and so on. This also means overcoming or avoiding fatigue and managing feelings so that emotion does not cloud decision-making. Needless to say, minimizing interruptions would also be of value.

Edward de Bono's tool called 'Consider All Factors' (CAF) is an important one related to biases. At least all the relevant stones need to be turned over and the decision-maker must recognize and be accountable for past errors. That reflection on past experience will inform current activities and allow time for questions and answers to enter into the diagnostic process.

There isn't any magic wand, incantation or elixir here, no secret sauce. We are all beset by biases that are sometimes very hard even to notice. What it really comes down to is thinking about one's thinking, taking time and being systematic.

---

99 https://first10em.com/cognitive-errors/. Accessed Sept 8, 2023.

Chapter 21: Deeper Thoughts About Diagnosis

KEYWORDS: Types of Diagnosis, Diagnosis with Known Causes, Descriptive Diagnoses, Rare Conditions, Common Conditions, Frequency of Diagnosis, Urgency of Diagnosis, Predictive Models

ABSTRACT: Physician-imposters are successful because they pronounce on, and make choices, that are usual and common, and they avoid harmful interventions. Sometimes clinicians just rename a problem and act as if it were a special medical diagnosis. We distinguish between those problems that are urgent because a delay in diagnosis and treatment might be harmful, and those that are less important because the results of delay are not very harmful, or because the condition is self limited. Everyone can contribute to making a diagnosis by providing essential information, or by looking for the possible causes of a problem.

Diagnostic terms (or labels) can be confusing. Some indicate an objective cause for the patient's complaints; others are just a fancy way of saying that we don't know the cause.

Introduction

It should be clear by now that a diagnosis is a label a doctor uses to explain why a person feels uncomfortable, cannot do as much as before to or why life expectancy may be limited. A diagnosis is a shorthand description of what the doctor believes is the cause of a problem. Well, that's the idea, anyhow!

Some 'diagnoses', for example, 'essential hypertension' (which means 'high blood pressure with no identified cause') masquerade as a diagnosis but the underlying cause of the high blood pressure is a mystery – the doctor has not figured out the actual cause of the problem. Other diagnoses, like 'breast cancer', indicate that the doctor knows the reasons for a lump, swelling or inflammation. Even that one, however, is a bit fuzzy as, at least initially, no one may know the specific type(s) of cancer cell(s) causing the cancer or what caused them to become cancerous. Both labels, essential hypertension and breast cancer, imply a range of solutions but especially the former one does not engender detailed guidance. Some diagnostic labels just suggest that further investigation to find a biological reason for the abnormality might be beneficial.

Diagnoses with Known Cause

A diagnosis means that the physician understands the actual biological mechanisms causing the problem. Normally, diagnoses grounded in knowledge like that have associated 'biomarkers'. A biomarker is an objective finding, such as a laboratory test result, an x-ray image showing an abnormality or any objective physical finding (such as the inability to bend a joint). In other words, there is 'incriminating evidence' of the perpetrator. Depressed feeling, consequent to a low level of thyroid (hypothyroid) hormone, is a problem where the diagnosis reflects the known cause.

Descriptive Diagnoses

Other 'diagnoses' (they don't really deserve that label) may just be mere descriptions and restatements of the problem, like the use of the words: 'depression' or 'anxiety'. They are symptoms, not causes – patients use these terms to describe how they feel. Some doctors incorrectly behave as if restating the description of the problem, for example 'anxiety' or 'depression', is the same as understanding the cause of the problem. It isn't and it serves little value.

A different but related problem is that some 'diagnoses' are really just saying that the cause of a problem is unknown. We mentioned 'essential hypertension' in that regard. There is also 'idiopathic pulmonary fibrosis', a chronic and usually fatal disease associated with the continuous decrease in lung function because of lung tissue scarring. That diagnosis is a description of the changes in lung tissue, not an explanation of the cause of those changes. 'Idiopathic' literally means 'a disease of its own kind', as if it caused itself. We just don't yet know the cause.

Essential hypertension is, despite its nebulous nature, a risk factor for other problems including heart attack and stroke and is sometimes a biomarker for kidney disease. It is also sometimes a signal that the patient's diet should be improved. Reducing weight and reducing salt intake help many people with essential hypertension reduce their blood pressure. But they don't help all.

Another good example of a descriptive 'diagnosis' is 'epistaxis'. It is just a fancy way of saying 'nosebleed'. The label itself does not suggest any of the possible causes of a nosebleed. Again, it is really a symptom – like 'sweating' but scarier. Interventions for nosebleed include treating an underlying clotting problem or a nasal tumor. It may also be that merely applying pressure or moisturizing ointments corrects it. Knowing (diagnosing) the actual cause would help in selecting the most appropriate of these interventions. Restating nosebleed as 'epistaxis', as if epistaxis is a diagnosis, does not help in finding an addressable cause. However, when someone has a severe nosebleed it is important to implement urgent solutions, including pressure to the nose or packing the nose with gauze, to solve the immediate problem.

The use of descriptive 'diagnoses' is, unfortunately, endemic in Medicine. Perhaps it provides comfort to physicians (and patients, possibly), giving them the feeling that they know something, when they don't and no one else does, either. However, sometimes a descriptive label can be camouflage or a distraction, resulting in the physician's abandoning the pursuit of the real cause. The doctor has arrived at an effect, not a cause, and treats this effect. This is called 'symptomatic treatment' and is sometimes all that the doctor can do.

Health services administrators, health informaticians, doctors and patients should critically review diagnostic labels, in order to identify ones that aren't truly informative. This can be a focus for research, correcting the situations where treatments are not tackling definitive causes, but are only addressing a placeholder or best guess as to what is going on.

FIGURE 1.21.1 lists the different types of diagnosis. The only valid diagnosis is the first one!

Types of Diagnosis Related to Our Understanding and Meaning of the Condition

TYPE OF DIAGNOSIS	EXAMPLE
Diagnoses implying underlying cause	*Hypothyroidism*
Descriptive Diagnoses	*Depression (really is a symptom)*
	Idiopathic Pulmonary Fibrosis (really is a sign)
	Essential Hypertension
	Hypercholesterolemia (is a symptom + risk factor)
Relabeling the problem as diagnosis	*Anxiety*
	Epistaxis - nosebleed

For most descriptive diagnoses, including depression and idiopathic pulmonary fibrosis, researchers are working actively to find the reasons for the problem. While they speculate on the reasons, they might suggest a variety of empirical solutions aimed at relieving the problem.

FIGURE 1.21.1 An Important Descriptive 'Diagnosis': Depression

Many people suffer episodically or chronically from feeling depressed. It is a prevalent symptom and can be debilitating. Being depressed or 'having depression' is how we describe someone who feels lethargic, fatigued, unmotivated and less energetic. There are, however, many possible causes of lethargy and depressed feelings, including hormone problems, cancers, cardiac and respiratory diseases, lack of sleep, infections, cancer, obesity and deconditioning and drug side effects. Treatments should be specific to the actual cause of the problem.

Regretfully, clinicians, health administrators and the public do not always distinguish their hypothesis regarding what is causing a problem from what the actual cause is. The effect and long-term value of an encounter with the health system for the patient only accrues from the positive identification of the actual cause. The only way that a diagnosis of 'depression' can be a valid diagnosis is if medical science can cite an objective cause (indicated by a biomarker of some kind). This biomarker could be, for instance, having a certain genetic make-up – researchers have sought this, but they have found nothing definitive yet. Another biomarker could be an indicative blood chemistry profile – ditto. Perhaps, maybe a specific brain electrical signal or MRI finding – ditto. Severe Depression may have been associated with blood chemistry changes but even these are not definitive. There just are no known biomarkers of depression, at least as of now.

In the absence of a biomarker associated with feelings of depression, we do not know the underlying physical causes of depressed feelings. The distinction between hypotheses and actual causes is not merely academic because how people think about a problem determines or at least influences their treatment recommendations and which treatments patients find acceptable. When physicians use the descriptor 'depression', it is as if it were a disease and a meaningful explanation for why we have certain feelings. Given that, physicians are more likely to inappropriately recommend antidepressant medication as a treatment to correct the cause rather than safer and more effective interventions like diet, exercise and lifestyle change.[100]

It would be nice if each of our problems had only a few possible causes or possible treatments, but most abnormal signs, symptoms or abnormal lab results have many possible causes. The challenge is to learn the specific and meaningful diagnosis that applies to each patient. In order to make a correct diagnosis, it is necessary to understand the nature and frequency of illnesses, to know and use structured approaches to identify both common and uncommon conditions, and to recognize which patient characteristics should prompt aggressive investigations that help determine a diagnosis that avoids serious harm.

A useful way to categorize diagnoses and their importance is to consider their frequency, urgency, and importance to life, comfort and function. The following table (FIGURE 1.21.2) lists several common and rare problems according to their severity.

	Urgent	**Non-Urgent**	**Serious**	**Less Serious**
Rare	Autoimmune Encephalitis[101]	Kikuchi's Disease[102]	Intermittent Porphyria[103]	Alopecia Areata[104]
Common	Pulmonary Embolus[105]	Viral Upper Respiratory Infection	Various Cancers	Contact Dermatitis

FIGURE 1.21.2: Different diagnoses, their urgency and frequency

100 Street vendors and the public know that drugs change thoughts, feelings and behavior in people who do not have a medical condition. When people feel tired for medical reasons, such as hypothyroidism, then drugs are the appropriate answer. When the cause is unknown, safer interventions are more appropriate as a first choice.

101 https://www.nytimes.com/2019/06/19/magazine/low-blood-pressure-seizures-diagnosis.html. Accessed Sept 13, 2023. A rare condition causing decreased blood pressure and mental problems. Delayed diagnosis could lead to death.

102 https://rarediseases.org/rare-diseases/kikuchis-disease/. Accessed July 19, 2022.
Kikuchi's disease is a rare condition that is self limited but presents with signs and symptoms compatible with more serious illnesses. The signs and symptoms include enlarged glands, mild fever, muscle pain, night sweats and joint pain. The problems usually resolve spontaneously but patients are at risk of the symptoms being misinterpreted as something more sinister and receiving possibly harmful treatments for the wrong condition.

103 https://rarediseases.org/rare-diseases/porphyria/. Accessed July 19, 2022.
Porphyria is a condition related to abnormalities in how the red bloods cells metabolize heme, a substance essential for the transport of oxygen in the blood. The condition can affect the skin and also present with symptoms of severe abdominal discomfort. People who suffer from delayed diagnosis of this condition sometimes face additional suffering because they have unnecessary exploratory abdominal surgery or receive psychiatric drugs that might worsen the condition.

104 Hair loss in a particular area of the scalp, thought to be related to an autoimmune response, sometimes regresses spontaneously and is not usually associated with other life-threatening or life-limiting conditions.

105 Pulmonary embolus is a common condition, important because delayed treatment can lead to death. Sometimes the symptoms of pulmonary embolus are mistaken for other conditions, including bronchitis and pneumonia. One third of patients with a pulmonary embolus who went to emergency departments received a misdiagnosis. H. Torres-Macho, Juan, et al. Clinical features of patients inappropriately undiagnosed of pulmonary embolism
The American Journal of Emergency Medicine, Volume 31, Issue 12, 1646 – 1650.

Why Physician Imposters are Successful

It might be illuminating to consider why people who fake being physicians seem to get away with it, sometimes for decades.[106] Physician imposters are often successful because they face problems and make choices that are usual and common. Basic doctoring is not rocket science – or even rocket engineering! Some imposters succeed because they just know to exhibit 'doctor-behavior' and how and where to look for the solutions to medical problems or when to defer to others.

ROCKET SCIENCE

Many years ago, a cartoon appeared in the 'Pepper and Salt' series in the Wall Street Journal. It showed two scientists in front of a door labelled "NASA". One scientist said to the other: "You know, this IS rocket science." Though it is really rocket engineering! Regretfully, we could not find the cartoon itself again.

Often, it is not even necessary to make a diagnosis. Acting the role that a patient expects is not difficult, nor is asking questions, making appropriate (grunting) sounds and comments, listening and doing a basic examination. What is important is that the imposter physician recognizes (and the patient accepts) when the body itself will solve a problem, without or despite an intervention. It may not even be necessary for the imposter to order esoteric tests. Sparing patients unnecessary tests and treatments may even be a good thing. The treatments, too, can be minimal, as unnecessary treatments place people at risk of adverse, unexpected and unnecessary complications. Actors on TV have mastered the basics and even a third-rate actor can get away with a lot.[107]

Many Medical Problems are Transient and Self-Resolve

From what we have touched on so far, the reader realizes now that many problems are transient and fade away on their own, even if no one ever finds an exact or satisfactory explanation. The imposter only needs to master the 'form' of the medical encounter and apply the minimum of the 'substance' of diagnosis and care. The mind and body of the patient can often take care of the rest. Of course, sooner or later, a real patient will need a real physician to find real cause for real problems and get a real treatment…or the patient may end up real dead!

Everyone Can Contribute to the Diagnostic Process

We are surely not advocating for the reader to become an imposter physician.

We believe that the tools of the future will make what we are advocating easier and more likely to succeed. As Health Informatics and information systems become more sophisticated, both doctors and patients will better understand the likelihood that a patient has a disease and will recover spontaneously and how to help those who won't. Predictive models already help Amazon forecast shopping behaviors and how best to influence them. Similar technology in the medical future will not only help patients to discern what is wrong with them, it should also help them learn which diseases they are likely to develop. Information like that may motivate everyone to engage in the behaviors that are most likely to prevent or at least delay problems.

These predictive models have the potential of working because the interpretation of the significance of a person's signs and symptoms depends on the individual's context. Context is

106 https://en.wikipedia.org/wiki/Frank_Abagnale. Accessed August 30, 2022.

107 https://en.wikipedia.org/wiki/Catch_Me_If_You_Can_(book), https://www.imdb.com/title/tt0264464/ (movie), Catch Me If You Can, F. Abagnale, 1980. Accessed August 30, 2022.

where you live, who you work and play with, what your genetic background is, your diet and exercise, what you are exposed to and the diseases that occur in your community. Context rules. When means exist to capture and analyze people's characteristics, predicting the future won't require seers, at least when it comes to medical diagnosis.

In this Section we have tried to give the reader some idea of the many diagnoses and conditions that may be responsible for treatable and preventable human suffering. Few normal human beings can remember all of them. However, anyone can review and use the lists of causes (See Appendix X) that various academics have created to help us determine the origin of medical problems.

VOLUME 1

Section 4

MEASURING HEALTH

PROGNOSIS

Patients often ask physicians how long they will live. At best the physician can provide a general estimate and it can be very wrong. This is called a 'prognosis'.

Here is an interaction with an imaginary patient:

Doctor: I have some bad news and some very bad news.

Patient: Well, might as well give me the bad news first.

Doctor: The lab called with your test results. They said you have 24 hours to live.

Patient: 24 HOURS! That's terrible!! WHAT could be WORSE? What's the very bad news?

Doctor: I've been trying to reach you since yesterday.

Source: http://www.jokes4us.com/medicaljokes/adoctorandapatientjoke.html. Accessed August 30, 2022.

A Story: Measurement and Ageism

Health workers are often accused of ageism, prejudice and discrimination against people based on their age. Some people are ageist, most aren't. Ageism cuts both ways, though, as the elderly are different... they are older and their remaining expected life before them is shorter than that of a youth! Sometimes, clinicians act against their older patients' best interests in order to show that they treat young and old people the same way. Another form of ageism is when people are treated based on their age alone, not on their needs – for example not providing appropriate care for a patient with a potentially (but not necessarily) fatal disease. Mary's experience was informative.

Mary, a 91-year-old youthful woman, drove to her family doctor's office and asked for a checkup. The doctor learned that Mary lived on her own, cared for herself, and occasionally had her great grandchild stay overnight with her. She was concerned she might be at risk of becoming sick and because she so enjoyed her life, she wanted to do whatever was necessary to maintain her health. The doctor, perhaps overly and harmfully conscientious, reviewed her bodily systems, and did a complete exam including her blood pressure and a urinalysis. He was surprised that her urinalysis showed microscopic hematuria – signs of a small amount of blood in her urine – and ordered further investigations. He found that she had a small cancer in her left kidney and sent her to a urologist (a doctor specializing in kidney and renal system surgery). Not being ageist, and not being sensitive or sensible, he surgically removed her left kidney. Five days later, despite technically excellent surgery, she died in hospital leaving her car in the parking lot. An autopsy did not reveal the cause of death.

The purpose of health care is to produce measurable improvements in comfort, function and lifespan. Mary, at age 91, had a life expectancy of about 4 additional years. She had normal function and comfort. Surgery for a hidden tumor was unlikely to increase her expected lifepan but would definitely lead to at least short-term postsurgical reductions in comfort and function. In this case, the ageism was to treat her like a young person, who might have a more resilient body and could expect to benefit more. The lesson is that it is important to assess the likelihood of measurable benefits and harms before undertaking aggressive testing or interventions. Perhaps learning about Dr. Max would drive this home.

Dr. Max, an excellent respirologist at a local hospital, quit and went to practice in another country. He was upset because administrators claimed that his patients with pneumonia were kept in hospital longer than necessary. The administrators criticized him because they found that Dr. Max's patients with pneumonia were in hospital on average longer than patients in other seemingly comparable hospitals. Well, no wonder! Because his colleagues regarded Dr. Max as exceptional, they sent him their most difficult patients, ones who were sicker and had less chance of survival. The problem arose because the administrators' data base considered all patients with pneumonia as if they were the same. Oddly, we all know people who have had pneumonia, were treated with antibiotics as an outpatient and had no need of a hospital stay. Many know people who were admitted to hospital with pneumonia for a short time, as well as people admitted for lengthier stays because their condition was more critical. Without adjusting for patient health, including their comfort, function and test results showing overall biochemical abnormalities (including low oxygen levels, high or low pulse rates and lung capacity), it is impossible to predict how long a patient might be in hospital or the expected outcome of their treatment. Comparing length of stay performance and health outcomes per physician, without adjusting for how sick the patients were before and after treatment leads to erroneous and disputed conclusions.

Chapter 22: ——— Introduction

KEYWORDS: Measurement, Use of Metrics, Gauges, Why Measure, Uses of Measures, Feedback Loops, Measures in Clinical Offices, Comfort, Function, Disease Severity, Predicting Lifespan, Health Status

ABSTRACT: Measurement is essential in health care and in everyday life. Clinicians capture objective information from clinical examinations and the results of laboratory tests and imaging studies. Measures include an estimate of comfort, assessments of function and the results of investigations. Together all these measures provide information about health status. Clinicians and researchers use this information to estimate health before and after care and to learn about the effectiveness of their interventions.

Measurement is a human process. Every day, humans measure, formally and informally, many characteristics of nature and aspects of their lives. Measuring goes back to human prehistory. Some will remember the ancient story of Noah whose measurements for the Ark were stated in 'cubits' (about 1.5 feet). Twenty-three centuries ago, the Greek philosopher Eratosthenes used some simple geometry to estimate the size of the Earth and got a circumference (in 'stadia', the definition of which we are somewhat uncertain) quite close to modern measurements. In fact, it seems more unusual when we do not measure than when we do!

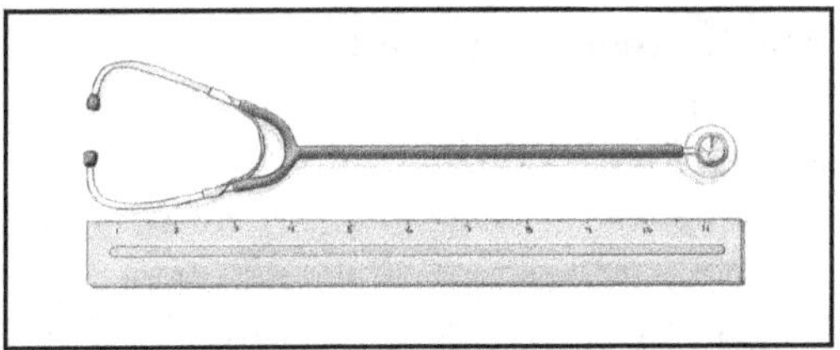

FIGURE 1.22.1: We need objective metrics

We measure things in our daily lives for many reasons.[108] Sometimes, we want to find out how big, heavy, fast, distant, valuable or efficient a thing or process is. Other times, we want to find out if things can fit together. It can also be that we want to discover if one thing is the same as, better, more valuable, or perhaps longer lasting or more powerful than another. An important reason for measuring related to health is to determine if something is happening that affects health, or if what we are doing about health improves it. We try to learn if people or groups of people are healthy or are sick and we want to determine how many, how much and why. When we then decide on treatments, we need to know if they lead to improved health and to what degree. We may also wish to learn if being close to a source of pollution, for example living near or working in a coal mine, impacts health.

In the case of health care, measurement and judgment are essential. Some estimates of health comfort, function and illness severity are informal but are used to evaluate performance, as alternatives do not exist. However,

108 https://mtiinstruments.com/knowledge-center/history-of-measurements/. Accessed July 19, 2022.

this isn't only true of health care; it's true of other service industries.[109] There is continuing research into formalizing and making assessment more objective. However, at least in the case of the assessment of comfort, subjectivity and human perception likely will limit achievements in that direction.

An oft-repeated management slogan explains why measurement is important to any process: "if you don't measure, you cannot manage". Management is precarious without measurement![110] It should be clear that we also must have measurements that are formal, stable and objective, as FIGURE 1.22.1 illustrates. This because both formal and informal measurements provide signals that encourage and enable participants to change their behavior or strategy when things are not going well and to continue on course when they are.

What We Measure

The kinds of things it is essential to measure and to make judgments about in health care include the following:

1. **The health of patients:** if we do not know how sick or well a patient is before, during and after a care process, we can have no idea of the quality or value of that process. Without formal and informal assessments of an individual's health, it is not possible to know whether to begin treatment, provide reassurance or alter an existing treatment plan.
2. **The function of the care system:** our healthcare system costs real money and lots of it. We need to know the value it delivers in improving the health of patients. Value in health care means that we all derive benefit and not harm from medical interventions. If the system does not work the way we want, we need to fix it so that it does. Health care is often the single largest expenditure of society and by individual patients.
3. **The performance of care providers:** within the healthcare system, many different professionals perform activities that are supposed to improve the health of patients. We need to know if these professionals add value, how much they add and if they improve health.
4. **The quality of the overall management of the care system by government or government-level agencies and its results:** here we look at the total system of systems and measure its performance and make judgments regarding whether or not it satisfies our expectations given what we pay for it directly or through our taxes.

Any entity that is not measured is essentially an unknown. We don't know what it does. We don't know if it delivers anything of value. We don't know if it wastes resources or helps or harms us. We don't know anything! Worse still, we may feel it is worthwhile when it is not. Measuring something recognizes we place value on that thing. Measurement is a proof of how important something is to us. The lack of measurement is proof that we don't care that something is just kind of there, that something isn't really necessary, or maybe that we don't want others to know. Furthermore, measurement enables us to enhance the

109 National Academies Science, Engineering, Math, Technology in Services: Policies for Trade, Growth and Employment, 1988 https://www.nap.edu/read/764/chapter/9. Accessed July 19, 2022.

110 For some, this statement is controversial. At a simple level, we all manage many activities without formal measurements. For example, parents don't generally do formal measures to learn if their children like or dislike foods. On the other hand, they pay attention to school report cards that provide some measures of a child's progress in learning. When dealing with larger groups, or when managing an individual's health, formal and informal measurement is essential to determine what to do. This section elaborates on the hows and whys of measurement in clinical care and health system management.

value of something or to decide to toss it into the dustbin.

As individual human beings, we are constantly measuring ourselves and the aspects of the reality in which we live. We sense and evaluate our feelings, make judgements about our weight, notice if our vision is sharp or fuzzy, take our temperature, see how much exercise we get (e.g., by counting steps), count our calories and perform many other measures. Based on these measures, we make assessments of ourselves. Similarly, we want the health system to be the vital, adaptive, useful, productive and worthwhile system it must be to keep us healthy or overcome sickness. To ensure that, we must measure it in all its aspects, all the time and make constant judgments and adjustments based on real knowledge of what it is doing. Without that, we lose our health system as a supporter of our lives.

Our Gauges

To measure something, we need some kind of a gauge or ruler. The fancy term for a 'ruler' is a 'metric.' A lot of things we measure in our daily lives use imprecise measurement tools. For instance, we may measure how far we walk by counting how many strides we take (a stride being perhaps a meter or 3 feet), or we give a guesstimate of how far away something is by noticing the height of a person in the distance. Let's call these things 'rubber rulers', meaning that they are affected by perception and even bias.

To measure health and health care, we need objective and reproducible measures. To be able to make long-term or inter-entity comparisons, these metrics must be reasonably firm and certainly repeatable by other people at different times.

There is the key challenge. We want to measure something like human health, something that is often subjective, by using a stable and repeatable metric. Many researchers have labored decades designing metrics that are at least approximations to stable measurement tools that produce repeatable results. Perhaps some have heard of 'pain scores,' which involve asking a patient to indicate the level of pain on a scale from 0 to 10. Another example is a 'satisfaction score' that asks patients to indicate how pleased they are with their care or other service. Metrics like these are imprecise and manipulation is possible by people with specific interests; they just give us an idea of what people feel. However, they are useful and may be the only way to get somewhat objective and reliable assessments.

INCREASING SATISFACTION

One administrator told DZ that the best way to increase satisfaction is to reduce expectations. Patients who have been told their respiratory infection might kill them are relieved even if they have a reaction to the unnecessary antibiotic.

There is a constant struggle to evolve metrics that provide repeatable, comparable, semi-quantitative or quantitative assessments of many aspects of the health system and of human health.

We will delve into the value that measuring health can have and provide some examples of what and how to measure.

Chapter 23: Bringing Measurement to Health

KEYWORDS: Objective Measures, Measuring Health, Measuring Health System Function, Evaluating Clinical Performance, Evaluating Health System Management, Feedback Loops, Informed Consent, Cost of Care, Importance of Accurate Measurement

ABSTRACT: Clinicians capture information about patient health. This information has many uses, including making diagnoses, predicting remaining life expectancy, supporting informed consent and estimating the quality of health care.

MEASURING HEALTH: IMPORTANT IDEAS

1. **Importance of accurate measurement:**
    a. Measuring Comfort.
    b. Measuring Function.
    c. Laboratory Investigations.
    d. Images.
    e. Predicting Life expectancy- in biomarker booklet.
2. **Health measures used for clinical purposes:**
    a. Predicting lifespan.
    b. Predict likelihood of treatment success or failure.
    c. Identify and modify patient risk factors.
    d. Support informed consent-treatment choices.
    e. Support end of life decisions – goals of care – young and old.
3. **Health measures used for administrative purposes:**
    a. Report benefits and harms of care.
    b. Assess costs of care.
    c. Sick people cost more than healthier ones.
4. **Health measures used for quality assessment:**
    a. Outcomes by severity level.
    b. Compare organizations one with another- Identify organizations or clinicians that have superb severity adjusted outcomes.
5. **Health measures used to assess government interventions on individual and community health markers.**

A TERMINOLOGY ASIDE

We have two words that express the general effects of processes: 'efficiency' and 'productivity'. Some have understood 'productivity' to be an expression of only the volume of things or services we produce. Similarly, some have understood 'efficiency' to just mean how quickly or cheaply something can be made or done. Regarding the words 'efficiency' and 'productivity', work on Economics applied to health care incorporates the assessment of the quality of what is produced into those definitions and relates costs to the benefits of what is produced.[111] *Most scientific and econometric work considers efficiency to be the cost for a benefit. Cost can be measured in financial terms or the hours of labor and consumables it takes to produce a result. The result in health care normally is the magnitude of the improvement in health. However, some administrators measure the number of events of care, not the health outcomes. They ignore the quality of the product.*

In earlier work with several economists, DC became convinced that there was still ambiguity in the terms and that there was the need for a term that explicitly expressed both these concepts. Therefore, we coined the term 'comprehensive productivity' in an article on the effects of information technology on health care.[112] *In healthcare research, however, many use the term 'efficiency' to cover both concepts, Therefore, we will use 'efficiency' herein despite the terminological ambiguity. In health care, people are buying changes in their health produced by their care. In Public Health, the measures are improvements in the overall health of the population as measured by decreases in illnesses, improvements in happiness (comfort) and increases in function.*

Why Measure Health?

As we mentioned in the last chapter, there are several areas that require constant assessment to ensure that we have an effective healthcare system.

Measuring health and changes in health is essential to learn about and understand the efficiency (cost for a benefit, which includes human outcomes) of healthcare activities. It is relatively easy to assess costs because individuals, governments, insurance companies and others paying for health care know how much money they spend on healthcare processes, how many workers are employed, and how much they spend on equipment, drugs and supplies. However, few have essential knowledge about how many people get better – or do worse – as a result of healthcare spending. Unless organizations measure health benefits, it will not be possible to learn which healthcare activities are helpful, harmful or merely superfluous. Most organizations, including government, would prefer to spend only on helpful activities, not ones that are harmful or wasteful.

Measuring the fate of patients, that is, are they better or worse after care, is essential for managing the care system. How sick are patients when they enter the system? How well are those patients when they leave the system? Is patient comfort enhanced by the care the system affords? How many people are healthier or worse off? How many survive care? We are asking here if the system is effective, a necessary measure to include in the estimation of efficiency. A factory can produce tons of widgets per hour, but are they usable widgets that suit their purpose? The healthcare system is supposed to produce healthier people. Does it?

We also need to look at the effectiveness of individual care providers to determine which kinds of and how many care providers of each type we need, what their competencies should be, how well they perform in improving patients' lives and what they do (like sending patients for tests or treating them) that is worthwhile, wasteful or harmful.

111 Palmer S, Torgerson D J. Definitions of efficiency BMJ 1999; 318 :1136. https://www.bmj.com/content/318/7191/1136. Accessed July 19, 2022.

112 Bodell, R, Covvey, H.D., et al. Achieving a "Therapeutic Dose" of IT Medinfo, 2004. https://www.academia.edu/9204936/Achieving_a_Therapeutic_Dose_of_IT. Accessed July 19, 2022.

So, there is a lot to measure! It is interesting that the healthcare system must do these measurements at the individual level (like for patients and doctors). It must also do them at the system level, such as in each area, at each institution or even in each department within an institution. And it must do them at the population level – the overall effect of health care on the population of an entire city, region, province/state or country.

In a greatly simplified way, one can think of measuring health care at each level being like observing and managing a boiler for generating steam. Without knowledge of the temperature and the pressure of the boiler, we have no idea if it is producing the desired amount of steam, doing so efficiently and doing so without danger of blowing itself apart. In the healthcare system, 'blowing itself apart' is where the expense becomes too great for a city or a region or even a whole society, where enough care isn't produced to address peoples' needs or where the system injures people, like an exploding boiler can do. The current controversy about health spending and controversies related to apparent shortages of specific types of healthcare professionals cannot be resolved unless we know something about the benefits to expect from each health professional and what communities need.

Why It's Important to Measure Changes in Health Associated with Care

To measure health care and its impacts, we need data. However, we need to realize that the care process routinely produces vast amounts of data that can be used to do measurements. This is both a blessing and a curse.

Clinicians capture, use and produce clinical data to support their care of patients and to communicate with others caring for the same patient. Health systems, using appropriate tools, can exploit this same data to measure their services (the effects of health services care and administration) and educate themselves and staff about what they are doing. The data clinicians[113] capture at each visit includes patient reports of comfort, lists of symptoms, assessments of overall wellness, the functioning of individual limbs and organs, the results of laboratory and imaging investigations, diagnoses and the treatments physicians apply.

Fortunately for patients, clinicians usually try to collect at least the type and amount of information necessary to solve or alleviate a patient's problems. Unfortunately for researchers and administrators, there is no real standard indicating how much information of what types a clinician must collect. Some clinicians collect and record lots of information, while others produce relatively sparse health records. The challenge is to develop useful methods to collect and use whatever information clinicians put in the record, including information about the patient's overall health.

Health informaticians are the experts who develop and foster the use of information systems that capture and provide this clinical information to support patient care, health services administration, research and provider and patient education.

Clinical information systems fielded by Health Informatics experts can capture and provide information indicating if care interventions do what they are supposed to do. A later chapter discusses how to evaluate and report the benefits and harms of treatment. The best information systems also help clinicians to identify people at risk of illness and help them plan and implement preventive interventions. This enables care providers to stave off or at least delay preventable illness.

Then there is the issue of how much money we devote to providing care. It is possible but somewhat challenging to measure how much we spend and what its effects are. Such

113 We use the term clinicians to mean anyone on the clinical team including nurses, physiotherapists, occupational therapists, social workers, psychologists, pharmacists and medical doctors.

information is necessary to evaluate the effectiveness (what we have termed 'efficiency': the benefits achieved and the speed and cost of a process) of care. North Americans believe they spend too much for healthcare. Data indicates that the U.S. spends more than any other country in the world on health care, twice as much as the average and about 50% more than Canada. However, there is no answer as yet to the question: is this too much and do Americans get their money's worth?

Consider, for instance, that Canadians spend on average over $5,600 per person per year for health care. This includes health insurance, pharmaceuticals, various aides and out-of-pocket costs. This means that a family of 4 has a health insurance cost of about $22,000 per year paid through taxes. We must face the reality that over 40% (!) of Provincial government spending is on health care. According to the Canadian Institute for Health Information, Canadian Provinces, in fact, spend more on health care than on any other government program! Americans, on the other hand, spend about $7,500 per person per year or about $30,000 for a family of 4.[114] With these significant costs in mind, it is essential that we evaluate whether or not the money is well-spent, meaning that it delivers the benefits we expect.

After all, we need to determine at least if certain tests and treatments are irrelevant or harmful. If they are, neither individuals nor governments nor insurers should pay for them.

To really understand the problem, we must recognize that how we support health care is somewhat disconcerting. For example, payers – individuals, private insurance companies and government insurers – compensate doctors and health organizations for their services. In the past, American payers reimbursed hospitals based on what the hospitals reported as the cost of the services they delivered. In Canada, hospitals were paid (and most still are) based on their ability to negotiate with government and associated hospital charities.[115] This means that the payers rewarded doctors and hospitals based on the invoices they submitted for services they provided, rather than for what they actually did and the health results they produced. That's like paying a plumber who shows up for work and usually, but not always, repairs the leak and sometimes causes a flood!

One reason that insurers, both public and private, do not pay for results is that many health services administrators do not know how to measure health and the changes associated with care. Or perhaps they do not want to; they may perceive that there is no incentive to do so! Consequently, systematic assessment is impossible. Unfortunately, those who know how to measure health rarely bother to collect clinical data in a systematic way that would enable them to aggregate the results of many patients and learn what works and what doesn't. Often, clinical groups are able to secure resources without collecting and showing information about the benefits or harms they produce. Allocating resources would be more rational if clinicians and clinical organizations provided funders with meaningful information about what they deliver. See the text box for an example.

114 https://www.brookings.edu/articles/with-health-care-costs-the-u-s-is-a-huge-outlier/. Brookings Institute. August 7, 2012. Accessed Sept 8, 2023.

115 Most Canadian health organizations have associated foundations that raise money over and above what government will provide. One consequence is that richer communities can support a wider range of services, and more modern equipment.

RESOURCE MANAGEMENT

DZ was an active clinician and chair of a hospital utilization committee. The head of the Psychiatry department complained about the lengthy wait times and asked for additional resources. Additionally, the departmental secretary complained that the waits were so long that when she called a patient after several months and offered an appointment, the prospective patients claimed to have forgotten that their family doctor had made a referral and they did not remember the problem they had. When the committee asked the psychiatrist for information about the consequences, harms and benefits, of extended waits no answer was forthcoming.

On the other hand, the Cardiology and Cardiac Surgery departments also complained and reported that resource shortages meant that patients suffered because they waited too long. The cardiologists and cardiac surgeons were able to obtain additional resources because they had tracked the fate of people who waited and knew the characteristics of people most likely to be harmed by waiting. They linked the characteristics of patients, waiting times and outcomes to show that additional resources would be clinically beneficial and also be cost beneficial by reducing hospitalizations during the waiting periods.

Recent research confirms this observation.[116]

There are many measures of care and of health. A representative catalogue of health measures is available in the interesting book "*Measuring Health: A guide to Rating Scales and Questionnaires*" by *Ian McDowell and Claire Newell.*[117] The material includes disease-specific and overall measures of comfort, function and feelings of well-being. Doctors and patients use measures of comfort and function along with the results of laboratory investigations to decide on how best to intervene. Administrators and clinicians can use health measures to assess their costs and compare their clinical outcomes with other organizations. Doing this, they can learn if one organization achieves substantially better results than others. Identifying organizations achieving outstanding results, encourages inferior performers to emulate the clinical and administrative practices of superior performing institutions.

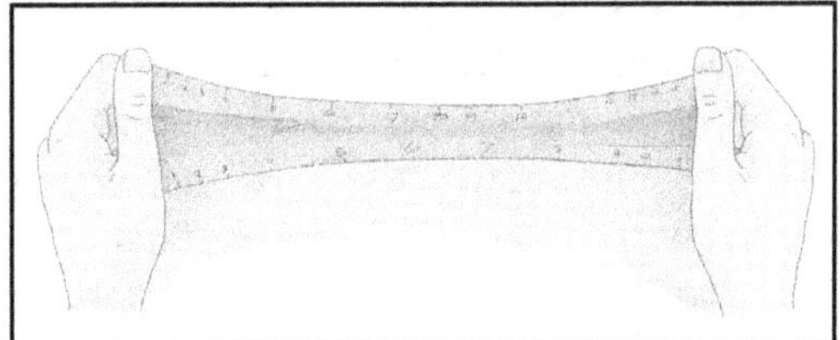

FIGURE 1.23.1: An unstable metric

Why It's Important to Measure Accurately

To understand the issue of accuracy related to measurement, it is useful to look at an example. Blood pressure (BP) is one factor that enters into predictions of health and life expectancy, augmented by other measures including pulse rate, waist circumference and walking speed.

FALLING FOR A DRUG

At a recent dinner, DZ met a woman who mentioned that her doctor had prescribed blood pressure medication because her blood pressure was "slightly elevated". The visit with the doctor was brief. Later she suffered an inconvenient side effect (frequent urination) of the blood pressure medication (a diuretic – often called a 'water pill') the doctor had prescribed. To address that problem, her doctor prescribed another blood pressure medicine. Regretfully, that medication led to an even more serious complication (a fall) caused by low blood pressure. (A later chapter discusses how to evaluate treatment suggestions.)

116 Ray, A.A., Buth, K.J., Sullivan, J.A.., et.al., Waiting for Cardiac Surgery Results of a Risk-Stratified Queuing Process, September 2001 Circulation 104(12 Suppl 1): I92-8 DOI: 10.1161/hc37t1.094904. https://www.ahajournals.org/doi/full/10.1161/circ.104.suppl_1.i-92. *Accessed July 19, 2022.*

117 http://www.a4ebm.org/sites/default/files/Measuring%20Health.pdf. Accessed July 19, 2022.

McDowell, I., Newell, C., MEASURING HEALTH: A Guide to Ratings and Questionnaires, New York, Oxford Press, 2006.

Now, thinking about blood pressure measurements, recognize that medical experts all agree that accurate blood pressure assessment requires more than one reading and that this should be done under certain conditions, like a rest of five minutes. They suggest this because the first blood pressure reading is often artificially high. Most experts recommend getting three readings at every visit because the first one or two are likely to be artificially high. This phenomenon is known as "white coat hypertension." What's more, a white coat is not even necessary! FIGURE 1.23.1 indicates that an unstable metric does not help much either. On the other hand, there are stable ones as shown in FIGURE 1.23.2.

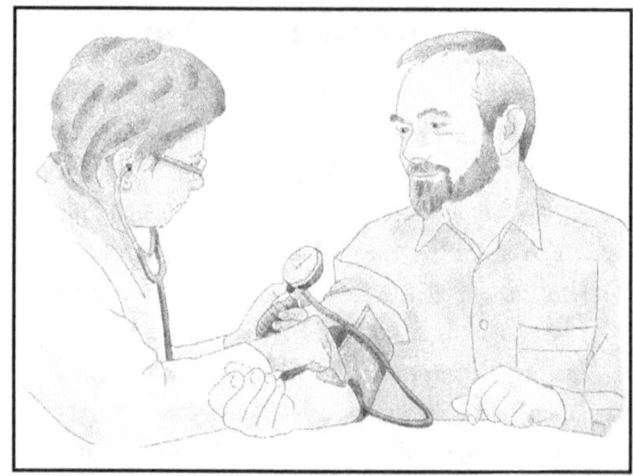

FIGURE 1.23.2: A sphygmomanometer used properly is a stable measuring device

A HIGH-PRESSURE GUY

DZ was at a drug store waiting for someone and decided to check his own blood pressure using the self-serve blood pressure machine. The first reading appeared to be dangerously high; the second was moderate. The third showed low normal blood pressure, a result more likely valid, as he was very fit at the time.

Patients might well try a BP machine when at a drug store or clinic. Many will be surprised to see how much higher their first blood pressure reading is compared to subsequent ones. Anxiety associated with the odd circumstance of having blood pressure measured may lead to a reading that is higher than usual. It is for this reason that experts suggest several blood pressure measurements on more than one occasion before considering blood pressure-lowering drugs.

Of course, the easiest thing to do is for patients to buy a battery-powered automatic blood pressure cuff and monitor their own blood pressures. Many cardiologists today expect this of their patients and ask them what their self-measured blood pressure has been. Many people being treated for hypertension may be surprised to find that they have normal blood pressure and that their blood pressure measured at home is lower than when measured in a pharmacy or a doctor's office.

There are problems with other measurements, too. For example, even supposedly objective laboratory results can vary for many reasons. Changes in diet, hydration, activity, moving from one lab to another and variations in the instrumentation used in the laboratory, all can have effects. Sometimes, different patients' results get mixed up. Human-to-human variation is also a factor. If one does a battery of 10 - 20 different tests on blood, it would not be unusual for one to give abnormal results due to simple statistical variation.

The accuracy of the results from the testing of specimens and the reliability of the reporting of laboratory test results challenge clinicians. In addition, there are the problems of ordering the appropriate tests, interpreting results properly and losing, confusing or misinterpreting test results.[118]

Looking at the latter point, every year in North America, people are harmed because an abnormal laboratory result was not reported. Misplaced or lost laboratory reports deprive clinicians of key information and, of course, cannot contribute to clinicians' estimates of a patients' health or support the clinicians' judgments of proper interventions. Patients cannot benefit if the doctor never finds out that the result was abnormal. Some patients, in communities where people do not have access to their own charts, will ask the doctor's staff if they should come in to review a lab result. Sometimes, staff reply "if no one called you the test is probably normal". Unfortunately, the absence of evidence that the test is abnormal, is not evidence that the test was normal. It could be that the result was lost or that the doctor and staff did not notice the abnormality. Consequently, patients should make sure they receive a thoughtful reply about the results of laboratory tests from someone who has seen the results. Better still, they should do that with the results in hand.

This book discusses test interpretation in a separate chapter. Our purpose here is to help people to be aware of false positive test results – those that are alarming but that do not really reflect an alarming event – and false negative test results – results that are reassuring when the patient really has a worrisome condition. However, we all must understand that people interpreting laboratory tests must first be certain that the laboratory reported accurate results.

SICK LAB RESULTS

DZ's clinical practice was very busy. One morning a patient presented with what appeared to be a seriously abnormal blood profile (unusual relative numbers of different types of cells). DZ requested further investigations to confirm and explore the reasons for the abnormal profile. Shortly afterward, another patient presented with the same abnormality. When a fifth patient arrived that day with the same abnormal results, DZ realized that, most likely, the lab was having a recurrent problem with the test and that the 5 abnormal results suggested a "sick" testing process and not sick patients. He called the lab and they confirmed the problems were with the lab testing processes and that there was not an epidemic of blood disorders in his practice.

118 Tarkan S, Plaisant C, Shneiderman B, Hettinger AZ. Reducing Missed Laboratory Results: Defining Temporal Responsibility, Generating User Interfaces for Test Process Tracking, and Retrospective Analyses to Identify Problems. AMIA Annual Symposium Proceedings. 2011; 2011:1382-1391. https://www.ncbi.nlm.nih.gov/pmc/articles/PMC3243200/. Accessed July 19, 2022.

Chapter 24: The Challenge of Measurement: How and What to Measure

KEYWORDS: Physical Characteristics, Clinical Signs, Function, Lab Tests, Social Characteristics

ABSTRACT: Evaluating health before and after treatment and predicting outcomes after treatments require measures of the health of the individual patient, laboratory investigations, imaging studies and the context of the person's life.

Introduction

The challenge for clinicians and everyone else, is knowing what to measure, how to measure that and how to respond to the measurements. Although physicians speak about the "complete history and physical" as part of the initial assessment of all patients it is not clear what anyone really means by "complete." Another chapter discusses the difficulties in knowing when any assessment is sufficient, especially since clinicians occasionally are trying to solve a problem caused by a known (at least to them) rare disease.

The first step in the journey, however, is to develop some understanding of how to assess each of the dimensions of health: comfort, function and estimations of survival.

Some things are relatively easy to measure. For example, we can easily measure someone's weight with a scale (although the accuracy of the scale, the presence or absence of clothes and so forth can be an issue). Height is also not a difficult measurement. However, many human characteristics are extremely difficult to measure. For example, getting a useful blood pressure, as we have shown, can be difficult and, certainly it is challenging to get a good and useful measurement of subjective parameters, like how one feels. It's worthwhile to look at some of the challenges. There are quite a few things in Medicine that can be reliably measures, as FIGURE 1.24.1 shows.

The kinds of things that we can measure objectively

- *Physical characteristics (size, weight, duration...)*
- *Clinical signs related to bodily location.*
- *Clinical signs related to function.*
- *Laboratory results, including medical image and signal characteristics.*
- *Some social characteristics.*

FIGURE 1.24.1: Things we can measure objectively

Estimating Symptoms and Feelings Including Pain

Most people have an overall impression of how they feel. They also know if they have aches, pains or other discomfort in parts of their bodies. Comfort measures are, however, necessarily subjective, that is, they are dependent on a person's self-reported perception and mostly are not measurable other than by asking and recording the patient's responses. Patients report how they feel. The reality is that their doctors cannot directly observe those feelings, except perhaps as they are reflected in the patients' demeanors, which can sometimes correlate with how they feel. Realize that some people are stoic – their external demeanor might not necessarily reflect the intensity of their pain, while others are more demonstrative and appear to be in distress when the pain stimulus or insult is minimal. None of us can get direct access to other people's perceptions of how they feel, though we might believe we can. Therefore, clinicians must sometimes accept, at face value, patient reports of how they feel and the intensity of pain.

The elements that contribute to semi-objective measures of comfort include:

1. Assessments of overall feelings of well-being.
2. Organ or site-specific evaluations, like the presence of a headache or a painful knee.
3. Appraisals of psychological well-being. Is an individual satisfied with his or her life? Is the person happy and content with relationships? Is the person copacetic about his or her financial and social state?

It is worth noting that all of these can be faked or dissembled about. Physicians who do insurance physicals use a variety of means to increase their certainty that what patients claim is valid. Insurance companies sometimes ask doctors if someone is 'really' having pain. Their premise is that if the doctor cannot identify the mechanism for the pain, then the patient must be lying. One danger of this approach is that some patients in serious pain will be undertreated. The doctor is not specially endowed with the power to read a person's mind or sense feelings.

Measures of comfort indicate patient's perceptions about themselves. It is in everyone's best interests, in most cases, if health providers assume that people, especially those looking for health advice, are telling the truth. But they must be cautious, as people sometimes display discomfort to obtain drugs, while others believe that showing discomfort implies weakness.

Generally speaking, effective treatment should improve overall comfort or at least trend in that direction. Medicine has not succeeded if a drug controls pain from an ankle sprain but produces moderate or severe abdominal pain and nausea or, even worse, bleeding in the stomach.

Most of us do not need formal scales to help us understand how we feel. However, health researchers and clinicians often want to find out if treatments or changes in lifestyle were worthwhile. To do that with some degree of consistency and assuredness, they use formal measures to assess changes in comfort associated with care.

Formal quizzes (using questionnaires that experts call 'instruments'), applied to document overall feelings of well-being or comfort, incorporate the types of questions most of us would expect. The questions, though, are very well-considered, carefully worded and tested to demonstrate that they are understood and will solicit reasonably consistent answers. For example: "Do you feel healthy enough to do the things you would like to do?"

Some instruments ask patients to rate on a numerical scale how they feel or how bad their pain is. Others ask about sleep and diet habits or ask focused questions about various organs or systems. For example: Do you feel sick at the stomach? Do you have a good appetite? (The chapter on mental health includes comments on evaluating emotions). Attempts to assess overall feelings of well-being or comfort generally have questions like: do you feel tired? Do you have any kind of pain?" Others ask about sleep habits, like how long do you usually sleep and how often do you wake up each night? The important thing to remember is that all measures of comfort or well-being ultimately rely on what the patient says.

Researchers are continually working to improve measurements of feelings. Interested readers can easily find several formal measurement tools.[119]

The key message here is that assessing the subjective perception of another in an objective way, like one might do with a scale, ruler or thermometer, is well-nigh impossible. Statements are always based on the patient's own, private, inaccessible feelings and depend on the patient's way of expressing them. We all know also that perceptions vary from person-to-person, perhaps the best example being the perception of pain. Many women claim that if they had a male's perception of pain, the human race would've ended a long time ago. We must recognize that all these instruments that assess subjective matters depend on the patient and sometimes on the interpretations of the physicians who apply them.

Measuring Objective Signs – Measures of Observable Patient Features Including Function

Signs are visible, tangible, audible and other observable attributes or characteristics detected during the physical examination of a patient. They include attributes of the skin that are visible to doctors, as well as measures like the range of motion of a joint that the doctor can observe and record without requiring laboratory tests. The knee reflex (tapping the knee causes the lower leg to move) is one example of a sign and blood pressure is another.

Psoriasis is a skin condition where skin cells grow more rapidly, causing skin cell build up on the skin surface. The objective signs of psoriasis include scales and red patches on the skin surface. Sometimes psoriasis is also associated with symptoms including itchiness and joint discomfort. Many people demonstrate signs of psoriasis, i.e., the skin lesions without any symptoms. Patients with very visible signs, like large psoriatic plaques, often desire treatment because of the cosmetic defect. They might also ask for treatment if they suffer from joint pain (psoriatic arthritis) even though the objective skin signs are not bothersome.

Measures of function are also objective; the physician can observe them, and they indicate what an individual can do. An external observer can easily tell if you can run a mile in seven minutes, the range of motion of your arms or legs, your visual acuity and how well you can remember a list of names or numbers.

Usually, we all have an idea of how well we function, and these personal assessments, usually, but not always, relate closely to objective measures.[120]

Measures of function include overall assessments represented by questions like:

1. Can you perform the normal activities of daily living?
2. Are you able to care for yourself or do you need help?

119 Pearson, E., Comfort and Its Measurement: A Literature Review, 2014 Disabil Rehabil Assist Technol. 2009 Sep; 4(5): 301-10. doi: 10.1080/17483100902980950. Pearson EJ. http://www.ncbi.nlm.nih.gov/pubmed/19565373. Accessed July 19, 2022.

120 Young Y, Boyd CM, Guralnik JM, Fried LP. Does self-reported function correspond to objective measures of functional impairment? J Am Med Dir Assoc. 2010 Nov;11(9):645-53. doi: 10.1016/j.jamda.2009.12.084. Epub 2010 Jul 1. https://pubmed.ncbi.nlm.nih.gov/21029999/. Accessed Sept 8, 2023.

3. Can you walk and how quickly up or down hill?
4. Can you climb stairs?
5. Can you feed yourself?

There may also be specific measures related to one or other body system, such as:

1. What is the range of motion of your knee? Of your elbow? Actual movement can be observed.
2. When the doctor taps the knee, is there a normal knee reflex?[121]
3. How long is the list of numbers you can remember for some time?

Measures of function include quantitative statements and physical measurements made by the clinician. Generally, even if the patient self-reports a certain level of function, the physician will check this, for instance, by moving the leg in a predetermined way.

Laboratory Investigations – Objective Measures of Patient Physiology

Physiology is the study of living things and biological processes. Laboratory tests measure the physiology of cells, organs and body systems. Lab test results contribute to estimates of a patient's current state of health and his or her life expectancy.

Objective clinical measures, such as laboratory investigations and medical images, produce objective diagnostic 'findings'. There are many sources of this type of information, including the analysis of bodily fluids (blood, mucous, saliva, sweat and urine), feces, tissue samples (biopsies) and medical images. The latter include x-rays, ultrasounds, computed tomographic imaging, nuclear medicine scans and many more esoteric imaging technologies (see below). We should also mention that it is possible to measure electrical signals produced by the heart (the electrocardiogram: ECG/EKG), brain (the electroencephalogram: EEG) and muscles (electromyogram: EMG). Lists of the full catalogue of laboratory tests and imaging studies are available in most medical textbooks and from the catalogues of medical laboratories.[122] Many things about the body, its organs and systems and its functions can be learned from these investigations. See, for example: https://www.amazon.com/DeGowins-Diagnostic-Examination-Tenth-Lange/dp/0071814477. Accessed July 19, 2022.

Physicians can make most diagnoses from their evaluation of patients' descriptions of they feel, how they function and their personal perceptions of overall health. Sometimes function alone provides a good estimate of the severity of illness. Someone who is bedridden and not able to speak is usually sicker and less likely to survive compared with someone who is active and coherent, regardless of the cause or diagnosis.

We all regularly make informal assessments of the health of colleagues, neighbors and even passersby. Sometimes we say, "He looks to be at death's door", meaning he looks very sick and might be dying. These informal assessments are often correct, but sometimes misleading. Many people are not able to make accurate predictions of even their own survival.[123]

Reliable estimates of survival encourage clinicians to pursue treatment options that are likely to be beneficial, while avoiding ones

121 Reflexes provide a measure of neurological function.

122 https://www.mayocliniclabs.com/test-catalog/. Accessed July 19, 2022.
Mayo Clinic Laboratories 3000+ tests and pathology services. Accessed August 29, 2019.

123 Romo RD, Lee SJ, Miao Y, Boscardin W, Smith AK. Subjective, Objective, and Observed Long-term Survival: A Longitudinal Cohort Study. JAMA Intern Med. 2015;175(12):1986-1988. https://archinte.jamanetwork.com/article.aspx?articleid=2463589. Accessed July 19, 2022.

that are more likely to produce even transient harm. Patients with a short life expectancy (for example, people over 90 and some cancer patients with multi-organ involvement) usually do not benefit from treatments designed to increase their life expectancy at the price of a time of decreased comfort and function.

Measures of comfort, function and the results of laboratory tests and imaging studies are all called 'biomarkers'. They refer to the existing, observable and potentially measurable characteristics of a person. They contribute to estimates of sickness and health including longevity. Other characteristics, including living and working environments, also contribute information that is useful.

Diagnostic Imaging

We mentioned imaging and a little detail may be informative. Diagnostic imaging is a major medical field dedicated to obtaining still or moving images of body structures beyond what we can see directly.

There are many kinds of diagnostic imaging technologies. Some are based on x-rays (high-energy light that can pierce the body and create shadow-like images). These include standard chest x-rays, Computed Tomographs (CT: the word literally means computer-generated pictures of horizontal slices through the body) that allow the reconstruction of three-dimensional images of internal organs, and several specialized x-ray technologies (such as those for breast imaging).

Images of internal organs can also be created using Magnetic Resonance Imaging (MRI), a technology that combines magnetic fields and radio technology to visualize bodily structures in 3-D. Another way of obtaining these images is through the use of radioactive nuclear isotopes and special cameras (gamma cameras) that can record images using gamma rays (another type of high energy light even more penetrating than x-rays) emitted by the radioactive isotopes.

X-rays and gamma rays damage cells in the body, as well as providing valuable images. Using sound to penetrate the body is far less dangerous. Ultrasound (high-frequency sound that is reflected by the acoustical differences between body structures; it's like sonar) can be used to image many parts of the body and has the advantage of not using high-energy (ionizing; it disturbs or removes the electrons in atoms), damaging radiation. MRI also has that characteristic; it doesn't damage cells. MRI and Ultrasound are particularly useful for imaging soft tissue (muscle and fat), which the higher-energy radiation (X-rays and gamma rays) simply passes through. The list goes on and on, including Positron Emission Tomography (PET), thermography (the use of infrared radiation – heat – to create images) and other highly esoteric systems.

The objective of imaging technology is to produce a picture of the internal body structures and/or their function that is normally invisible to the eye. These technologies allow the clinician to see and measure tumors or the state of organs, broken or damaged bones, injured muscles, collections of fluid, ruptured blood vessels and many other goings-on and their effects deep in the body.

The risk associated with producing diagnostic images is a consideration in making the decision to subject the patient to imaging. Unfortunately, in the case of x-ray and nuclear isotope studies, they can cause significant harm through radiation exposure and must be applied very carefully and conservatively. Imaging also engenders the same issues as are associated with the performance of other laboratory investigations. For example, technical staff might mislabel images with another patient's name, imaging reports could get lost (physically or in a computer system), or a Diagnostic Radiologist might misinterpret the images. In addition, the patient's physician or the office staff might fail to receive or may ignore or forget an imaging report showing a serious problem.

The quality of images is important. The technical abilities and perceptiveness of the imaging specialist (e.g., a Diagnostic Radiologist) or the patient's physician reading (interpreting) the reports, influences the quality of the eventual report or action taken based on it. Consequently, researchers in academia and industry are working to develop automated and computer-assisted systems to help in the interpretation of images. For example, Densitas[124], a software company based in Halifax, Nova Scotia, has developed a program that reads digital mammographic (breast) images and produces a reliable report on each patient's breast density, which can indicate or camouflage cancerous tumors. IBM and many other companies are also working on programs to interpret and report on other types of digital images.[125]

One other kind of imaging is performed using microscopic images of very thinly sliced tissues to detect cellular pathology. These images are challenging for pathologists to 'read' (determine normal versus abnormal cells and classify them). One reason is that there are so many cells requiring examination. As a consequence, computer-assistance has become very important.

A serious effect of all these different imaging technologies has been the creation of vast stores of digital images requiring significant computing, storage and communications facilities (these are called 'Picture Archiving and Communications Systems': PACS).

Computer-Assisted Test Result Interpretation

There is hope that automated or computer-assisted systems will eliminate the anxiety and worry that come from the misreading of medical images and other test results, including reducing the reporting of worrisome problems that the patient does not have (reducing false positives). Another hope is that computer-based systems will reduce the number of times that Diagnostic Imaging physicians miss an important finding. This hope is well-based. Decades ago, researchers produced systems for interpreting electrocardiograms (ECGs or EKGs: tracings of electrical signals generated by the heart). It took a while, but now these systems are embedded in electrocardiographic machines and used in virtually every emergency department and cardiologist's office. They have dramatically increased the reliability of electrocardiogram interpretation. Work is also underway on the automatic or computer-assisted interpretation of pathology images, such as those produced to detect early cancer (e.g., in the case of Pap Smears).

Treatment in health care relies on the capture and accurate reporting of information and its reliable interpretation. Making sure that clinical investigations, including both the subjectively reported history and the more objective physical and laboratory examinations, are accurate is vital. Other chapters discuss important issues related to the interpretation of clinical findings.

124 http://densitas.ca/about/. Accessed July 19, 2022.

125 https://www.technologyreview.com/2016/02/04/246748/ibms-automated-radiologist-can-read-images-and-medical-records/. Accessed Sept 8, 2023.

Chapter 25: Uses of Health Measures in Clinical Care

KEYWORDS: Trade-Offs, Health Measures, Biomarkers, Surrogate Biomarkers

ABSTRACT: Health care often requires trade-offs or compromises and the assessment of the benefits of an intervention against possible harms. Measures of health, including overall health and function, as well as the health and function of body parts are necessary to provide care and predict the overall outcomes of treatment.

Taking a drug to "make you better" always involves trade-offs. As we have written, you are making a wager. The wager is that the benefits of the drug will outweigh the harms. After every treatment, comfort, function or life expectancy change for the better, for the worse or remain the same. Evaluating benefits and risks requires measures of gain and loss. How different is each person's health after treatment? How many people improve or are worse after treatment?

Trade-offs in Health Care

We have seen that, at every visit, clinicians collect important information about how comfortable patients are and how well they function. They use these, along with the results of laboratory and imaging investigations, to make informal or formal estimates of your health and longevity.

Ideally, doctors would prefer to improve comfort AND function AND lifespan at the same time. However, that is not always possible. Sometimes patients must make trade-offs and decide which of these is most important to them. People in pain may find they feel less alert with painkillers. They may be more comfortable but function less well. The patient is the person who must decide which to choose.

Unfortunately, some tests and many treatments can themselves cause harm, as we mentioned. Doctors do sometimes prescribe treatments that may be harmful or at least hurtful. They do this if avoiding treatment inevitably leads to more serious discomfort, dysfunction or death. Cancer care is one example. Chemotherapy agents are poisons that are more damaging to cancer cells than normal cells but are damaging, nonetheless. Hair loss indicates this.

Most treatments and diagnostic tests harm only some of the people some of the time, and mostly help most people most of the time. However, very few tests or treatments always improve or always harm everyone. This is a crucial fact – a reality that patients must understand and address if they wish to be active participants in their care. Patients should know the possible health outcomes of each intervention and the chances that it will help or harm.

The Medical Algorithm Company[126] provides a comprehensive suite of tools for various medical specialties, including Internal Medicine, Surgery and Pediatrics, which supports predictions of what patients with particular characteristics can expect from treatment. The site includes tools that may be useful to reduce mistakes related to the mishandling, misinterpretation or misunderstanding of laboratory information.

Using Health Measures to Assess Trade-Offs

As we mentioned, a very useful concept is that of 'biomarkers'. These are the crucial, objective health measures that influence assessments of current health and predict future health status. A later chapter discusses biomarkers in detail and illustrates how some are used.

We also noted that many clinical choices and interventions have unwanted consequences for some people and some treatments cause health problems for almost everyone.

Consider one common medication: statins. Doctors recommend statin drugs (e.g., Lipitor, Crestor) to reduce cholesterol levels, because high cholesterol is considered to be an indicator or predictor of cardiovascular disease. People with high cholesterol have an increased chance (which increases with the cholesterol level) of suffering from a heart attack or stroke. Consequently, patients and doctors use cholesterol levels as a surrogate marker (see below) and a contributor to predictions about having a heart attack or stroke. However, for some people, statins may cause serious liver and muscle problems.

Patients who exercise and have normal cholesterol are medically different from those whose cholesterol level is only normal when they are taking drugs. In the latter case, the lowering of cholesterol may not have addressed the primary blood vessel problems; it may have just lowered the cholesterol. It is possible the correction of the indicator (high cholesterol) does not correct the root cause of the problem that causes both high cholesterol and fatty plaques in blood vessels that interfere with circulation. Lowering cholesterol seems to help only people between 40 and 75 years of age who also have other risk factors.[127] There is real question about the value of prescribing statins for anything but extremely high levels of cholesterol in other groups of patients.

Surrogate Biomarkers

'Surrogate biomarkers' are indicators intended "to substitute for a clinical endpoint", the latter being "a characteristic or variable that reflects how a patient feels, functions, or survives".[128 129] Experts caution that the use of surrogate biomarkers may be useful, but might be misleading, depending on the marker.

Consider, for example, for diabetics, glycated hemoglobin (HbA_{1c} – read this as "Hemoglobin A one C", a measure of the average level of blood glucose – sugar) is a surrogate biomarker. If it is elevated, it predicts poor outcomes for diabetic patients. Clinicians believe that treating the surrogate marker and achieving a normal level of glycated hemoglobin is an indication that the patient will avoid important complications of diabetes such as blindness, kidney disease or limb amputation.

126 https://www.medicalalgorithms.com/browse?tab=specialty. Accessed July 19, 2022.

127 Preventive Services Task Force, Statin Use for Primary Prevention of Cardiovascular Disease in Adults: Recommendation Statement, Am Fam Physician. 2017 Jan 15;95 (2) online. https://www.aafp.org/afp/2017/0115/od1.html U.S. Accessed July 19, 2022.

128 NIH Definitions Working Group. Biomarkers and Surrogate Endpoints. Amsterdam: Elsevier; 2000. Biomarkers and surrogate endpoints in clinical research: definitions and conceptual model; pp. 1–9.

129 Aronson JK. Biomarkers and surrogate endpoints. Br J Clin Pharmacol. 2005;59(5):491–494. doi:10.1111/j.1365-2125.2005.02435. x. https://www.ncbi.nlm.nih.gov/pmc/articles/PMC1884846/. Accessed July 19, 2022.

Unfortunately, reducing the level of surrogate markers is not always associated with an improvement in outcomes that are important to patients. *"There are the oral hypoglycemic drugs that reduce HbA_{1c} but increase the risk of cardiovascular events, antihypertensive drugs that do not reduce the risk of stroke, and drugs that improve cholesterol profiles but do not reduce cardiovascular events. Explanations for such phenomena include unwanted effects of the drug or an incomplete understanding of the pathophysiology of the disease.*[130] In other words, using drugs to change biomarkers is not always associated with changes in health that are meaningful to patients. The treatment may not address the underlying cause of the patients' problems. Think of it this way. Suppose your car has a light that goes on if your oil is low. Removing the bulb will not address the oil problem!

Again, patients who are on drugs to improve cholesterol levels or to reduce blood glucose are different from patients who have the same cholesterol or blood sugar levels but who are not taking drugs. The drug does not magically change them into patients who have natural cholesterol or sugar levels. If a predictive model, a formal method of predicting the risks and benefits associated with using certain drugs, is being relied on, one must be cautious. We must adjust the predictive model to reflect the additional risks and benefits that come with the use of the drug. The drug does change the patient, but not necessarily into a normal one. It gives the patient another characteristic that must be considered, namely, the presence of the drug used to change the cholesterol or blood sugar level. That should be obvious, but it is not.

People with the same cholesterol or glucose level are different if they achieved reduced blood glucose or cholesterol levels by using drugs versus doing so through diet and exercise. Drug-assisted patients are at increased risk, even if surrogate biomarkers like cholesterol level or glycated hemoglobin level are normal or even sub-normal. This is because they are exposed to possible drug side effects and their physiology is altered.

Doctors and patients must include the fact of drug treatment as a factor in their informal or formal predictions of patient outcomes. Drug-taking is not a formal indicator of health status like comfort, function and the results of lab tests are. However, clinicians trying to predict changes in short- and long-term health must take account of drug use, prescription or not.

We must recognize that most investigations and treatments involve trade-offs. Sometimes, people trade off benefits in one dimension of health for possible discomfort or harm in another. Some treatments might help a person live longer or improve function, but the person may feel worse during or immediately after treatment. Chemotherapy and radiation therapy may extend life, but patients might feel nauseous and be prone to bacterial and viral infections from treatment. Patients do it anyway for the long term: to live longer. Consequently, it is necessary to track the outcomes of people who have had any tests or treatment.

CONTROLLING HODGKIN'S

A 38-year-old relative of DZ's, (who is currently an energetic, well and healthy mother to a healthy daughter) had Hodgkin's disease treated with radiation. She had presented with a small lump on her neck but otherwise felt totally well. She was energetic and fully functional. At the time of her diagnosis, she was working and attending university. Twelve years later, it appears that the radiation therapy cured her. However, when the treatment started, she suffered from a dry mouth and fatigue, so much so that she had to reduce her work activities in order to continue her university education. She presented material at a professional seminar and was forced to carry a water bottle because the radiation treatment reduced

130 Yudkin John S, Lipska Kasia J, Montori Victor M. The idolatry of the surrogate BMJ 2011; 343: d7995 http://www.bmj.com/content/343/bmj.d7995. Accessed August 31, 2014.

the effectiveness of her salivary glands, giving her a constant dry mouth. She decided that this short-term harm was worth the long-term benefit. Her lifespan would have been dramatically shorter without treatment. With treatment, she is now healthy, expects a normal life and is a top-notch professional and mother. The tradeoff of a near-term reduction in comfort and function for a dramatically extended life expectancy was well worth the physical, emotional and financial costs of treatment.

Sometimes a successful surgery aimed at treating an orthopedic condition, for example, a fractured hip or a knee replacement, will be successful. However, another person might suffer a disastrous complication such as a heart attack or stroke or other adverse event during or immediately after surgery. The patient's hip or knee might be cured, but the patient ends up disabled in another way. This is one reason why efforts to evaluate the value of each treatment must consider not only the condition-specific results (the improved knee), but also the effect (the disabling stroke) of the treatment on overall health and on other organs.

Medical treatment frequently involves compromises, but the primary purposes are always the same: to improve comfort, to improve function and to increase life expectancy. Measuring health before and after interventions is essential if we are to know what works and what does not. Better decisions only flow from measurement!

Chapter 26: Administrative Uses of Health Data

KEYWORDS: Information, Measures, Administrative Use of Information, Cost of Care, Effectiveness, Efficiency, Administrative Evaluation

ABSTRACT: Administrators use health information to assess the effectiveness and efficiency of care. It's not enough to assess the cost of diagnoses. It's also essential to estimate the cost for caring for people with a diagnosis who have different levels of illness. We expect patients who present with more serious illness and more comorbid conditions to stay in hospital longer, to use more resources, and to have worse clinical outcomes.

Wait a minute! Aren't clinicians the only people who need clinical information? Nope! In fact, unless others can get access to and analyze clinical information, the healthcare system will diminish in value. Let's consider healthcare administrators.

Why Administrators Need Health Information

Assessing health is necessary to learn if medical services, like a surgicenter or a diagnostic imaging department, provide overall benefit, inflict harm or just waste time and money. Healthcare administrators track and analyze clinical data because they, like all managers, recognize how important measurement is to management. Responsible and accountable organizations need to understand what they are doing and producing. They need to assess how efficient they are, what their costs are, what effects they are having (for example on patient outcomes), where they need to make changes, what the effects of those changes are and if it is worthwhile to continue with what they are doing or alter course. That is a substantial job and a great challenge.

To accomplish their goals through competent management, leaders of health organizations need several kinds of data. Of course, they need fiscal or financial data: what processes cost, how much money is or should be made available and how their expenditures compare to similar organizations. But administrators also need to get and use other kinds of data: process data and clinical data.

Process data are used to understand what the organization is doing and to measure how well and how efficiently (including quality) various healthcare functions operate. How many patients of what kind and over what time does the organization see? How long does a patient have to wait for service? How much time does it take to handle a patient in the Diagnostic Imaging or other department? How satisfied are our patients with their care? What are staff assessments of their own morale and of departmental function? These and much more are daily concerns.

In addition to process data, it should be obvious to the reader that clinical data is the most important element. What good is it to operate a health institution, department or a follow up program for diabetic patients, unless we know the health of individuals entering the program, their health during the course of their care and their health on leaving and over time?

Perhaps it is worthwhile to think about something simpler than health care. Consider a widget factory. How could a manager successfully manage that factory without objective and quantitative information about what goes into the factory (the types and quality of metals and components, for example), what goes on in the factory and what the quantity and quality is of the widgets the factory produces? Without that information, it is really not possible to ever be sure that what the factory produced would be affordable, useable and valued.

MEASURING PIZZAS

One day, long ago, DC dropped by at a local pizza store in Toronto. A young couple ran it and they made delicious pizzas – so they got the quality right! DC, while waiting for a pizza, learned that the young entrepreneur had taken a job at a nearby meat-packing plant. That was surprising, so DC asked why he'd done that. The wife said that they were not making ends meet in their business and the job had been necessary for financial stability. As the business seemed to always have a lineup, DC, being nosey, asked where their problems were. The wife said that they were losing money; they just never seemed to catch up. So, DC asked to see what it cost them to make different kinds of pizza. They had absolutely no idea! It turned out they had never looked at costs and had simply set their prices to be super-competitive with other stores. They were in fact donating a part of each pizza to the community. How can one run a business without knowing at least one's costs? They also didn't really want external advice and went on to fail a few months later. Management requires measurement!

DOES OUR TOASTER PRODUCE TOAST?

An interesting aside is a novel called 'Mockingbird' by Walter Tevis. A very brief overview of a story within the novel involves a toaster factory. It is set in a society where people have not been able to purchase toasters for a very long time. No one knows why; there just aren't toasters on the market. A person wandering around the country comes across a totally automated factory in the middle of nowhere that produces toasters. He notices that no toasters are coming out of the plant. He starts at the end of the assembly line and notices that an automated quality assurance device turns on each toaster the plant has produced, it fails to turn on and the flawed toaster goes into the recycling hopper. The hopper's contents eventually are transported to the start of the line. The flawed toasters are disassembled, and the parts put back into the assembly process. The wanderer walks down the assembly line noting the addition of each part. At one point along the line, he discovers that an electronic component is stuck in a stack feeding a machine that inserts one part into the toaster. He jiggles the stack and notices that the machine now properly installs the component. He then follows the toaster down the line, noting that, at each stage, the toasters are now being properly assembled. He gets to the end of the line, sees that when the quality assurance unit tests it, the toaster functions properly and it is boxed for shipment. Now toasters will be on the market! The moral of the story is that by paying attention to processes, departments or organizations can assure that they at least produce something for all their effort and cost. In health care, we are also interested in knowing if we produce something that is of value: healthy patients!

So, administration has a fundamental interest in clinical data. These data indicate that a quality means turning sick patients into healthier ones. Otherwise, health care is just a sink for money.

Assessing the Cost of Care for Competent Administration

Unfortunately, getting actual clinical data for the administration of health care is not easy. Some administrators believe that administrative data (like the activities performed and their volumes) can serve as proxies for actual measures of health outcomes – the objective changes in health associated with care.

In the 1980s, healthcare administrators developed the concept of Diagnosis-Related

Groups (DRGs).[131] The idea was that payers would remunerate health organizations and physicians based on the types and volumes of services they provided. The belief was (and to some degree still is) that a patient's diagnosis – remember that this is defined before the patient is treated – would provide a useful indicator of the value of the services provided. For example, there would be a price associated with the treatment of the patient with simple pneumonia and another price for the care of someone with complicated pneumonia.

Great idea but it just doesn't work! For example, in Pennsylvania in 2009, the average charge for treating pneumonia at one Community Hospital in Pennsylvania was $6,772. On the other hand, according to the Pennsylvania Health Care Cost Containment Council, the average charge for treating pneumonia for another Hospital in Pennsylvania was $88,447.[132] That's a difference of about 1300%! But both organizations provided the same type of service. Maybe pneumonias at the latter hospital were much more complicated or maybe they just wasted money, but we don't have information that could confirm either hypothesis. Understanding what happened to cause such a difference would require detailed examination. In fact, such a large difference in cost demands more detailed analysis.

A Detailed Example of Pneumonia and the DRG Idea

Most readers know someone who has had the misfortune of suffering from pneumonia. The term pneumonia describes a lung infection with an associated x-ray picture showing a buildup of material (a 'consolidation') in the lung. You do not have to be physician to realize that some pneumonias might involve more of the lung, other pneumonias, less. Some patients have only pneumonia, while others also have other conditions (called 'co-morbidities'). Some patients with pneumonia are obese, others have a normal weight. Each patient has different characteristics that influence how sick they may become, how aggressively treatment must be pursued, how difficult and time-consuming it will be to treat them and how much it will cost.

When you consider your acquaintances with pneumonia, a few may have been very sick and required hospitalization. Others continued most of their daily activities and took antibiotics by mouth ('PO': 'per os' or 'per orem') either at home or in their workplace. We must conclude that, for some people, pneumonia is a serious problem, while for others it might be a mere inconvenience.

Treating pneumonia in an intensive care unit (a pricey place!) with intravenous fluids (IV: fluids introduced into a vein via a tube – a catheter) and oxygen therapy with careful monitoring, is more expensive than giving someone an oral antibiotic to take at home. Therefore, in order to determine an appropriate price for care of an individual patient, it is necessary to determine how sick the patient was to start, his or her other conditions and health status and also how healthy the patient was after treatment.

Labor is the largest cost in hospitals. The amount of labor it takes to care for patients relates to their level of function (such as if patients can feed themselves) and to the intensity of treatments. The costs can be much greater if patients need oxygen, regular IV therapy and close monitoring. Care and cost vary with disease severity.

At first, most people, including many administrators, expect there would be a uniform cost to treat most patients with the same diagnosis. This rationale suggests that hospitals should get about the same amount for treating similar patients. In the case of pneumonia, however,

131 http://www.aaos.org/news/aaosnow/dec13/advocacy2.asp. Accessed May 7, 2015.

132 Pennsylvania Health Care Cost Containment Council. http://www.phc4.org/hpr/Results.aspx?Years=20084-20093&CC=Pneumonia&CID=0&Facilities=Pennsylvania. May 7, 2015. Accessed August 25, 2022.

it is clear that reimbursement should be based on what actually happens to patients, assuming this is in proportion to how sick they are. It turns out that the same is true for virtually all diagnoses. Severity is crucial information additional to the diagnosis and, without it, we can make no judgment about the appropriateness of either of the Pennsylvania organizations' costs.

So, reality is that remuneration based on DRGs alone does not make any sense. It does not take into account disease severity. Indeed, the International Classification of Diseases (ICD) classifies pneumonia using information about the site of the pneumonia and the infectious organism (bacterium, virus, fungus) causing pneumonia but does not capture objective estimates of illness severity. The DRG classification also does not consider the patient's state of comfort or function. Nor does the classification capture information about the laboratory information that contributes to clinical assessments, and these can vary vastly according to severity. Also, hospital patients who can function independently are less expensive to treat when compared with patients less able to function, like bed-ridden patients in an intensive care unit.

Another issue is the effectiveness or the value of the services. Anyone who buys goods or services knows that price alone does not determine value. People also consider the quantity and quality of the goods and services they buy. The value of health care should relate to what we might call 'comprehensive efficiency' (the magnitude of health benefit per unit of cost). When we buy health services, we hope that the result will be improved health as measured by improved comfort, improved function and increased longevity. That's what we expect, anyway.

The average cost of a day in hospital does not provide sufficient information for us to determine if an organization is efficient or inefficient, unless there is accompanying information revealing the sickness of patients the hospital treated and what the hospital accomplished. We must measure how sick the patients were when they were admitted and how healthy they were when discharged or shortly after. Dumping people who are still sick back onto the street is not a good thing – and today's institutions already recognize that they often discharge patients now at a level of sickness that would have been the basis for admitting them in earlier times.

Although paying doctors and hospitals based on diagnosis had intuitive appeal, on reflection it is clear that to get the remuneration right, we need to know both the diagnosis and the severity in addition to the kind, level and cost of services and the outcome of patients.

Measures of severity also provide an adjustment needed to predict chances of surviving the disease episode. When diagnostic labels are used for costing there is perverse incentive to admit the healthiest patients with a condition because they are the ones who cost the least to treat. But that is cheating!

Measuring health is essential to assessing the quality of the care provided and the magnitude of the rescue achieved for all the investments in the care of every patient. When the care process fails and a patient is injured or dies, it is also crucial to know that everything possible was done and that there were no medical misadventures.

Assessing Quality for Administrative Competence

The fact that people are sick, sometimes seriously so, means that death will occur in the healthcare system. However, excessive death rates (more than the number that usually occur by sheer chance) for patients admitted with relatively minor problems are a reason to flag those medical charts for review. Yes, that is important, but what frustrates many clinicians and some administrators is that the information about disease severity they capture as a matter of course is usually wasted and not used to relate costs to health benefits.

Much of the debate about the organization of health care is mundane; it's about dollars and cents. This reflects underlying beliefs about the kinds of systems that will produce the best health results for people at the least cost. As we have stated again and again, measurement is essential for management! Because most Canadian and American health organizations do not routinely measure health and track health outcomes, cost has become a proxy for the value, efficiency and effectiveness of care. This is despite the fact that cost alone does not say very much at all about the quality of care. Hospitals could make patient's sheets out of $100 bills and it would have no impact on their care (although there might be many quicker self-discharges and missing blankets)!

DUST BUNNIES AS CARE FOCUS

The HAY group, in Canada, routinely used information collected by the public system to opine confidentially about health system performance. Years ago, one hospital CEO crowed to DZ about how efficient her organization was. She remarked that her cost for cleaning per square foot was the lowest in the country but neglected to note anything about infection rates or dust bunnies proliferating in the corridor. Having the shortest length of stay for a diagnosis or the lowest cost means little without the results the organization achieves in terms of improving health.

Does the private sector provide better care than the public sector? This important question is the foundation of contentious arguments in the United States and Canada about which type of organizations should provide health care and about how to pay for it. Does my doctor get good results or not? Is the hospital in my neighborhood terrible or terrific? Unfortunately, no one really knows, so resolving the argument is impossible. Absent data, we are operating in the dark!

Clinicians, researchers and health services administrators cannot even start to answer questions like these unless they first link healthcare activities to healthcare results. This means measuring, capturing and using information about sickness at the time of admission, during care, at discharge and after. For all patients, it means linking prescribed interventions with the changes in health that follow these interventions.

Quality must be our most important product!

Chapter 27: How Measurement of Care Helps Choices About Treating the Elderly

KEYWORDS: Eldercare, Fairness, Life Expectancy, Algorithms to Measure and Predict Longevity

ABSTRACT: Communities expect that the healthcare system will treat both young and old people fairly and that they will experience the care they need. However, it's important to realize that what is appropriate for young person may not only be inappropriate but also contraindicated for an older individual. This chapter describes ways to make fair decisions for old and young and to avoid implementing treatments that are more likely to harm than help.

Care of the Elderly Involves Conundrums

Sickness of the young, especially mortal sickness of the very young, puts us and the health system into high gear. Our goal is to preserve the opportunity for a healthy and long life. Sickness in the elderly, though, especially the very elderly, has different impacts and goals. If we are smart, we will focus on increasing comfort and function and not as much on longevity.

CASE STUDY OF DECISION MAKING FOR OLDER PEOPLE

The story about Mary at the start of Section 4 (pg. 136) illustrates the issue of appropriate treatment of the elderly.

Aggressive treatment for older people who feel well and who are functioning is rarely a good choice!

Most surgery creates an immediate decrease in comfort and function. Post-anesthesia complications add additional risk and surgical complications are another worry. Sometimes it is best to leave well enough alone, especially when a problem poses no immediate risk. Older people suffer from increased chance of death and complications following surgery.[133] Frail older people have even a lower probability of a successful surgical outcome. Measures of frailty include measures of mental and physical function, including movement, and measures of physiological status, including heart and kidney function.

When an intervention is not meant to change comfort and function, it is important to estimate the chances that the treatment will increase the patient's lifespan.

FIGURE 1.27.1: Decision making regarding the elderly

133 Monson, K., Litvak, D.A., and Bold, R.J., Surgery in the Aged Population, Archi Survey, Vol 138, Oct 2003, 1061-1067 http://archsurg.ama-assn.org/cgi/reprint/138/10/1061.pdf. Accessed July 19, 2022.

Thinking About This Case

(See FIGURE 1.27.1)

Understanding the purposes and measures of care and the potential benefits and harms of treatment helps people make complicated choices. In many countries there are raging and sometimes acrimonious debates about end-of-life care. Some have called quality review agencies "Death Panels" because they raise questions about the appropriateness of interventions. Some claim they are driven by cost and trade lives for dollars. However, not undertaking useless or harmful care is important for medical reasons, not only financial ones. Understanding the promises and perils of treatment is essential if we are to be able to choose useful treatments and avoid harmful ones.

Older people, like our parents and grandparents, should receive the care they require, not too little and not too much.[134] The opportunities available to young people should be available for the care of the elderly. No one should be deprived of access to care simply because of age. However, some apparently life-prolonging treatments are simply not appropriate for older people and are a sign of poor quality of care. They represent a casual and somewhat thoughtless, albeit good-intentioned, approach to care because they cause discomfort and dysfunction, while offering little promise of life extension. And sometimes they accelerate demise. FIGURE 1.27.2 gives an idea of potential predicted lifespans.

At advanced age, physicians should aim treatments at improving comfort and function, not primarily at increasing lifespan. Regardless of treatment, a 95-year-old cannot expect to live much longer. But that person should be helped to live in comfort and be able to function as well as possible. Treatments that attempt to increase lifespan, but simultaneously reduce comfort or function, are a poor wager for the elderly.

Year of Birth	Male	Female
1944	63.6	66.8
1945	63.6	67.9
1946	64.4	69.4
1947	64.4	69.7
1948	64.6	69.9
1949	65.2	70.7
1950	65.6	71.1
1951	65.6	71.4
1952	65.8	71.6
1953	66.0	72.0
1954	66.7	72.8

This selection from a longevity table shows that a male born in 1954 will most likely live for 66.7 years, while a female will live for 72.8 years.

FIGURE 1.27.2: A longevity table

Old people and young people are different because of marked differences in the number of years we would normally expect them to live. Many aggressive treatments are just as likely to shorten an older person's life as to lengthen it. Thinking about the effects of attempting to increase longevity is important. We must consider that older people do not heal as quickly as younger ones, nor return to normal as quickly or completely when their body suffers a traumatic event, like surgery or radical chemotherapy. Older organs, like the liver, kidneys, and pancreas are not as tolerant of toxic influences, including anesthetics, as younger ones are. Older people do not do as well and do not recover as quickly as the young when exposed to many powerful drugs. Even body temperature regulation is not as effective in older people as in the young.[135]

134 People should be investigated and treated in proportion to the seriousness of problems and the threat they represent, as well the possible impacts of interventions.

135 Blatteis CM. Age-Dependent Changes in Temperature Regulation. Gerontology. 2011 Nov 11. [Epub ahead of print] PubMed PMID: 22085834. http://www.ncbi.nlm.nih.gov/pubmed/22085834. Accessed July 19, 2022.

To summarize: since aggressive treatments often reduce comfort and function, it is inappropriate, in general, to subject elderly people to such treatments. Except in very unusual circumstances, treatments for older people should be aimed at improving immediate comfort and function, rather than extending future life.

Not Depriving a Person of Care—

The other side of the coin needs to be considered as well.

Patients should not be denied care just because they are dying. We are aware of many circumstances where those suffering from the throes of cancer have been denied interventions that would reduce their suffering. In one case, an elderly patient with liver cancer was denied, at least before vigorous argument, the placement of stents (devices to keep blood vessels in the liver, in this case, open). This intervention was initially refused because, as the physician said, the patient was dying anyway. The patient's father-in-law, a veterinarian, protested and the physician eventually altered his decision. In this instance, the patient lived an additional four years in relative comfort after the procedure was finally performed.

Many other examples relate to the relief provided by opiates in terminal cancer. They are sometimes denied because death is inevitable or there is the concern – an absurd one – that the patient will become addicted. Most patients would be happy to live a life of addiction as long as that life went on and was livable! Comfort and even function can be extended despite the reality that a disease is bringing life to a close after Medicine has done its best. FIGURE 1.27.3 will give an idea of the most appropriate goals of care at different times of one's life.

GOALS	YOUNG	MIDDLE-AGED	ELDERLY
Increase Life Span	YES	YES	NO
Improve Comfort	YES	YES	YES
Improve Function	YES	YES	YES

Goals of care differ for young and old because, for the oldest segment of the population, most medical treatments rarely increase lifespan, but rather cause immediate reductions in comfort and function. Radical treatment of the oldest segment of our population is appropriate when the goal is to increase comfort and function.

FIGURE 1.27.3: Treatment goals differ according to age

No one would argue that patients or insurers should pay for unnecessary or harmful care. Implanting a cardioverter-defibrillator (an electronic device to sustain or alter the hearts rhythm of contraction) in an older person who does not need one, is not only a waste of fiscal and professional resources, but also exposes the person to harm. Yet, a recent article in the Journal of the American Medical Association (JAMA) suggested that as many as 22% (more than 1 in 5) of patients who received an implantable cardioverter-defibrillator did not satisfy evidence-based criteria for implantation.[136] Implanting a cardioverter-defibrillator offers hope of improved life span, but there are immediate consequences, including discomfort, possible infection and dysfunction associated with the procedure. It is interesting to note that those who have experienced a device defibrillating (changing the heart's rhythm to a positive one) their hearts have

136 Al-Khatib, S.M. et. Al, Non-Evidence Based ICD Implantations in the United States. JAMA. 2011;305(1):43-49. doi: 10.1001/jama.2010.1915 http://jama.ama-assn.org/content/305/1/43.short. Accessed July 19, 2022.

said that it feels like someone kicked them in the chest. For older people whose life expectancy is short regardless of health, betting that implanting a cardioverter-defibrillator will increase life expectancy is usually not a worthwhile wager.

Treatments that offer the illusory possibility of prolonging life are not signs of caring. They are the hallmarks of a poorly thought-through and sometimes financially motivated approach to care. Another example might be an 89-year-old woman who is comfortable and functional who notices a breast lump. She is probably better off leaving well-enough alone. The exceptions might be if offered treatment as a part of a research trial, or the doctor can give reasonably accurate assessments of the chances of benefit or harm following the treatment. This is because the immediate treatment for an asymptomatic breast lump in an 89-year-old is likely to cause an immediate reduction in comfort and function and expose the patient to the risk of immediate infection, without promising a corresponding increase in lifespan.

As of 2020, people who are 90 or more can, on average, expect to live about another 3 or 4 years. Treatments that reduce their comfort and function are unlikely to increase their life expectancy and are not usually warranted. Age often is the measure most predictive of remaining years of life.

Comment on Physician-Assisted Death

Canada's Supreme Court ruled that Canadian doctors must participate in physician-assisted death. The raging argument following this decision suggests that this matter is something very new. However, doctors have always used drugs, appropriately, to alleviate suffering. Often, the doses required to reduce pain and suffering may also hasten death. Until recently, this has not been controversial. Communities expected doctors to alleviate suffering, even if the treatment might shorten life. Now, however, providing this comfort has become more complicated and subject to unproductive intrusion.

Measuring Health to Enable Truly Informed Consent

Being able to measure health, before, during and after any significant treatment is essential to a patient's giving informed consent to the treatment. When patients agree to treatment or undergo a test, they are accepting the idea – and making a wager – that they will be better off as a result. In other words, they believe that their health will be better in some measurable way, or that they will know more about themselves and their health after the intervention.

To estimate if patients will be better off or worse off after a test or treatment, they and their doctors must have some idea about what happened to other people who, like them, had the same test or treatment. For that information to be available, someone had to follow up on and assess previous patients' outcomes. Then it would be possible to find out how people fared after care. Patients should accept a treatment only if most of those previously treated were better off, few people were worse off and hardly anyone had a serious complication. The bad news is that such data is seldom available. Sometimes, there are even upsetting reasons it is not, like burying mistakes (sometimes, literally).

KILL THE MESSAGE

DC was establishing medical-surgical databases quite a few decades ago. At the time, patients were invited to come into several clinics, such as those for the follow up of implanted cardiac (heart) pacemakers, prosthetic heart valves (replacing natural, but worn-out or damaged ones) and coronary bypasses (surgery to improve blood circulation to the heart muscle). He had the hypothesis that patients who came into the clinic were relatively well, while those who were sick stayed away. Instead of just waiting for patients to come in (and many didn't), we developed a process to interview patients via phone to find out how they were doing.

Interestingly, at that time, the clinic did not even know which patients were alive, dead or lost to follow-up. Patients who revealed they had bothersome symptoms were asked to come to the clinic for further assessment. In addition, we followed up on patients we could not reach to see if they had possibly died. It is particularly disturbing that in these cases of relatively serious surgical interventions, little data was available and what was available was incomplete or unconfirmed until this program.

When the process was extended to other major institutions in the city, it could easily be seen that there were differences in the results at different hospitals. One might think that this would stimulate further data collection and documentation. Instead, it was perceived as being a threat to the reputation of the primary institution and the project was unceremoniously terminated. The mechanisms for the collection of data in this process were documented in articles in major journals.

One wonders if the fear of being compared to other institutions causes information to go undocumented or to be suppressed. It sometimes has taken a law or a mandate from a quality assurance organization to force data collection.

In Canada, when disease severity indices were mandated, rather than information being suppressed, it was used "creatively" and led to the overstatement of severity to justify the cost of care. In the United States, this activity has been called 'DRG Optimization'. We call it the 'game of fish' (as tools called 'groupers' – a type of fish – are used), where an institution 'fishes' for additional information to allow it to justify a higher fee. It's not illegal, as it is simply taking advantage of the rules. All games have rules and a lawyer or accountant will tell you that taking the greatest possible advantage of the rules is fair game! The problem is the rules.

A later chapter discusses how to choose and assess proposed treatments, specifically, what patients should ask for as they decide whether or not to have tests or treatments.

Physical Measures of Health/Handicap

The PULSES[137] profile is one tool for measuring physical function. It asks questions about a patient's overall physical condition, upper and lower limb function, sensory capabilities (touch, feeling, hearing, vision), excretory function and mental and emotional state. It helps capture what people can do and how well they function in terms of the working of body parts, including arms, legs, senses, bowels and bladder.

A variety of other indices exist (see, for example, the Barthel Index).[138] Some rely on subtle findings, such as the state of reflexes. Others address broader interpretations of health, including the ability to walk upstairs, go to the bathroom and to dress and feed oneself.

Patients can apply overall measures like these to their own circumstances. The worth of more subtle measures collected by doctors is not always known because no one knows how often these tests lead to accurate predictions. This points out yet another need for discovering outcomes.

A later chapter discusses the sensitivity and specificity of various tests, which are measures of their ability to detect and predict problems.

Most people assume that early detection of illness will increase survival. Yet, early detection also exposes patients to the possibility of overdiagnosis from false alarms and the possible adverse effects of unnecessary treatment. A very important example is screening men for prostate cancer. Interestingly, research has shown that those who are regularly screened are no less likely to die from prostate cancer[139] compared with those who are not screened, nor are they likely to

137 http://www.physio-pedia.com/The_Pulses_Profile. Accessed July 19, 2022. Physiopedia The Pulses Profile.

138 https://albertahealthservices.ca/assets/about/scn/ahs-scn-bjh-hf-barthel-index-of-adls.pdf. Accessed July 19, 2022.

139 Andriole GL, Grubb RL III, Buys SS, et al. Mortality results from a randomized prostate-cancer screening trial. N Engl J Med 2009; 360:1310-1319. http://www.nejm.org/doi/full/10.1056/nejmoa0810696. Accessed July 19, 2022.

live longer overall.[140] What should we think, then, of the public awareness campaigns to get more men to undergo screening?

SOME ALGORITHMS TO MEASURE HEALTH

http://www.medicalalgorithms.com/browse?tab=specialty. Accessed July 19, 2022.

From Medal the Medical Algorithms Company.

http://www.a4ebm.org/sites/default/files/Measuring%20Health.pdf. Accessed July 19, 2022.

McDowell, I., Newell, C., MEASURING HEALTH: A Guide to Ratings and Questionnaires, New York, Oxford Press, 2006.

Studenski, S., Perera, S., Hushang, P, et. Al., Gait Speed and Survival in Older Adults JAMA. 2011;305(1):50-58. doi: 10.1001/jama.2010.1923 http://jama.ama-assn.org/content/305/1/50.short. Accessed July 19, 2022.

Harmon, K., Walking Speed Predicts Life Expectancy of Older Adults, Scientific American, January 4, 2011, http://www.scientificamerican.com/article.cfm?id=walking-speed-survival. Accessed July 19, 2022.

http://www.mdcalc.com/ Many Medical Calculators. Accessed July 19, 2022.

http://cvrisk.mvm.ed.ac.uk/calculator/calc.asp Cardiovascular Risk Calculator – Smiley Faces. Accessed July 19, 2022.

140 Recommendations of the U.S. Preventive Services Task Force 2010-2011. http://www.ahrq.gov/clinic/pocketgd1011/pocketgd1011.pdf. Accessed August 27, 2012.

Chapter 28: Understanding Medical Records

KEYWORDS: Medical Record, Information Contained in Health Records, Cost of Complete Records, Value of Complete Records, Understanding the Medical Record, Components of the Medical Record

ABSTRACT: The medical record contains information about the patient, the patient's context, and the treatment and outcomes the patient experiences. This chapter discusses the elements and structure of the medical record, the cost and time required to capture complete information and the value of the information collected. Sometimes those collecting the information do not find it valuable, while others believe complete information is essential for analysis. We have not yet realized the full benefits of automated, computerized capture and analysis of medical records.

The Nature of the Medical Record

A picture might be worth a thousand words, but it may take many more words to capture 'pictures' of a person's health and sicknesses over a lifetime. Those words reside in the patient's medical record – often accompanied by medical pictures, like X-rays.

It is crucial that we understand the nature of medical records: what they are, what they are not, who uses them, and why and how they are used. Medical records support not only clinical care, but also health services administration, research and education.

The Data and Information for the Record

Every patient has a set of relevant characteristics starting from identification and location information and including signs, symptoms and findings acquired during care. These descriptors include words (like 'flushed' – having hot and red skin), numbers (like a blood chemistry test result), images (an x-ray), signals and graphs (an ECG) or data in other forms (formal diagnostic terms, reports from other physicians, et).

Familiar patient characteristics include height, weight, temperature, heart rate, and blood pressure. In addition, there are numbers derived from these, like BMI (Body Mass Index – a calculation using weight and height to estimate obesity). The set of characteristics is virtually without limit. Each human has, literally, millions of characteristics including genetic information.

To understand the nature of the medical record, we must realize that the patient's physician, another clinician or even the patient determines which of these many characteristics will be recorded. Some physicians will consider certain patient characteristics crucially important, while others will not. Moreover, different physicians may even measure these characteristics differently, such as blood pressure, for example, and this can be a problem. It's almost as if some clinicians do not recognize that what they record must be readable, understood and used by other clinicians.

ISSUES IN RECORD COMPLETENESS

Some clinicians write shorter, less complete notes when they believe there is a small chance that other clinicians will need the information in the future. Others do that because they believe there are better uses for their clinical time. They deal with the competing responsibilities of lengthy waiting lists and patients' need for immediate and adequate care. They have decided that other patients will be better off if they receive more timely care, versus writing comprehensive records that might never be used..

Clinicians must constantly balance the time they have to do direct patient care while dealing with all the other demands of practice. Keeping proper records is essential. However, the patients' circumstances dictate the amount of recordkeeping that is required. Each clinician strikes a balance. Some are virtually (hopefully, non-fiction) authors describing whatever happens in the office. Others keep focused, pithy records that directly support care. There are professional standards of recordkeeping, but each physician has latitude within those standards. At some point, record keeping can become an end in itself and can negatively impact care. Dr. Campbell comments on this in Volume 2 on Mental Health.

Well, there are many views about what should be in the record. In addition to the directly relevant patient state and physician interventions information, there may be medical-legal requirements or regulatory protocols that demand other information. Regarding legal stuff, in some jurisdictions, patients may sue physicians for what the patients perceive as mistakes or deficiencies in care. The insurance companies, which back-up the physician financially related to litigation, may require additional information, such as any indication that the patient was intoxicated, under the influence of drugs or suffering from a problem irrelevant to the current visit but that the agency feels should be noted by the physician. In addition, medical professional organizations, like medical colleges or boards, may set minimum record standards. Clinicians are under pressure to record these additional pieces of information despite their peripheral nature to the immediate and future care of the patient.

Who is Served and Who Does the Recordkeeping Work?

The pressure on record contents originates in the colleges, boards, insurance companies and others that place demands on physician time – the time associated with data capture and entry. The problem is that these demands can quite dramatically increase the length of the medical visit but without additional benefit to the patient. This is a serious problem. In a certain sense, these external agents transform the physician into a data entry clerk serving their interests. Furthermore, getting that data into the record becomes a major logistical and financial issue. Research indicates that using existing eHealth systems to record all this information can easily double the time the physician must spend in recordkeeping. Just imagine if a home renovations contractor had to document all the leasehold improvements performed for a client as well as their visual effect. If that were the case, we would expect for the contractor to charge for that time and get far less construction work done in a day. The problem is that physician fees are typically fixed and not time dependent. The result: the physician is serving as an unpaid data clerk. Perhaps even worse is that the system steals time that could be invested in patient care and interferes in the intimacy of the encounter.

PERSONAL EXAMPLE

DZ, as a patient with a knee problem, recently saw a dramatic illustration of the problems of recordkeeping. In the early days of his practice, if a patient needed a referral for an x-ray or to a consulting specialist, DZ would ask his secretary over the intercom to book the x-ray. The request would be of the nature "Ms. X has a cough and peculiar breath sounds. Please order an x-ray." Now doctors use electronic information systems and must enter some of the information manually. When the secretary wrote the requisition, a copy became part of the record and the doctor didn't have to write it. Now the doctor must select from lists or manually enter the information necessary. A process that took about 30 seconds before has become a 3 to 4-minute exercise. Similarly, for requesting that a specialist see a patient (called a 'consultation'), the secretary used to be able to write the patient information necessary for the consult based on phone instruction from the doctor. Moreover, the secretaries who made and booked appointments knew one another so they could negotiate priorities for the appointments based on patient severity. Now, it has become more difficult to accelerate care even when important.

These are unintended consequences of the way health record information systems have developed.

There are other arguments for more detailed recordkeeping that may be more cogent for the physician, however. If medical records are sparse then Public Health surveillance can be impaired. Also, many have very convincingly argued for the assessment of the effectiveness of care. A 2010 study of Carotid Endarterectomy surgeries[141] found that some records, depending on patient complexity, were inadequate to support accurate coding, a process crucial for assessing care. Effectiveness studies are rendered impossible unless physicians accurately record, and health record systems accurately capture, details of the patient's health status, testing, interventions and resultant patient state.

Therefore, many physicians find themselves in a bind.

Technology Comes to the "Rescue"

Over the last six decades, researchers and companies have worked to design, develop and implement computer-based information systems for medical recordkeeping. In the United States, the Obama administration funded a tens of billions of dollars effort to acquire and implement these systems. The idea was that eHealth systems would assist physicians in producing comprehensive, usable and shareable records that could be subject to analysis and used to predict the patient's course. What a great idea! Regrettably, it may have produced a far greater ability to bill for healthcare services, but the effect on medical recordkeeping was not the one desired.

RECORDKEEPING TIME

This study found that ophthalmologists spent a median of about 11 minutes per office visit in recordkeeping, resulting in almost 2 hours of use during a half-day clinic session. The study also examined how billing level and clinic volume impact EHR time per office visit (positive correlation with billing level and a negative correlation with clinic volume).[142]

Today's computer-based systems in effect interrogate a physician for information and thereby increase the time it takes to produce records. This is because these systems implement record content standards. Physicians may perceive these standards to be in excess of what may be appropriate for the immediate care of the patient.

Then there is the problem of the 'data entry bottleneck': we have only a limited set of ways to get information into a computer system. For instance, we can type it in, select options from

141 Chart Documentation Quality and its Relationship to the Validity of Administrative Data Discharge Records, L. So et al., Health Informatics Journal, pp. 101-113, 2010. https://journals.sagepub.com/doi/10.1177/1460458210364784. Accessed August 25, 2022.

142 Read-Brown S, Hribar MR, Reznick LG, Lombardi LH, Parikh M, Chamberlain WD, Bailey ST, Wallace JB, Yackel TR, Chiang MF. Time Requirements for Electronic Health Record Use in an Academic Ophthalmology Center. JAMA Ophthalmol. 2017;135(11):1250-1257. https://pubmed.ncbi.nlm.nih.gov/29049512/. Accessed August 25, 2022.

lists (e.g., the names of drugs) by pointing or using a mouse or we can dictate the information to the computer. However, every one of these data entry methods is problematic.

Consider the options. Typing, for most people, is slow and error prone. On the other hand, selecting items from lists using a mouse means that the clinician must scan many very long lists of drugs, for example, choose the desired item and sometimes slip from one item to the next, resulting in errors that are easily overlooked. Furthermore, the route of drug delivery (such as by mouth, injection), the dosage and the frequency all need to be selected. Each step affords the physician of opportunities for errors. Dictation may be a better option, but existing computer-supported dictation software's abilities to recognize speech is still imperfect and speaking out loud in the location where the clinician works may be inappropriate for privacy or other reasons.

The information relevant to the encounter, the information demanded by external agencies or for other purposes, the corrections and even the mistakes all contribute to a lot of data entry. Worse still, the clinician only has a very restrictive 'funnel' for getting information into the record. This causes widescale frustration with and even rejection of quite a few of the existing record capture systems.

The Real Nature of the Medical Record

Maybe looking at a well-known process will help us understand the nature and limitations of the medical record. Refer to Diagram A. Imagine the patient to be like a detailed scene we wish to capture in a picture. Think of the physician as being a camera acquiring the image through a lens specific to that clinician. The medical record captured by the physician is like the picture recorded by a camera on film or an electronic sensor.

Those who take photographs with electronic cameras will realize that different camera systems will have the ability to pick up more or less detail (they will have higher or lower resolution), have greater or lesser light and color sensitivity, and will be able to record a photograph, versus continuous or video images. In this analogy, the patient is like the detailed scene. The physician is like the camera and the medical record is like the photograph, at least in the case of the medical records we have today. It's just that physicians act differently from cameras. They can focus on only certain aspects of the patient and ignore others. Some physicians focus on the patient 'landscape' as a whole; others focus on the specific details. The most talented physicians can capture relevant detail in the record but also perceive the whole person.

If the camera is not designed to capture fine-enough details, then some important characteristics will not appear or be fuzzy in the photograph. In the same way, if the physician chooses not to observe and measure certain characteristics, or doesn't pay attention to them, those characteristics will not be in the record or the information may not be detailed enough to comprehend the full extent of the patient's problems. However, just like when interpreting a picture, incomplete information about a patient might be sufficient to enable physicians to recognize the problem. At other times, the lack of detail could lead to delayed or mistaken diagnoses.

How carefully the physician reviews the patient and records what he or she finds will determine the adequacy and quality of the record. For example, the physician's measurement of the patient's blood pressure may not be accurate, because the physician does not do it in the accepted way. The fact is, that in today's systems, the medical record is like a poor, sparse and instantaneous image of the patient acquired during an office visit. Another image/record will be made at the next office visit, of course, and the new image might capture or ignore additional important information, including changes between visits.

It should be obvious that the medical record is not a continuous view of the patient. That's why we likened it to a photo instead of a video. Particularly, it only measures characteristics captured at the time of the encounter with the physician. This should bother the reader who is aware of the continuous variability we exhibit. However, the good news for the instantaneous medical record is that the variation of some patient characteristics does not matter much. The bad news is that the variation of some characteristics, for example blood pressure, is important.

An interesting question is: for whom is the physician capturing this 'image' of the patient? Is it for him or herself only, or for other care providers or researchers, as well? It may be that the record will be adequate for the originating physician. However, it may fall short of the needs of other care providers. This reality creates a constant tension regarding the setting standards for the completeness and quality of medical records. This is important, as the record may also be used for research, as a source of information about the benefits and harms of care and as the basis for studying the epidemiology (kind, prevalence and spread) of illness in the community.

A Framework for Understanding the Medical Record and its Limitations

If we look at the patient-observation-recording system a bit more abstractly (See Diagrams A and B), it is quite revealing. Think of the patient as a real-life, almost infinitely detailed composite of characteristics. Let's call this the 'Reality Model' of the patient. In observing and measuring this Reality Model, the physician perceives or captures a description of it as what we will call the limited 'Observed Model' or 'Descriptive Model' of the patient. This Descriptive Model is the one that exists in the physician's mind. Anything the physician missed observing or ignored will not be in that Descriptive Model. Anything the physician did not measure in enough detail will be kind of fuzzy in the Descriptive Model.

Next, the physician will record information in the medical record a variety of patient characteristics observed and measured, limited by the choices the physician makes as to what to record, as well as biases, inaccuracies, misstatements and misperceptions. In other words, the limited Descriptive Model in the mind of the physician will not be the same as the 'Recorded Model' captured in the record. It will be a sketchier-still version of reality.

These points are illustrated in FIGURE 1.28.1.

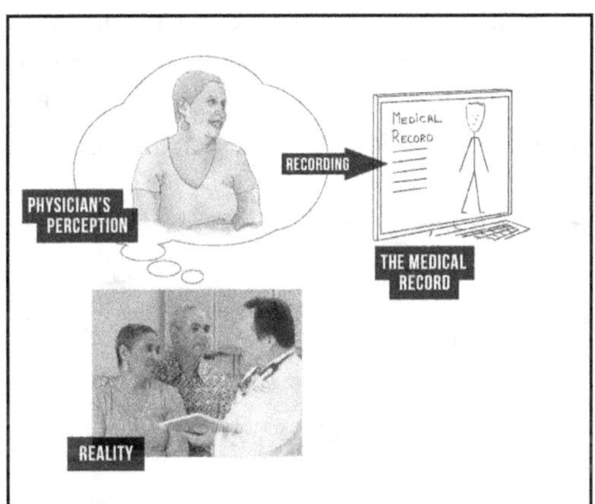

FIGURE 1.28.1: Medical Record Information is based on perception

There are interesting consequences of this way of looking at the medical record. For instance, the medical record is limited not only by what the physician has chosen to observe and measure (or has mis-observed or mis-measured). The medical record is also limited by what the patient reveals or keeps secret and which observations and measurements the physician has chosen to record. This means that the 'image' of the patient – the degree to which the record represents the real patient – is very limited in content, detail and in its temporality. The limitation in temporality refers to the fact that the observations recorded are instantaneous ones that occurred during the visit with the physician and ignore what happens between visits.

In optical science (See FIGURE 1.28.2), the study of lenses or equivalent modes of acquiring images has led to the definition of 'filtering'. Every lens to some degree 'filters' (enhances, blurs or eliminates) what's really out there in the scene. Furthermore, the recording mechanism, such as film or a digital imaging array must be recognized as doing filtering of even what comes through the lens. The imaging array or film may not be sensitive to certain levels and colors of light, for example. So, the image recorded is twice filtered. This is the exact situation that occurs in the patient-physician-record situation. It is even possible to apply some of the same theory to it. But we will spare you that for now!

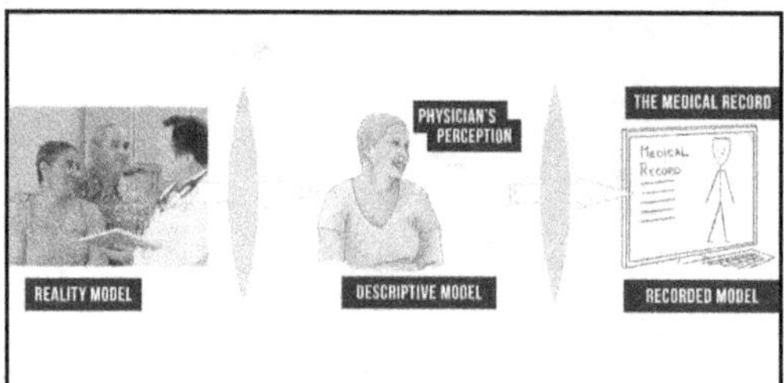

FIGURE 1.28.2: Record information is a filtered representation of reality

Recognizing the capabilities and limitations of the total 'imaging chain,' as it's called in optical science, is crucial for understanding the value of the medical record. The ultimate worth of the record is the productive use to which it is or can be put. The record, for example, of a specialist will be considered and used by the originating – 'referring' – physician (e.g., a General Practioner). If the referring physician goes back to the record at the next visit, the information from the specialist, that in the physician's memory and new statements by the patient at the follow up visit might augment what is actually in the record through the processes of recall and association. The problem is more acute in determining the real value of the record when used by other physicians, other care providers and researchers.

Others who use the record, do not have direct knowledge of the patient and cannot embellish what's in the record from recollections. Furthermore, other record users may color what's in the record with their own biases and misunderstandings, as well as recollections about their own patients, misinterpreting what's there.

There are Other Record Users and Interpreters

Researchers and health services administrators can use information in the health record to learn the relationships between clinical findings, the interventions applied in clinical care and the resultant health outcomes. However, what is actually included in the record constrains the researchers or Public Health analysts, for example, in their conclusions. If a patient died after being admitted for pneumonia and was treated with an antibiotic, but the physician treating the patient did not consider and document other possible causes, researchers will have no way of knowing that the cause of death might have been a pulmonary embolus or a reaction to the prescribed drug. On the other hand, conscientious clinicians may be reluctant to spend a lot of valuable clinical time including what for them might be superfluous detail in the record if there is little evidence that researchers or administrators make worthwhile use of the record.

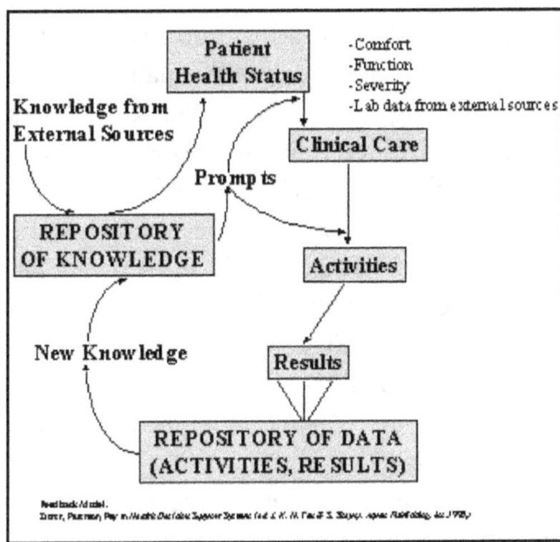

FIGURE 1.28.3: This diagram represents what happens in the doctor's office

SEE FIGURE 1.28.3

Data is collected by clinician on comfort, function and test results, which contribute to a severity estimate. Prompts to action are provided by electronic information systems or obtained from other sources (e.g., clinical guidelines or standards). The doctor makes clinical recommendations to the patient to undertake health care and personal activities. These recommendations influence the patient's health status and will ultimately generate a new set of information (results) about the patient's health. These results are later observed as changes in comfort, function and test results. All interventions and results from patients are captured and stored in a repository. Analytical methods are used to generate new knowledge based on the linking healthcare activities with healthcare results. This new knowledge contributes to a growing repository of knowledge about effective care. This repository of knowledge along with knowledge from external sources is used to generate new and more sophisticated prompts.

Detailed Structure of the Medical Record

In the days when medical records were on paper (and many records still are!), there were probably as many different ways of organizing the record as there were record keepers. Through time, however, it became clear that there should be standards as to what the contents of the record should be, how the record should be structured (like which sections, in what order), and even as to how certain meaningful connections (the fancy way of stating this is 'semantics') among record elements should be expressed. A great example of the latter was the work of Dr. Larry Weed on the Problem-Oriented Medical Record (POMR[143]), which he eventually embodied in an electronic system (PROMIS[144]) and application tools (Problem-Knowledge Couplers[145] – PKCs). His work enabled inter-record element references. He promoted the idea of making it clear as to which findings stimulated the physician to order a specific lab test and which symptom or finding a prescription targeted. He called the historical paper record a "medical-legal dumping ground" – sort of CYA for the physician – and described the POMR as enabling "records that guide and teach." Dr. Weed's life and its impacts merit a whole other book. There have been other like efforts, especially in the era of electronic records.

For our purposes here, refer to the list of record sections that follows. It contains common examples of contents.

143 Jacobs L. Interview with Lawrence Weed, MD — The Father of the Problem-Oriented Medical Record Looks Ahead. The Permanente Journal. 2009;13(3):84-89. https://www.ncbi.nlm.nih.gov/pmc/articles/PMC2911807/. Accessed July 19, 2022.

144 Schultz J. A History of the PROMIS Technology: An effective Human Interface. A History of Personal Workstations. 1988. New York. PP. 44-46. Available from: http://www.campwoodsw.com/mentorwizard/. Accessed July 19, 2022.

145 Burger C. The Use of Problem-Knowledge Couplers in a Primary Care Practice. The Permanente Journal. 2010;14(1):47-50. https://www.ncbi.nlm.nih.gov/pmc/articles/PMC2912707/. Accessed July 19, 2022.

Solutions Regarding the Use of Computers in Recordkeeping

When it comes to figuring out solutions to the productive use of computerization, we must realize that there are a lot of smart people working on the problem. They have recognized that the capture of medical records requires more robust methods.

Clearly, one partial solution is the implementation and use of dictation systems that are highly accurate, being particularly capable when it comes to medical terminology, drug names and doses. This will not help when the clinician is in public circumstances, however.

Some have suggested the use of machine learning or artificial intelligence capabilities (Can AI Fix Medical Records? C. Willyard, Sci Amer, pp S13-S16, Feb 2020). Properly implemented, these technologies might be able to locate information and extract it directly from other sources, such as laboratory and consultation reports coming from elsewhere. These tools could conceivably dissect out the specific information of relevance to the patient and place it into the record of the encounter. There is also the possibility that the system could, in the 'background' (processing independent of the user), analyze the existing patient record in the light of new information acquired during the encounter. It could use this to suggest specific investigations and even to propose a differential diagnosis to the clinician. One system (Saykara virtual assistant "Kara", www.saykara.com) already 'listens' to conversations, turns them into notes, diagnoses and orders that are put into the record. Robert Wachter at the University of California has pointed out that, regretfully, it and similar apps are "probably not quite ready for prime time" (ibidem, pg. S15). At the very least, tools like this could make the effort of data entry easier.

Work we have previously done suggests that we think through and specify the kinds of information needed at each patient encounter and create focused data collection efforts rather than either accepting arbitrary information or requesting masses of information. The magnitude of the kinds of information is a bit overwhelming, as FIGURE 1.28.3 shows. This would involve determining who will be using the data, what uses will be made of it and which information is most critical in achieving the effects desired. We have called this the "User, Uses, Effects Model" (Covvey, H.D., Berry, D., et al., Formal Structure for Specifying the Content and Quality of the Electronic Health Record", Requirements Engineering 2003, September 2003).

Short of brain-computer interfaces, which are actually being explored in research labs, one of the above suggestions is likely all we have to work with at this time. However, we need better than what we have!

The typical components of the health record include[146] the following:

1. **Patient Demographics:**
   - Age, gender, location.
2. **Chief Complaint:**
   - What the patient describes as the reason for the visit.
3. **History of the Presenting Illness:**
   - When it started, what seems to have brought the problem on, changes in environmental factors.
4. **Past Medical History: Medical Events in the Past.**
5. **Family History.**
6. **Social History.**
7. **Current List of Medications and Past Medications.**
8. **Allergies to Medication.**
9. **Other Allergies.**
10. **Review of Body Systems:**
    - Anatomical review, functional review, e.g., endocrine, reproductive system....
11. **Physical Examination.**
12. **Thoughts on Possible Reasons for the Patient's Problems.**
13. **Laboratory Tests Ordered to Help Support or Disprove the Diagnosis.**
14. **Diagnostic Test Results:**
    - Including results of biopsies and x-rays in order to help support or disprove the diagnosis.
15. **Problem List:**
    - List of patient's existing problems, list of ideas about diagnosis and treatment the clinicians plan to explore.
16. **Ongoing Clinical Notes:**
    - Progress notes describing course in hospital, reports from consultations, medications ordered, description of surgical procedure, description of other treatments including radiotherapy.
17. **Notes from Other Clinicians Including:**
    - Psychology, respiratory therapy, occupational therapy.

FIGURE 1.28.3: An overview of the content of a medical record

146 http://samples.jbpub.com/9781449652722/9781449645106_CH02_037_064.pdf. Accessed July 19, 2022.

Chapter 29: Addressing Differing Purposes for the Record

KEYWORDS: Medical Vocabulary, Standard Medical Terminology, Health Record Users

ABSTRACT: Researchers have made many efforts to develop standardized vocabularies to capture and code the information in medical records. The problem of efficient and reliable data collection and storage has not yet been adequately solved.

Users of the Medical Record and their Purposes

Those who care for patients will typically access the record using personal identifiers such as the patient's last and first name, perhaps augmented by other information to differentiate one patient from another (e.g., gender, date of birth, address). There is also usually some form of 'medical record number'.

The primary purpose of the health record is to document the continuing health status of the patient, the cause(s) of illness and the care provided to the patient. However, there are many other uses of the record. One example would be for a national healthcare monitoring agency to get information on large numbers of patients regarding events during visits or hospital stays. Another is for a Public Health agency to get information regarding the prevalence of disease, why and how patients were treated or how many were injured or died in the hospital. Yet another example would be for government administrators to obtain financial information, such as what patient care cost. To address the needs of these different types of users, a variety of 'Classification Systems' or terminologies have emerged.

Classification Systems and Coding

Each classification system serves a particular purpose, like the ones we mentioned. It should be obvious that these classification systems differ quite substantially from one another. Each of them has guidelines and criteria for the application of the terms in the system. One example is the International Classification of Diseases, or ICD in one of its versions, such as ICD-11[147], which the World Health Organization (WHO) uses.[148] A lesser-known one is the International Classification for Primary Care, ICPC[149], for primary care – the care doctors provide in general or family medical practice.

The inclusion in the record of terms from the ICD classification system allows governments, for example, to count how many patients have specific diseases and to determine

147 https://www.who.int/standards/classifications/classification-of-diseases. Accessed July 19, 2022.

148 Centers for Disease Control and Prevention, International Classification of Diseases, Ninth Revision (ICD-9). https://www.cdc.gov/nchs/icd/icd9.htm. Accessed July 19, 2022.

149 https://www.who.int/classifications/icd/adaptations/icpc2/en/. Accessed July 19, 2022.

how many patients have been treated for each disease. This means that researchers can enter a term into a computer and determine how many patients' records fall under that term, i.e., how many patients have a particular disease.

It is crucial that the terms of each classification system be very precisely defined and that the record is reviewed by a person or by a computer program to determine if those criteria have been satisfied. The patient's record must contain data that qualifies that record to be indexed under that term. Humans who carry out this task are called 'Coders' and typically have a formal background in Health Records Management (sometimes called 'Health Information Management'). They review the patient's record in detail and then associate one or more terms with that record or verify that a term included in the record was the correct one. As records have come to be recorded digitally, and as Natural Language Understanding (NLU, a sub-topic of Natural Language Processing – NLP) software has evolved to a state of usefulness, it is possible to use a program (software) to carry out the same task. A program of this type is called an 'Autocoder'. More and more examples are accumulating where autocoders demonstrate that they are, in many cases, at least as capable as the average human Coder in indexing a record.

One problem is that the information necessary to code a record and confirm diagnosis and treatment is often more than the information that clinicians needed to reach an appropriate diagnosis and prescribe treatment, so it wasn't recorded. This makes it difficult for researchers and administrators to mine clinical charts for reliable and useful information.

To appreciate this, consider the people whom you know and saw today. If someone asked you for a list of those people, it would not be difficult to create it by writing; "I saw Mary, Jane, Fred and Constance". However, if the person countered: "I want to confirm that it was really Mary you saw, please describe her ears, eyes, hair color and lips". That would be more difficult and certainly more time-consuming.

Similarly, clinicians can recognize many common clinical entities using pattern recognition, without the need to document a lot of data to help them come to that judgement. Indeed, excessive data capture might even interfere with pattern recognition[150] and sometimes increases the chances of an incorrect diagnosis. The downside is that no one else would be able to verify the full basis for the decision, potentially inhibiting the oversight of the clinician.

As clinical time becomes scarcer, clinicians resist taking the time to capture information for coding that is superfluous to care. For example, a clinician might recognize a benign, self-limited cold or upper respiratory infection without acquiring and recording all the information necessary to corroborate that diagnosis.

One solution is for assessors and researchers to form agreements with physicians to more thoroughly and formally document records on patients with problems of specific interest. Some researchers and private sector (drug companies and data collection companies like IQVIA) pay clinicians to capture very complete and detailed records on a small sample of their entire practice. They use statistical techniques to make inferences about the practice as a whole.

Formal Medical Vocabularies

It is clear that, for a person or a program to do proper coding, the record must contain the specific information required to justify the use of the index term (or sufficient other information exists in the record that implies the term). The closer the information in the record is to a formal terminology, the more likely it is that a Coder will properly associate terms with that

150 A. Schattner, Teaching clinical medicine: the key principals, QJM: An International Journal of Medicine, Volume 108, Issue 6, June 2015, Pages 435–442. https://academic.oup.com/qjmed/article/108/6/435/1548582. Accessed July 19, 2022.

record. In other words, it cannot be a guessing game, as it often is in the case of older patient records. This has led to efforts to have terms from standard vocabularies of medical terms be used in the record. Perhaps the best-known example of that is something called 'SNOMED', the Systematized NOmenclature of MEDicine, which uses a highly structured clinical vocabulary to record clinical information about patients. We are still quite a way from such formality, however. One study done in recent times indicated that Introducing SNOMED as a formal vocabulary into a single province of Canada would have a price tag of at least $65 million. A significant component of the cost is addressing physician education and guidance and the additional time it would take clinicians to complete a record. The best we can hope for now is that physicians use relatively standard wording. This would at least get us closer to the ability to index records using the most common classification systems.

The problem is that there is large variance in the use of terminology and many issues that frustrate the use of standard terminology, such as when we are still learning the underlying causes of some diseases.

Unifying the Babel of Terminologies

The fact that there are many different purposes for which different types of users actually use the record, has led to the emergence of tens of classification systems. An incredible piece of work has been carried out by the National Library of Medicine (NLM) in the United States to define and document the terms of these different classification systems and then to relate them to each other wherever that is possible. The product of this latter work is the Metathesaurus.[151] The Metathesaurus links terms in one classification system to terms in other classification systems using sophisticated language technology called 'Semantic Networks'. A semantic network expresses the relationship between one term and another. An example might be how a term in ICD-11 corresponds to a term in SNOMED. Another example of this is that a disease will be linked to the symptoms of the disease, and anatomical components (e.g., of the heart) will be related to each other, like that the heart valve is a <u>part of</u> the heart. This work is based on Artificial Intelligence and Computational Linguistics research and a rather esoteric area called 'Ontologies'. It is beyond our objectives here to get into details.

It is interesting to note that, today, we have programs that can access the world literature in Medicine indexed under key terms or 'keywords'. In addition, significant progress has also been made in Natural Language Processing to automatically index and summarize that literature. A person interested in medical records research will necessarily become an expert in Natural Language Understanding and its application to records, what we called 'autocoding'. This is an example where, when fully implemented, computerization will make medical records dramatically easier to access and analyze.

A PERSONAL STATEMENT BY DC AS A CLINICAL INFORMATICS RESEARCHER - ALBEIT RETIRED

Suggested Principles:

1. *Adequate (a fuzzy criterion) recordkeeping is essential for the care of the patient by the physician, by others and by the patient by him/herself. It is the communication nexus for continuity of care.*
2. *Taking adequate time and making an adequate effort (also fuzzy criteria) to care for the patient are also essential. Recordkeeping is the objective documentation of that care.*
3. *Accreditation agencies have a logical and defensible fiduciary responsibility and authority (by law) to define criteria as to the adequacy of*

151 https://www.ncbi.nlm.nih.gov/books/NBK9684/. Accessed July 19, 2022.

the record relative and certified physicians must accept this.

4. *Dealing with other matters like calming and comforting and otherwise accommodating the patient is surely at least important.*
5. *Similarly, enabling the physician to have an adequate level of practice to secure a living wage and still retain a sustainable personal life is also important.*
6. *Physicians deliberately chose and trained for this difficult career and must develop appropriate attitudes and skills to have a viable practice, care for patients and document that care.*

Position:

The physician must constantly strive to achieve a sustainable, dynamic balance influenced by all these factors. Sometimes records will need to be detailed/more comprehensive/deeper and sometimes not. The brevity of the record cannot be the objective nor an excuse. Nor can attention to the physician's record be permitted to compromise care.

Conclusion: *This is one (of many) of the reasons I am glad I am not a physician!*

Chapter 30: Performance Measurement

KEYWORDS: Performance Measures, Patients, Politicians, Journalists, Insurers, Educators, Lawyers, Health Services Administrators.

ABSTRACT: Many disciplines expect, report and use estimates of performance measurement. They need to understand and what is necessary to have reliable and meaningful assessments of overall institutional performance and the performance of clinical decision makers. Misusing the available data leads to unstable and possibly harmful assessments of institutional and individual performance and can lead to changes that might cause more harm than benefit.

Who Needs to Understand Health System Performance Measurement?

Everybody does!

And we mean everybody: doctors, patients, administrators, insurers, politicians, journalists, educators and lawyers are or should be interested in learning how the health system performs.

- Doctors want to learn how often patients are better or worse after treatment.
- Patients want to know if the doctors they choose are giving outstanding advice and realizing excellent results. Doctors also want to know this and be able to assure their patients about being well-served.
- Health services administrators, who allocate human, physical and financial resources to the health system, need to know if their spending is worthwhile and is achieving improved and not worse patient outcomes.
- Insurers and other agencies that pay for healthcare services share this need to know.
- Politicians need to know if their policies, plans and funding strategies for health care enhance or harm the health of their communities.
- Journalists and educators, who are watchdogs and who educate the public about health care, need to understand the nature and performance of the care system and its providers in order to critique the correctness of claims regarding individual and population outcomes and the efficiency and effectiveness of the health system.
- Last, but not least, lawyers need to know how one evaluates health system performance in order to participate in legal actions for any of the above.

All these stakeholders need a framework that helps them understand if a health outcome represents good or poor health services or merely luck.

What may be less obvious is that, despite good intentions, it is difficult to find reliable information about the performance of individual clinicians or of the health systems they work in. One reason is that most people working in health care are not particularly interested in the technicalities of performance measurement. Some cynics might even suggest that many clinicians and administrators don't benefit personally from performance measurement. Those systems or clinicians that are mediocre, or worse than mediocre might even feel threatened if the public knew how well or poorly the system works. Canadians and many Americans don't really have choices about which health system cares for them and knowing a system is doing poorly might make patients feel worse.

Performance Measurement AWOL

The cost and quality of health care are major issues in the United States and Canada. In America, people focus on what amounts to superfluous care, the increasing costs of care and health system error; in Canada, the focus is cost, rationed access and errors in care.

Yet, thoughtful, intelligent and well-meaning administrators and government regulators lack the information they need to evaluate the care of individuals, the efficiency of health system constituents and the impact of changes in policy on health care and health. Instead of having access to meaningful information, system decision-makers must use seat-of-the-pants determinations about how to organize or reorganize health care. The result is care that is expensive and often delivers results that leave lots of room for improvement.

What is the Origin of Information for Performance Measurement?

The goal of health care is to improve or maintain the health of individuals. At every medical visit, it is natural that clinicians assess and note the health of their patients. Evaluating health before, during and after treatment is the essence of clinical practice because clinicians cannot make recommendations to start, stop or continue treatments unless they know the current state of health of each patient.

Consequently, at each clinical visit, doctors gather information about their patients' comfort, function, life context and the results of investigations.

We lay this out in detail elsewhere in this book. See Chapter 15, for example, expands on the possible choices physicians can make at each visit. The Section on Measuring Health (Section 4) describes how we assess and quantify health, and the chapters on health records (Chapters 28 and 29) report the types of information clinicians usually collect and store.

Accurate performance measurement relies on:

> Doctors asking pertinent questions.

> Patients responding candidly to questions and providing complete accurate information.

> Clinicians capturing accurate information.

> Clinicians recording that information in a form accessible and analyzable later.

> Clinicians storing the information in record systems that enable them, colleagues who also care for the patient, researchers and administrators to aggregate the information from the patients treated by them and other clinicians.

> Decision-makers accessing that information and using formal methods to analyze, interpret and report it.

In addition, various entities (Public Health agencies, for example) do occasional surveys of communities to develop estimates of population health, including those who rarely see a clinician.[152] These surveys estimate the overall

152 https://www23.statcan.gc.ca/imdb/p2SV.pl?Function=getSurvey&Id=3359. An example is the Canadian Community Health Survey. Accessed July 19, 2022,

health of people in the community and the prevalence of various diseases.

Do we have any proxies that might at least give us an estimate of the performance of various population level health-related interventions?

Earlier, we recognized that that community context profoundly affects the health of people living in each community. We also realize that most of our taxes are not spent on the direct care of sick people but on other important community services (such as social programs, education, housing and economic development) that affect health.[153] Another chapter in this compendium includes more information on the determinants of health. Can we use the health of the community to get a measure of the effectiveness of these programs? Surely, the overall health of a community does provide at least an estimate of the effectiveness of this spending. For example, we know from studies that people who live in services-deprived communities often have higher levels of sickness and reduced lifespan. Governments are attempting to moderate these impacts through spending on those indirect services that influence health. The trick is to have some means of getting a first order assessment of community health that does not depend on mass data collection during the care process.

It may be that we can assess the status of health in communities indirectly in this information age. For instance, Google, Amazon, CVS Pharmacy and other companies that serve consumers, learn what people want or are worried about by analyzing what they search for and the types of health products they buy. We can do the same by analyzing illness-related purchasing in communities, thereby getting valuable insights into the epidemiology of illness. An increase in Google searches for flu symptoms, for instance, might suggest an increase in the prevalence of or at least concern about influenza in the community.

Considerations in the Use of Performance Measures: Overview

Clearly, patients and their doctors need to know about direct patient care. Specifically, they want to appreciate if their health results are better, worse or about the same compared to the results patients realize from other doctors and care agencies or compared to people who don't receive treatment.

Comparing clinicians with other clinicians and health systems with other health systems enables individuals and organizations to learn if they could or should do better. In the case of healthcare processes, copying – condemned as 'plagiarism' in the scientific literature but commended in healthcare administration – what other organizations do. Learning from what successful clinicians and excellent health organizations do is not merely acceptable, it's laudable! Imitation is not only the sincerest form of flattery; excellent performance is often the quickest path to being flattered.

The challenge comes in the development of reliable methods enabling comparisons that help us learn which individuals, health agencies or health systems achieve better results than others (FIGURE 1.30.1 emphasizes the need for formal measurement methods). Remember that the results of interventions relate not only to the intervention, but also to the initial health status of the people doctors treat. An obese individual with high blood pressure will generally be less healthy after treatment compared with a fit athlete who receives the same treatment for the same condition. A 95-year-old, regardless of the outcome of immediate care, will still have precarious health.

153 In 2021, the Nova Scotia government spent about 45% of its budget on health care, 14% on education and the remaining 41% was distributed among 19 other departments. Each department, including education, has some influence on community health.

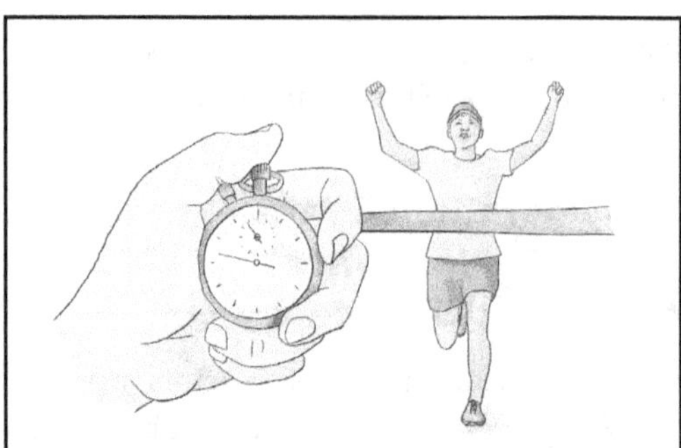

FIGURE 1.30.1: There are formal methods for measuring performance

Doctors and health organizations treating healthier people should expect to have better health outcomes. Useful comparisons must adjust for the initial health of the groups of people each organization treats.

ON READMISSION

Some health services administrators believe that patient readmission shortly after discharge is a marker of incomplete care or hurried discharge. However, unless there is an adjustment for the initial condition of the patients, the readmission rate information is not useful.

We would expect few otherwise healthy 42-year-old men to return to hospital soon after treatment for a simple or serious pneumonia. On the other hand, we might be surprised if an 88-year-old man with multisystem disease, also treated for pneumonia, did not return to hospital for something or other shortly after discharge. In fact, when very few older people return to hospital shortly after discharge, most would wonder if the low return numbers were not a marker of poor treatment or follow-up. Older people with complex disease who die before discharge cannot return to hospital shortly after discharge. Success in treating sick people with multiple conditions virtually guarantees that some will require readmission.

SEVERITY ADJUSTMENT PNEUMONIA AND DIABETES

Years ago, a system organized by the Canadian Institute for Health Information (CIHI) suggested that the in-hospital outcomes DZ achieved as a family doctor treating patients with pneumonia were better than those that several respiratory specialists achieved. More of his patients survived and those who lived had shorter stays in hospital. He was able to see these results because he chaired the hospital's quality committee.

DZ appreciated the seeming compliment, of course. However, he knew the real reason his patients were more likely to survive. DZ usually referred to specialists those people who had complicated or very difficult-to-treat pneumonias. Sometimes, the people he referred were patients who were not responding to conventional treatments. The Respirology specialists ended up responsible for the sicker patients who were more difficult to treat and therefore more likely to die. DZ's apparently better results were merely an indication that his own patients were less sick to begin with.

Similarly, DZ's results for diabetes seemed better than those achieved by an astute endocrinologist because he referred the sickest patients to the astute endocrinologist!

These results tweaked his interest in learning better ways of assessing health outcomes and determining how to adjust for illness severity.

The crude and minimally valuable measures of performance used by many health services administrators include such proxies as: how long people are in hospital, patient satisfaction, number of visits per patient, the number of prescriptions written, the number of patients the doctor cares for, readmission to hospital after discharge and survival. These measures are not useful unless there is a serious effort to measure and adjust for severity before treatment and to evaluate overall health after care. None, however, truly get at the actual results of treatments on the patients.

UNEXPECTED READMISSION TO HOSPITAL

The Canadian Institute for Health Information (CIHI) created a report titled "All-Cause Readmission to Acute Care and Return to the Emergency Department."[154] CIHI argued that unplanned readmissions to hospital have been identified as common, costly and potentially avoidable. However, CIHI recognizes that people who are sicker to begin with are more likely to require readmission. Patients most likely to be readmitted are older and sicker as validated by the number of previous hospitalizations and the number of illnesses they have. The unexpected readmission rate to a large extent reflects how sick patients are to begin with. Hospitals admitting healthier patients will have a lower readmission rate compared to hospitals that admit sicker patients. Sometimes readmission rate is an indicator of how sick people were when they were admitted to hospital and not necessarily an indicator of quality of care.

It is easy to understand that many of these proxies of performance do not relate to the most important questions, which are:

Are people healthier, sicker or the same after treatment and did the treatments make the difference?

Did patients achieve the best possible outcomes given their initial circumstances?

We often use indirect measures such as satisfaction, visits, length of stay in hospital or direct measures of changes in health associated with care. However, it is always essential to establish the person's health before treatment in order to predict and measure what health outcomes to expect. The patient's health has a major influence on the final result. It should be obvious that people who are near death are more likely to spend more time in hospital and receive more drugs and other interventions. People who have minor ailments are likely to spend little or no time in hospital, take fewer and less noxious drugs and have fewer investigations, particularly invasive ones. Consequently, evaluators must include health measures and risk factors at least before and after therapy. (This Section addresses Measures of Health. Also, Chapter 32 discusses the measures of risk and Chapter 37 addresses the expectations for the results of treatment especially related to age).

154 All-Cause Readmission to Acute Care and Return to the Emergency Department CIHI 2012. https://publications.gc.ca/collections/collection_2013/icis-cihi/H118-93-2012-eng.pdf. Accessed Sept 8, 2023.

Chapter 31: Understanding Medical Vocabulary

KEYWORDS: Medical Vocabulary, Jargon, Understanding Medical Vocabulary, Decoding Medicalese

ABSTRACT: Often clinicians use words that are difficult for patients to understand. However, most medical vocabulary is based on logic and the use of common roots. This chapter describes our methodology for understanding most medical words and presents a sampling and translation of the components of most medical words.

When we first look at the words of Medicine, they may seem to be hopelessly out of our reach. With a little understanding of how medical words are composed and why, however, medical vocabulary can be quite easy to understand.

However, communication in Medicine is crucial, as FIGURE 1.31.1 illustrates.

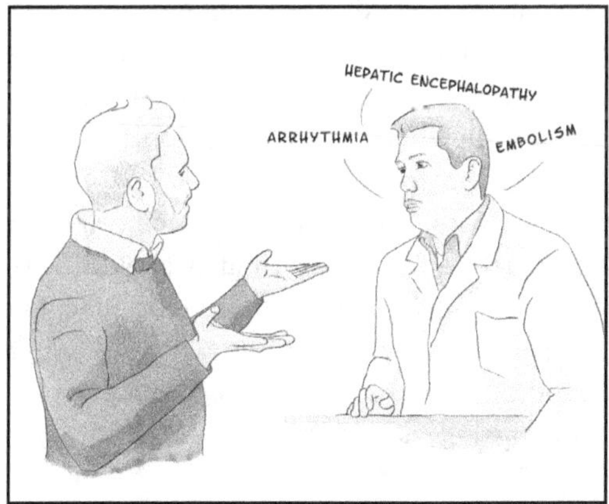

FIGURE 1.31.1: Communicating clearly with a patient can be challenging

A MEDICAL VOCABULARY LEARNING STORY

When DC left the physical sciences (Physics and Astrophysics) and worked as a grad student and then researcher in the medical sciences (cardiovascular mechanics), it was like going to a foreign country – the vocabulary, especially of Cardiology, seemed impenetrable! Worse still, the medical articles in the late 1960s and early 1970s were descriptive and quite vague and uninteresting to a researcher compared to Physics articles. He remembers many hours with dictionaries and medical texts trying to decipher the content of the literature. He was, however, fortunate (in more ways than one), in that he married a radiologist. Suddenly, he had a flesh and blood dictionary to which he could refer. Dinner became a vocabulary-learning experience, as well as the end of day recitation of the workday's events that had occurred in the Diagnostic Imaging department. This massively enhanced the process of learning medicalese. There is no better way to become familiar with a vocabulary than to be immersed in it. Perhaps the message is: marry into Medicine! It worked for Dominic.

The Foundations for Medical Vocabulary

First of all, it is enlightening to understand why medical words are composed of Latin and Greek parts. The truth is that, way back, only the highly educated, such as physicians, were able to read and write Latin. Having the vocabulary of Medicine in Latin placed it beyond the understanding of ordinary, pedestrian mortals. That allowed physicians to have a kind of secret code that not everyone could access unless they had special training or at least advanced education.

This is not so different from the way the Catholic Church originally treated the Bible. It, too, was in Latin, making it easy for the Church to keep to itself the reading and interpretation of the texts. Then Luther came along and translated the Bible into the vernacular German, causing incredible tumult in the world and leading to his being cursed by Rome. The intent of this little section is to show how anyone can figure out what medical words mean instead of having to depend on a medical expert – someone who speaks 'medicalese', as we say. There is a good reason, however, that some words remain in Latin to this day. The reason for that is to ensure precision in medical statements. Indeed, it would be hard to come up with words (or it would require many more of them) in English that carried the same density of meaning as typical medical terms.

A typical medical word is not so different from German words. It is commonplace in German for words to be composed of shorter words. Our favorite is 'Eisenbahnwagon.' This word in German is the concatenation of three smaller words 'Eisen' that means 'iron', 'bahn' that means road and 'Wagon' that means 'coach', producing the German word for a railroad car.

In the case of medical terms, typically they have a root, which is often anatomical and a prefix and a suffix that modify that root. A table is provided below that gives very common roots, prefixes and suffixes and, if you read it a few times, you will probably remember and understand a high percentage of the words you will come across in looking into Medicine.

Perhaps an example would be useful. 'Encephalitis' is a medical term, meaning an inflammation of what we call the 'encephalon', which includes the brain and the spinal cord. This term concatenates the root 'encephal' (for encephalon) with the suffix 'itis', which means inflammation. So, the word very precisely describes the inflammation of the brain and/or the spinal cord. Of course, the description can become more specific by prefixing the work 'viral' or 'bacterial', as in 'Viral Encephalitis', indicating the cause of the inflammation, a virus or a bacterium. One more well-known example is the medical term 'appendectomy.' This concatenates the root 'append' (for appendix) with the suffix 'ectomy' which means removal or extraction. So, an 'appendectomy' is the removal of the appendix. By the way, 'appendicitis' is the inflammation of the appendix. It's as simple as that!

Perhaps the easiest way to learn these words is to look up some examples of medical words and dissect them or try creating some of your own words (fun can be had doing this! Consider words like: 'spouse-ectomy' – divorce; 'bronchodilator' – device for fattening a horse; 'supraman' – you have to look up to see him. You can do the rest).

We do not intend that you memorize the table in FIGURE 1.31.2, but it should help. Together with looking up words you come across, the table will serve as your secret decoder ring – removing a barrier to understanding the nature of Medicine.

Same for All Systems		Vary by System		Same for All Systems	
Prefix	**Meaning**	**Root**	**Meaning**	**Suffix**	**Meaning**
a/an	Without, Absent	**Nervous System**		aspir/o	Removal
ab		auro/oto	Ear	ectomy	Removal, Excision, Resection
andro	Male, Masculine	encephalo	Brain, Spinal cord	gram/graphy	Recording process
anterior	Front, Nearer the front	meningo	Membrane covering brain and spinal cord	genic	Produced by or in
articular	Joint, Relating to joint(s)	neuro	Nerve	iasis	Abnormal condition
auto	Spontaneous, Self-caused	oculo/ ophthalmo	Eye	itis	Inflammation
carcino	Cancer, Cancerous			megaly	Enlargement
con	With	**Respiratory System**		osis	Abnormal condition
costal	Ribs, Related to the ribs	broncho	Bronchial tube to lung	otomy	Cut into, Make incision
dorso, dorsal	Of, to, or on the back	naso	Nose		
endo	Within	respiro/ pulmono	Breath, Breathing, Lung		
gyneco	Female, Related to women				
idio	One's own, Private, Personal, Peculiar to one	**Cardiovascular System**			
medio	Middle	aorto	Aorta (largest artery)		
mega	Big, Abnormally large	arterio	Artery		
muta	Change, Genetic Change	cardio	Heart		
posterior	Back of, Behind	hemato	Blood		
pyo	Pus, Infection	vasculo	Blood vessel		
stenotic	Narrowed, Constricted	veno	Vein		
sub	Under, Below				

supra	Above, Upper	**Digestive System**			
tempo-ral, temporo	Pertaining to the temple (head), or to time	ano/ recto/ procto	Anus, Rectum		
ventral, ventro	Front-side of body	dento/denti	Teeth		
		esophago	Esophagus		
		gastro/ entero /viscero	Stomach, Intestines, Internal Organs		
		hepato	Liver		
		oro	Mouth		
		pancreato	Pancreas		
		Urinary System			
		reno	Kidney		
		Reproductive System			
		genito	Reproduction-related		
		masto/mamo	Breast		
		testiculo	Testicles		
		utero	Uterus		
		Endocrine System			
		endocrino	Endocrine system (hormones)		
		Immune + Lymphatic System			
		immuno	Immune, Protection		
		lympha	Lymphatic		
		Muscular System			
		ligamento	Ligament		
		myo/musculo	Muscle		
		tendino	Tendon		

		Skeletal System			
		arthro	Joint		
		brachio, brachi	Arm		
		carpo	Wrist bones		
		cranio	Skull, Head		
		phalango	Finger, Toe		
		spin/o	Spine		
		tars/o	Foot, Ankle		
		Integumentary System			
		dermat/o	Skin		
		sarc/o	Flesh, Connective tissue		
		General Anatomy			
		abdomen/o	Abdomen		
		thorac/o	Thorax, Chest		
		Miscellaneous			
		caries	Cavities		
		Path/o	Disease		

FIGURE 1.31.2: Understanding medical terms

VOLUME 1

Section 5

HEALTH PREVENTION AND MAINTENANCE

A CHECKUP

An 80-year-old man is having his annual check-up. The doctor asks him how he's feeling. "I've never been better!" he replies. "I've got an 18-year-old bride who's pregnant and having my child! What do you think about that?" The doctor considers this for a moment, then says, "Well, let me tell you a story. I know a guy who's an avid hunter. He never misses a season. But one day he's in a bit of a hurry and he accidentally grabs his umbrella instead of his gun. So, he's in the woods, and suddenly a grizzly bear appears in front of him! He raises up his umbrella, points it at the bear, and squeezes the handle. The bear drops dead in front of him." That's impossible, said the 80-year-old! Someone else must have shot that bear." "Exactly!" The doctor replied.

Source: http://www.jokes4us.com/medicaljokes/80yearoldjoke.html. Accessed July 19, 2022.

What Did Monica Gain or Lose?

Everyone wants to stay healthy and avoid disease. We believe that disease prevention is better than cure and most believe that screening for disease leads to early detection of potential disease and reduced harm. Monica's experience with screening raises concerns.

Monica, a sunscreen-wearing, energetic, fit, 55-year-old senior executive walked or ran regularly in the California sunshine. She was part of a community that was concerned about health and determined to retain fitness and function while aging well. She went for medical check-ups, once or twice a year, more when suggested by her doctor.

She told me that on her doctor's advice, and despite a well-balanced diet, she routinely took Vitamin D and Calcium supplements. She understood the supplements would improve bone fitness and help her avoid osteoporosis. Several years previously she said her doctor remarked that a blood test showed she had decreased levels of Vitamin D. (Something that is possible but highly unlikely in a healthy woman who spends lots of time outdoors in the California sun).

After taking Vitamin D and Calcium for several years her doctor recommended screening for heart disease and found evidence of calcification in her coronary arteries. Her doctor correctly noted that coronary artery calcification "is often associated with major adverse cardiovascular events".

Monica related her story because she was frightened by her doctor's recommendation that she had become a candidate for cholesterol lowering medication and possibly for a coronary artery stent.

Monica did what was necessary, she ate well, exercised, and did not smoke or drink much alcohol. She believed that medical screening would be beneficial. The result was she took Vitamin D, a supplement we now know, is of little or no use in preventing osteoporosis or fractures.

Worse still, and apart from the issue of how Vitamin D and Calcium supplementation contributes to coronary artery calcification there is the question of whether the coronary artery calcification is important for an athletic person like Monica.

One recent study, for instance, reported that people with a life-long history of exercise had increased signs of coronary atherosclerotic plaques with a more benign composition. They concluded endurance athletes have increased longevity despite "the presence of more coronary atherosclerotic plaque in the most active participants."

Chapter 32: Health Promotion, Disease Prevention and Health Maintenance

KEYWORDS: Risk Factors, Biomarkers, Health Maintenance, Disease Prevention, Health Promotion, Cholesterol Paradox, Accumulation of Deficits, Apache System for Neonatal Assessment

ABSTRACT: People want to understand, maintain and improve their physical and mental health. Many tools, some examples of which we include in this chapter, enable clinicians and patients to estimate their own health. We also address the changes in lifestyle or treatment that can help to maintain and improve health.

Why We Go to Doctors

Sometimes people go to a doctor for what amounts to a social visit: they need human contact! However, most people visit a doctor because they want to live longer, be more active or feel better. People also go to learn what to do to maintain their health, hoping that a physical exam, questions – and answers – from the doctor and appropriate laboratory tests will find hidden problems that will be resolved before causing serious damage. In other words, they are worried about the unknown.

Although everyone knows that researchers are still dreaming of discovering a latter-day version of Ponce De Leon's fountain of youth, some believe that doctors have access to a reasonable facsimile of its waters. They believe that regular and comprehensive checkups are always good and that the doctor can usually do something to help maintain their health and prolong their lives. Quite a few also believe that various nutritional compounds, marketed and sold by health food stores, drug stores and some clinics will prevent and cure illness.

Sadly, doctors do not always help. Something as simple as a checkup or screening test for a disease might, in fact, cause harm. In the real world, screening and diagnostic tests sometimes produce worrisome false alarms – indicating that a healthy person is sick – or mistaken reassurance that someone is healthy despite having a medical condition.

Then there is all the hype about preventing disease. This hype often side-steps valid preventive interventions like stopping smoking or becoming fit. Instead, much propaganda about disease prevention is based on untested commercial tonics, guru-sourced 'secret ingredients,' potions or even strongly held beliefs that lack research support. We all see this in TV ads: diet supplements for enhancing memory, a rare vegetable or a veggie extract only available from a certain company, a treatment that reverses your chromosomes' age. Think of it and someone's already marketing it!

OK: AN EXAMPLE

Are you 'Eyelash Impaired'? People noticed that a drug used to treat glaucoma, a disease of the eye that can cause blindness, stimulated the growth of eyelashes. Its generic name is 'bimatoprost'. However, it is now marketed as a cosmetic. 'Latisse' is its brand name – it can treat "inadequate eyelashes" (there is even a medical term for that: hypotrichosis), which for some might be a problem. Not being able to bat one's eyelashes could ruin an attempt to initiate a relationship, for sure! This drug is used as a cosmetic despite side effects, including inflammation, dry eyes and hair growth around the eyes.

Usually, the advertisements for these agents include the disclaimer "not evaluated by the Food and Drug Administration or Health Canada," but not always. However, there are some well-tested and proven recommendations regarding what people can do to maintain their health and overall energy. They only require discipline, and the savings from avoiding useless nostrums may help preserve your retirement funds.

It turns out that annual checkups are the most frequent reason for visits to a doctor. Here again, though, there are issues. Checkups have major time and money implications, despite the evidence showing they are usually of little or no benefit.[155] [156] FIGURE 1.32.1 drives this home.

The best reason for going to a doctor is obvious. Patients with a problem or those with risk factors for an illness should see their doctor. However, seeing your doctor because of a problem is very different from seeing the doctor for a checkup just in case you have a hidden problem. The process of having a medical assessment when people have no signs or symptoms that concern them is called 'screening'. A chapter in this book discusses issues in screening and the differences between cause-finding and screening tests. The gist is that only some screening is of objective value.

This chapter relates to the things people must consider when they are motivated to maintain or improve their health while avoiding an unnecessary medical visit.

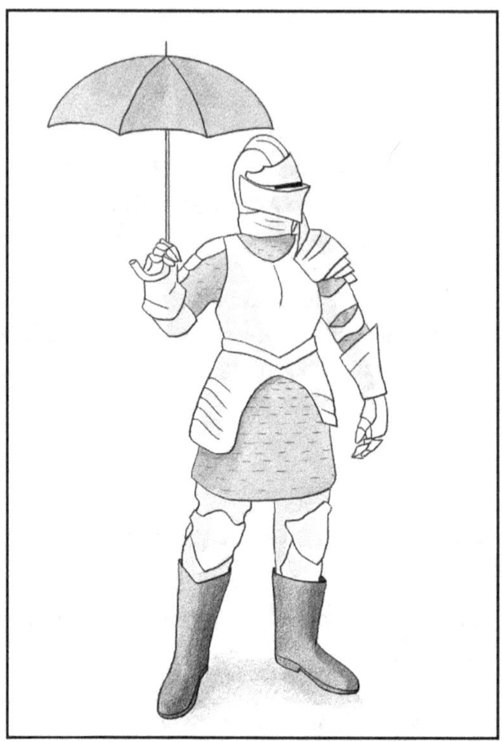

FIGURE 1.32.1: One can overdo self-protection

Understanding Risk Factors is Key to Maintaining and Improving Health! What are Risk Factors?

Risk factors are measurable characteristics of people or their environment that influence their health. They include measures of biology, comfort, function, mental status, community

155 Annual check-ups aren't needed, US study says; BMJ: British Medical Journal. Sept 29, 2007; 335(7621)631 http://www.ncbi.nlm.nih.gov/pmc/articles/PMC1995475/. Accessed July 19, 2022.

156 Mehrotra A, Zaslavsky AM, Ayanian JZ. Preventive Health Examinations and Preventive Gynecological Examinations in the United States. Arch Intern Med.2007;167(17):1876-1883. doi:10.1001/archinte.167.17.1876. http://archinte.jamanetwork.com/article.aspx?articleid=486857. Accessed July 19, 2022.

context and laboratory and imaging. To be as clear as possible, we really should distinguish the 'factor' from the 'risk'. Blood pressure is a factor, while high blood pressure or low blood pressure are the risks. We call the high BP or low BP 'risk factors'. The same applies to cholesterol.

Risk factors have many names. These include deficiencies, failings, hazards, perils, dispositions, vulnerabilities and susceptibilities. A risk factor is a characteristic, behavior or a condition that can dispose an individual to a disease, disability, discomfort or death. There are also 'health factors'. These are characteristics of an individual that predispose to longer, more functional and happier lives. Genetics, home environment and personal habits contribute to measures that predict health including lower cholesterol, lower weight and lower resting pulse rate.

Medications are often used to moderate risk factors. Unfortunately, medications are risk factors on their own because they expose people to possible harm. People who have normal blood pressure and normal cholesterol levels without needing medicine are generally healthier compared with those who must take medication in order to achieve the same normal values.

We have touched on these before. Examples of risk factors or deficits include increased waist size, abnormal pulse or respiratory rate, abnormal laboratory test results, fatigue and slow walking speed.[157] Many of these measures, along with objective signs, symptoms and the results of laboratory tests contribute to the information that Rockwood and Mitniski[158] include in their frailty index and use to predict survival or death. Their predictive models provide formal assessments of health and survival. Informal measures can use the same basis.

Statisticians have developed several ways to estimate survival including "Cox's Proportional-Hazards Model,' Cumulative Hazard Function H(t), hazard ratio, Kaplan–Meier Method, and a Log Rank Test".[159] It is not the purpose of this book to describe statistical methods in detail. However, it is useful for everyone, especially clinicians and health informaticians, to understand that these methods exist and how they are used.

The simple idea is that health care and a person's own actions, behavior, heredity and nutrition influence the chances that person will develop a 'defect' or condition.

How Do Doctors Assess Health and Risk?

When people ask for information about their health, they are pursuing the conclusions that doctors reach from an understanding of risk factors. At each visit, doctors obtain information about one or more risk factors.

Doctors collect information about risk factors the first time they see a patient and at each subsequent visit. The information is necessary to inform diagnoses and to formulate treatment strategies at every visit. Depending on the risk factors assessed at each visit, doctors will adjust their diagnoses and decide which treatments to start or to continue and which to stop or modify.

Most people are familiar with the important risk factors that influence their own health. Other, more obscure information, including

157 Middleton A, Fritz SL, Lusardi M. Walking speed: the functional vital sign. J Aging Phys Act. 2015 Apr;23(2):314-22. doi: 10.1123/japa.2013-0236. Epub 2014 May 2. PMID: 24812254; PMCID: PMC4254896. https://pubmed.ncbi.nlm.nih.gov/24812254/. Accessed Sept 8, 2023.

158 García-González JJ, García-Peña C, Franco-Marina F, Gutiérrez-Robledo LM. A frailty index to predict the mortality risk in a population of senior Mexican adults. BMC Geriatr. 2009; 9:47. Published 2009 Nov 3. doi:10.1186/1471-2318-9-47. https://www.ncbi.nlm.nih.gov/pmc/articles/PMC2776593/. Accessed July 19, 2022.

159 Statistics Review 12: Survival Analysis, Bewick, V., Cheek, L, and Ball, J., Critical Care, 2004, 8(5), 389-394. (http://www.ncbi.nlm.nih.gov/pmc/articles/PMC1065034/. Accessed July 19, 2022.

laboratory test results are not easily accessible to most people.

Obesity is an important risk factor (obesity is a high value of the factor 'weight'). People who are obese, with a large waist and who do not exercise, know they face an increased risk of heart attack, stroke, diabetes and the full list of lifestyle diseases. A visit to the doctor might reinforce the notion but most people know what they need to do. Some risk factors are just plain obvious.

RISK FACTOR ANECDOTE

Recently, someone asked DZ if her relative should have a "check-up" for heart disease. The relative, in his early 60's, is a smoker who does not exercise and wears 44-inch waist-size pants. He does not really need a "checkup" because everyone knows he is a ticking time bomb and that lifestyle changes are necessary. However, seeing a doctor might reinforce the time bomb notion, and the doctor could screen for other conditions, including thyroid disease, which lead to lethargy and obesity.

On the other hand, people who are lean and energetic in their daily life are less likely to develop heart disease, diabetes or respiratory conditions. People like this, even with high cholesterol and no other risk factors, have only a remote chance of experiencing a heart attack or stroke and treating raised cholesterol will not make much of a difference for these people.

The Cholesterol Paradox

High cholesterol is considered to be another risk factor, and low cholesterol can be as well. An interesting analysis, published in the Journal of Insurance Medicine[160] by Drs. Wesley and Cox, reported excess mortality not only for people at the highest level of blood cholesterol but also at the lowest level. Insurance companies make financial bets (read that as 'sell insurance at a given price') based on their beliefs and knowledge regarding an individual's expected longevity. Their financial success depends on accurate assessment of risk, so it is important for them to know which groups of people are likely to have the longest or shortest survival.

The authors of the article reported the paradoxical finding that people with very low cholesterol levels also have increased mortality! It seems that both high cholesterol and low cholesterol are accepted risk factors for illness. Usually, clinicians tell patients about the risks of high cholesterol, not low, although research suggests that patients with low cholesterol may also be at higher risk for accidental or violent death.[161] [162] [163] Community studies and meta-analysis (a formal comparison of the data and results of multiple high-quality clinical trials) of many research reports, suggest that "adjusting for other factors, low cholesterol is associated with increased subsequent criminal violence".[164] Of course, it could be that criminals who are lean and energetic also have low cholesterol and are more able to be violent compared

160 Wesley, D., Cox HF., Modeling total cholesterol as predictor of mortality: the low-cholesterol paradox, J Insur Med. 2011;42(2-4):62-75. Accessed Aug 4, 2014. http://www.ncbi.nlm.nih.gov/pubmed/21888191. Accessed July 19, 2022.

161 Golomb, B.A., Stattin H., Mednick, S., Low cholesterol and violent crime. J Psychiatr Res. 2000 Jul-Oct;34(4-5):301-9.http://www.ncbi.nlm.nih.gov/pubmed/11104842. Accessed July 19, 2022.

162 Neaton JD, Blackburn H, Jacobs D, et al. Serum Cholesterol Level and Mortality Findings for Men Screened in the Multiple Risk Factor Intervention Trial. *Arch Intern Med.* 1992;152(7):1490–1500. http://www.ncbi.nlm.nih.gov/pubmed/1627030?dopt=Abstract. Accessed July 19, 2022.

163 Repo-Tiihonen E, Halonen P, Tiihonen J, Virkkunen M. Total serum cholesterol level, violent criminal offences, suicidal behavior, mortality and the appearance of conduct disorder in Finnish male criminal offenders with antisocial personality disorder. Eur Arch Psychiatry Clin Neurosci. 2002 Feb;252(1):8-11. https://pubmed.ncbi.nlm.nih.gov/12056583/. Accessed Sept 8, 2023.

164 Golumb, BA, Stattin, H., Mednick, S., Low Cholesterol and Violent Crime J Psychiatr Res. 2000 Jul-Oct;34(4-5):301-9. https://www.ncbi.nlm.nih.gov/pubmed/11104842. Accessed July 19, 2022.

with obese criminals with high cholesterol. It's hard to know.

This increased chance of death in people with low cholesterol appears might also be associated with poor nutritional state (that can also cause low cholesterol), such as found in some cancers.

BRAIN EFFECTS OF CHOLESTEROL-LOWERING DRUGS

In 1995, as a family doctor, DZ, was able to introduce Dr. Sethu Reddy, an endocrinologist, to Dr. Pat McGrath, a research psychologist working with Dr. Karina Davidson. The group explored changes in the mood in patients who received cholesterol-lowering drugs and found evidence that some people suffer from increased feelings of depression when they use these drugs.[165] *Recently, the American Food and Drug Administration (FDA) commented: "Cognitive (brain-related) impairment, such as memory loss, forgetfulness and confusion, has been reported by some statin users."*[166] *The brain is 60% fat and most of it is cholesterol. So, it is not surprising that investigators are interested in the influence of cholesterol levels on brain function. It is always important to weigh the possible benefits and risk of drug interventions and the chances of each outcome with and without the drug.*

Some have claimed that criminals with low cholesterol are more likely to die from accidents and violence. So, another possible cause for the increased death rate is the influence of low cholesterol on mood. However, it is also plausible that people with anti-social and violent tendencies who have low cholesterol – sometimes thought to be a marker for fitness – are more fit, and consequently can more easily participate in risky behavior. You can see the challenge of coming to conclusions about causality.

Personal Devices Provide Feedback

Entrepreneurs build fortunes on tools that satisfy our need for timely information about our health. Academics, including health informaticians, continue to develop techniques that capture information about people and use the information to measure their current health, as well as to predict their futures.

The Fitbit is a popular device that measures activity (required to stay healthy) and provides timely feedback on measures of health, including the quality of sleep and pulse rate. Sleep quality[167] and resting pulse rate[168 169] are important measures of health – poor sleep or high resting pulse are risk factors. These factors make important contributions to assessments of current health and to predictions of life expectancy. Remember, people who regularly partake in rigorous exercise are more likely to

165 Behav Med. 1996 Summer;22(2):82-4. Increases in depression after cholesterol-lowering drug treatment. Davidson KW[1], Reddy S, McGrath P, Zitner D, MacKeen W. http://www.ncbi.nlm.nih.gov/pubmed/8879460. Accessed August 26, 2022.

166 http://www.fda.gov/forconsumers/consumerupdates/ucm293330.htm. FDA Expands Advice on Statin Risks. Accessed June 7, 2015.

167 Pilcher JJ, Ott ES. The relationships between sleep and measures of health and well-being in college students: a repeated measures approach. Behav Med. 1998 Winter;23(4):170-8.http://www.ncbi.nlm.nih.gov/pubmed/9494694. Accessed July 19, 2022.

168 Hsia J, Larson JC, Ockene JK, Sarto GE, Allison MA, Hendrix SL, Robinson JG, Lacroix AZ, Manson JE. Resting heart rate as a low-tech predictor of coronary events in women: prospective cohort study. *BMJ*, 2009; 338: b219. https://pubmed.ncbi.nlm.nih.gov/19193613/. Accessed August 26, 2022.

169 Li YQ, Sun CQ, Li LL, Wang L, Guo YR, You AG, Xi YL, Wang CJ. Accessed July 19, 2022. Resting heart rate as a marker for identifying the risk of undiagnosed type 2 diabetes mellitus: a cross-sectional survey. BMC Public Health. 2014 Oct 9;14:1052. http://www.biomedcentral.com/1471-2458/14/1052. Accessed August 26, 2022.

have the lower resting pulse rates[170] [171]and that is associated with greater longevity.

Everyone recognizes that efforts to improve health are successful when they reduce or eliminate the risk factors that predict sickness and improve the factors that predict health and greater longevity. Exercise is an activity that is clearly associated with an improvement in markers for better health and fortunately also with improved comfort, function and lifespan.

Accumulation of Deficits with Age

We have cited the work of Drs. Ken Rockwood and Arnold Mitniski who used elegant statistical methods[172] to demonstrate how to estimate health and to predict and improve life expectancy. Rockwood, a Geriatric Medicine expert and Mitniski, a mathematician, suggest that as people get older, they accumulate defects in an unpredictable way. As the number of defects increases, the chance of accumulating even more defects increases, as does the chance of death and disability. Some of these defects are controllable by changing what we do and how we live and, sometimes, by taking medication.

Capturing Information Like This

Capturing information from clinical encounters supports communication between providers. This information is the essential contributor to models that predict which treatments are most likely to be effective. Just as retailers learn about their customers to predict what they will buy at Christmas time, so health researchers try to capture information from population surveys and from clinical encounters to learn about patients and to understand and predict future health.

Health researchers and informatics experts capture longitudinal measures of health (health factors) and link them to present and future health status. The essence of the process of developing each method is learning how various factors contribute to increases or decreases in medical events and survival, what happens when people have several risk factors and when prescribed treatments produce better or worse overall health.

Researchers produce predictive models by noticing that events, like strokes, are correlated with sets of human variables (like being overweight or having diabetes) and then encoding that correlation in mathematical functions. Values from other patients can then be entered into the model to obtain an estimate of the probability a new patient will experience similar events. The common element of each model is a reliance on signs, symptoms, lab values, cultural and community factors and the health history of relatives. Models like these were extraordinarily important in the recent COVID-19 pandemic. They were used to predict mortality of the population and how measures like wearing masks might save lives.[173]

170 Oh D-J, Hong H-O, Lee B-A. The effects of strenuous exercises on resting heart rate, blood pressure, and maximal oxygen uptake. Journal of Exercise Rehabilitation. 2016;12(1):42-46. doi:10.12965/jer.150258. https://pubmed.ncbi.nlm.nih.gov/26933659/. Accessed Sept 8, 2023.

171 Cornelissen, V A Verheyden, B Aubert, A E, Fagard, R H, Effects of aerobic training intensity on resting, exercise and post-exercise blood pressure, heart rate and heart-rate variability Journal of Human Hypertension-2009/06/25/online. https://www.nature.com/articles/jhh200951. Accessed July 19, 2022.

172 Arnold Mitnitski, Le Bao, Kenneth Rockwood "Going from bad to worse: A stochastic model of transitions in deficit accumulation, in relation to mortality, Mechanisms of Ageing and Development 127 (2006) 490–493. https://www.sciencedirect.com/science/article/abs/pii/S0047637406000273. Accessed July 19, 2022.

173 https://covid19.healthdata.org/global?view=total-deaths&tab=trend. Accessed July 19, 2022.

Some Examples of Tools that Use Risk Factors to Monitor Sickness and Predict Health

The APACHE (Acute Physiology and Chronic Health Evaluation) score is used in intensive care units. It measures factors such as age, temperature, blood pressure, respiratory rate and the level of various substances in the blood and computes a severity score and the chances of mortality. The 'md+calc' website[174] shows APACHE and many other useful medical calculators. The common feature of these calculators is the ability to take information about a person and to generate predictions about their future health.

The md+calc website (http://www.mdcalc.com/) will be of particular interest because it includes a number of calculators that enable clinicians to estimate the chances that a patient has a particular diagnosis. The system works, like most others, by encouraging the user to insert patient characteristics and then using this information to calculate a probability score for health or survival.

In addition, the American Heart Association provides a spreadsheet for patients and clinicians (https://professional.heart.org/professional/GuidelinesStatements/ASCVDRiskCalculator/UCM_457698_ASCVD-Risk-Calculator.jsp) that enables people to enter the measures of their own risk factors including cholesterol levels, blood pressure, treatments for blood pressure, smoking history and presence or absence of diabetes to get an estimate of their chances of developing cardiovascular disease in the next 10 years or over their lifetime.

Thinking About Risk Factors and Their Treatment

Understanding the meaning and value of risk factors and their treatment can be complicated. Let's consider cholesterol as a case in point.

On its own, lower cholesterol is associated with lower risk of heart attack and stroke. However, as we have mentioned, many people, especially younger adults who are physically active and of normal weight, have a very small chance of suffering from a heart attack or stroke even if they have high cholesterol levels. Starting cholesterol medication (called 'statins') in a physically active young person may not be of any benefit and prolongs their exposure to the drug. This may even apply to older people (unless their blood looks like a milkshake – blood with really high cholesterol looks like that). Furthermore, it will likely be many years before we know through research if the benefits of statins outweigh the harms.

For active, otherwise-healthy people (those without 'serum milkshake'!), the potential benefit from a cholesterol-lowering medication does not warrant the risk of muscle inflammation, liver disease or diabetes, which can be consequences of taking the drug. To rationally justify taking a medication to reduce risk, it is necessary to know about the risk at the start and the change in risk from taking a drug. If the cholesterol is very high, the risk of a heart attack or other major event is high and taking the drug is indicated. If it isn't and if there is a reasonable chance or the occurrence of an adverse event (like muscle damage), it does not make sense to take the drug. Absorbing the cost of the drug in that case also makes no sense.

Assessing the benefits and harms associated with taking a drug to reduce cholesterol is not simple because a drug may (or may not) reduce the risk of a major medical event. Moreover, the person taking the drug is subject to a different risk, the one associated with the medication. It is a balance of probabilities. People must ask: what is the chance of having a heart attack or a stroke and what is the chance of the drug harming them? They must decide if they will be better off overall or worse off.

174 http://www.mdcalc.com/. Accessed November 8, 2014.

Some will come down in favor of the medication because the harm of taking it is perceived to be less than the harm of not taking it. It is unfortunate that, sometimes, the harms caused by drugs are pretty significant, like triggering diabetes. However, there is one more important consideration: the evidence, especially in asymptomatic patients, that the drug will actually prevent the feared major medical event. Regretfully, this evidence is often lacking! Evidence may, for instance, indicate the drug might help people who have had a previous heart attack but be lacking for someone who has not already had a heart attack.

This is another example of patients making a wager. Should they bet on the benefits of the drug (i.e., that it will prevent a heart attack) and that there will be no or minimal harm from it? Or should they bet that they won't have a heart attack or that the drug will harm them or might not work? Of course, like in a casino, there are no guarantees whichever way we bet. To make a safer bet, people must consider what research reveals are their odds. Does the drug 'load' the dice in their favor? Or should they not take chances by avoiding the craps table? At the very least, patients should ask their doctors about the evidence indicating the risks associated with accepting or rejecting an intervention. How many people in their circumstance benefited and how many were harmed?

Patients rarely ask and doctors usually do not volunteer the chances of benefit and harm from taking cholesterol-lowering medication, for example. Most regard low cholesterol as better than high and never bother to ask about the expected effects.

More About Cholesterol

The cholesterol story is an excellent example of how important it is to consider the overall promise of benefit and harm when clinicians suggest treatment. The following is one answer to the question of the value of statins for people who have high cholesterol but lack other risk factors.

Research[175] shows that, over 5 years: (1) no deaths are prevented if people with high cholesterol take a cholesterol lowering drug, (2) that about 1 in 100 patients (1%) will avoid a non-fatal heart attack and (3) about 1 in 150 patients (0.6%) will avoid a non-fatal stroke. On the other hand, 1 in 50 patients (2%) are harmed because they develop diabetes and one in 10 people (10%) are harmed because they develop muscle damage. Remember that some patients may have fatal strokes and that a non-fatal stroke isn't something to be joyous about either.

Another consideration is that the brain produces and uses more cholesterol than most other organs. Therefore, it is hardly surprising that recent research suggests that drugs, such as statins, which reduce cholesterol production are associated with reduced brain function as measured by tests of short-term memory.[176]

175 http://www.thennt.com/nnt/statins-for-heart-disease-prevention-without-prior-heart-disease/. Accessed July 19, 2022. Statins given for 45 years for heart disease prevention (without known heart disease).

176 Statins given for 45 years for heart disease prevention (without known heart disease). Strom BL, Schinnar R, Karlawish J, Hennessy S, Teal V, Bilker WB. Statin Therapy and Risk of Acute Memory Impairment. JAMA Intern Med. Published online June 08, 2015. doi:10.1001/jamainternmed.2015.2092. June 8, 2015. Accessed August 4, 2022. http://www.thennt.com/nnt/statins-for-heart-disease-prevention-without-prior-heart-disease/. Accessed July 19, 2022.

Chapter 33: Prevention

KEYWORDS: Primary Prevention, Secondary Prevention, Self-Sufficiency

ABSTRACT: Primary prevention is in the patient's hands and reflects the ability to do things like dieting and exercising, while as much of possible living in a healthy environment to maintain health. In other words, acquiring healthy habits. Secondary prevention refers to efforts to detect disease at an early stage before it can cause substantial harm. Screening can be helpful for illnesses where early detection leads to a better result. However, it can be harmful if screening itself causes injury or results in anxiety-provoking false positives.

Smokey the Bear is the symbol of prevention. His objective is to prevent of forest fires, a bit different from ours, which is to prevent of sickness or other disability. However, the message is the same. Prevention of forest fires takes a genuine effort on the part of campers and others who use or maintain our woodlands. If we do have a conflagration, moreover, it can be extremely difficult to control or extinguish. Vast forest fires during the period of global warming illustrate their catastrophic human and fiscal impacts. Health prevention is quite like that and risk factors serve as the alarms that we might have a problem.

The Nature of Prevention

The detailed nature of prevention is worthy of a few words.

Prevention may be direct or primary, such as giving warnings to avoid a poison or a situation that can cause injury. The idea of **primary prevention** is to <u>avoid</u> disease or other insults to our bodies or minds. We do primary prevention of injuries through education, such as learning to wear and actually wearing protective footwear and headwear around construction sites or personal flotation devices when boating. Primary prevention involves taking steps even when there is no immediate threat. A good example of this is not smoking and avoiding smoke-filled environments. Lung and other cancers are far more likely to occur in those who smoke or who are exposed to second-hand smoke. The occurrence of cancers may be delayed for decades, so the need to take preventive steps today is not obvious in real time. Vaccination is another form of primary prevention, not absolutely guaranteed to work, but reasonably effective against a wide variety of diseases and especially important when these diseases can result in serious impairments or death.

Secondary prevention refers to trying to detect a disease and, if it is incipient, attempting to avoid its consequences. This may be the reason many people undergo screening – detecting early on an asymptomatic problem or noting a risk factor connected to a problem. Elsewhere in this book we address the realities of screening and its propensity to detect problems that aren't there – false positives – that engender further testing that can harm (think: x-rays). The expense and risk can be significant!

However, there is a less direct form of primary prevention: maintaining one's fitness, nutrition and hydration. These less direct preventive activities are often the subject of what we call 'health promotion'. The idea is that we can take positive personal steps to reduce the likelihood of problems in the future.

Perhaps the most difficult preventive measures are the ones that relate to our emotional state or mental stability. Prevention in this case means taking steps to strengthen our character and to avoid putting ourselves or being put into an emotionally compromising position. This implies psychologically preparing for those unexpected traumata that seem to occur in every life, sometimes when least expected.

Prevention Mechanisms

We have evolved a variety of means for preventing disease.

Health promotion efforts involve the publication of guidance by various health organizations at the federal state/provincial and local levels.

At the federal or national level, the Center for Disease Control and Prevention (CDC) in the United States and Health Canada are crucial sources for and promoters of health guidance. They address every aspect of preventing disease. They educate people so they avoid unhealthy behaviors, assist those who have undertaken unhealthy behaviors to stop those behaviors before they cause problems and provide motivation for undertaking steps like these.

Similar organizations exist at the other two government levels through the efforts of state and provincial governments and cities. There are also local organizations and even academic centers. So, a significant capacity exists to prevent the health equivalent of a forest fire. A major issue, however, moderates the impacts of all these agencies, which is that funding is often minimal or lacking. Personal health insurance programs can fail in that regard as well by not paying for prevention-related visits to healthcare providers.

Another vector for disease prevention is the commercial world. One only needs to watch TV to note advertising regarding weight reduction, smoking cessation, and dangerous behavior avoidance. Individuals can respond to these promotional efforts by purchasing a wide variety of programs. It is somewhat tragic that the weight of paying for things like this rests on the individual, but we do live in a capitalistic society. It may also be that there can be many non-health-related motivations for participating in commercial programs. For example, one might purchase a smoking intervention medication because there is the desire to prevent wrinkles or to still the comments of friends. Similarly, weight reduction may focus on appearance, rather than being a step to becoming fit.

The promoters of these commercial programs use a variety of psychological tools that build on personal needs. For example, there is a dietary program that claims to be based on Cognitive Behavioral Therapy (see the section of Mental Health). Reality is that individuals and companies earn money from these programs. Clearly, this can be good or bad. In our society, anyone has the right and the incentive to build businesses that fund their desired lifestyle. In some instances, this can be good because a program may actually help people to avoid obesity. However, it is quite unfortunate that there is no true regulation. Anyone can claim that something or other will improve buyers in some way, make them feel better or even save their lives. The bad is that commercial organizations sell countless programs, devices and substances that are totally ineffective, no better than eating Mom's soup, or even harmful. Nonetheless, companies have a role in prevention. The key is being an informed consumer or, in other words, "let the buyer beware".

The Ultimate Prevention is Within Us

At the base of all prevention is the individual. A major purpose of this book is to awaken the realization that health is a personal responsibility and well within the realm of individual prerogative and action.

Many of us have thought about our lives and our bodies and recognized that our bellies are growing disproportionately to the rest of us. Some have sensed that activity simply makes them feel better. Others have recognized that plain old good hygiene is socially beneficial, to put it mildly. Still others having noticed the negative effects of poverty or living in a polluted area, have pulled themselves up by the bootstraps and have corrected that. Each of us has a built-in prevention mechanism that some call a conscience. We think about ourselves and our immediate surround and take measure of it. On seeing opportunities for improvement, we attempt corrections and sometimes we succeed.

Sometimes insight comes from outside. Most of us have someone with access to our ears. It might be a spouse, a friend, Mom or a drill sergeant. It might be that we read a book or saw a TV program or took in one of those ads or a government prevention video. Whatever the stimulus, it comes back to self. We have our own internal promotional voice to which we must tune in, listen to, and recognize the value of what we hear. Then we must apply the willpower to do it.

The most crucial starting point is education. Once people understand the messages of this book, for example, it is really hard to ignore them. Perhaps some lack access to education or they read comic books during class. Perhaps others simply follow mistaken or perverted beliefs and overcome what their mind, their conscience, is telling them. However, for those who learn, pay attention and do not permit their or others' opinions to mind-wash them, education is the key and motivation is the fuel.

Many billions of dollars are invested at every level of society to make it clear how people can prevent disease and other problems. It is interesting to recognize that the primary source we can all depend on for prevention is right there within us and costs almost nothing to use.

Chapter 34: Maintaining Health

KEYWORDS: Determinants of Health, Physical Determinants of Health, Social Determinants of Health, Community Context and Behavior to Maintain Health, Vitamins, Diet, Exercise, Placebos

ABSTRACT: Research has clearly established that healthy behaviors and some modifiable elements of how and where we live can contribute substantially to living longer and healthier lives. The chapter discusses those elements.

Introduction

How can a person stay healthy? Is it just a matter of not getting sick?

Health Canada and the United States Institute of Medicine recognize that individual actions and behavior, including how we exercise and what we eat, importantly influence our health. However, they also recognize that other influences, what we call the 'social determinants of health', additionally influence not only how we feel and how we function but also how long we are likely to live.[177] Where we were born, where and how our parents lived and how wealthy they were all have a major influence on our opportunity to live a healthy, satisfying life. So does being fit, as FIGURE 1.34.1 points out.

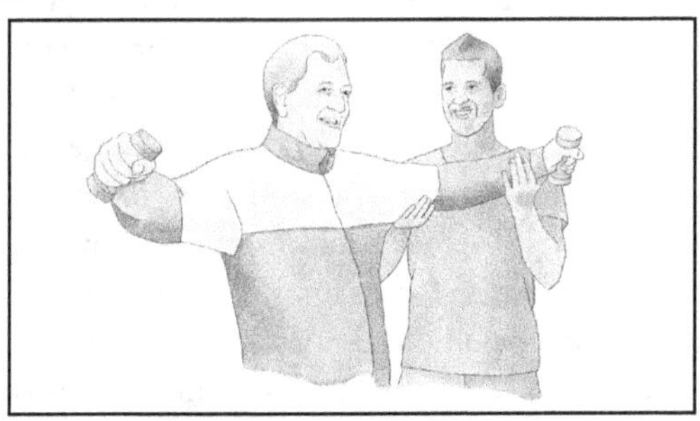

FIGURE 1.34.1: The fit patient

Health Canada[178] recognizes the following 12 determinants of health (in addition to access to health services):

"Many factors have an influence on health. In addition to our individual genetics and lifestyle choices, where we are born, grow, live, work and age also have an important influence on our health.

***Determinants of health** are the broad range of personal, social, economic and environmental factors that determine individual and population health. The main determinants of health include:*

1. *Income and social status.*
2. *Employment and working conditions.*
3. *Education and literacy.*
4. *Childhood experiences.*
5. *Physical environments.*
6. *Social supports and coping skills.*
7. *Healthy behaviours.*
8. *Access to health services.*
9. *Biology and genetic endowment.*
10. *Gender.*
11. *Culture.*
12. *Race / Racism"*

177 MIT News April 11, 2016. In the US the richest 1% of men live on average 14.6 years longer than the poorest, and for women the difference is 10.1 years. http://news.mit.edu/2016/study-rich-poor-huge-mortality-gap-us-0411. Accessed July 19, 2022.

178 Accessed July 19, 2022. Government of Canada Social Determinants of Health and Health Inequalities, https://www.canada.ca/en/public-health/services/health-promotion/population-health/what-determines-health.html. Accessed October 2, 2018.

The **'social determinants of health'** (see FIGURE 1.34.2) refer to societal and economic factors within the broader set of determinants of health. These are associated with an individual's place in society, which often depends on income, education or employment. The effects of discrimination or historical trauma are also important determinants for certain groups such as Indigenous Peoples.

Political-Social-Economic Context
Healthcare + Other Institutional Context
Community Context
Living Context
Relationship Context
Personal Risk Factors Context
Biological Context
Individual + Public

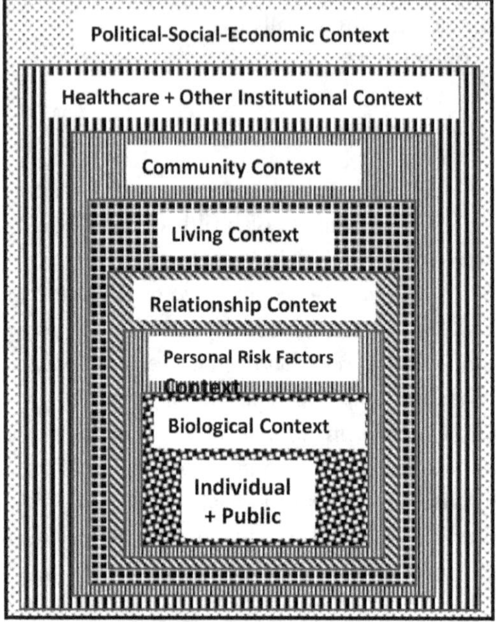

FIGURE 1.34.2: A graphical depiction of the determinants of health

CONTEXT is CRUCIAL: Our health exists within a nested set of interdependent contexts, all of which must be addressed if each of us is to be as healthy as possible.

Nevertheless, regardless of your parentage, how wealthy you are or where you were born, there are some actions you can take today to maintain and improve your health.

Actions to Maintain Health

Many providers, including clinicians, pharmaceutical companies and nutraceutical manufacturers, market products they claim to hold the key to a long and healthy life. Some may help and some do not achieve that lofty goal. For example, taking vitamin D may help if one lives in the far north deprived of regular exposure to sunlight. But dietary supplements and some vitamins can harm when they create unintended metabolic imbalances, cause toxicity or interfere with the metabolism of worthwhile medication.

However, we know that good old excellent diets and an active lifestyle have profound positive influences on overall health and survival.

Dr. Preetha Anand[179], publishing in Pharmaceutical Research, reports that lifestyle plays a larger role than heredity in influencing the chances of developing cancer. People who have a genetic predisposition to certain illnesses can avert the harmful consequences predicted by genetic makeup because lifestyle and environmental factors have profound influences on the expression of genetic characteristics.

According to Dr. Anand only 5-10% of cancers can be attributed to genetics. Environment and lifestyle play a major role in 90-95% of cancers. Living in healthy environments (low in pollution) and engaging in healthy lifestyles (eating well and moving more) are important approaches that everyone can adopt to maintain health and prolong life. Many of the factors that influence health are reflections of the community in which people live. Toxic substances are endemic in industrial areas, for example. Environmental pollutants include lead, mercury, many cyclic hydrocarbons and herbicides. Sometimes it is difficult to avoid environmental toxins because smokestacks, meat treated with hormones and

179 Anand P, Kunnumakkara AB, Sundaram C, Harikumar KB, Tharakan ST, Lai OS, Sung B, Aggarwal BB. Cancer is a preventable disease that requires major lifestyle changes. Pharm Res. 2008 Sept 25(9):2097-116. https://pubmed.ncbi.nlm.nih.gov/18626751/. Accessed Sept 8, 2023.

antibiotics and poor water quality are a part of the community context.

Dr. Anand and colleagues report that the major causes of cancer deaths are: "... cigarette smoking, diet (fried foods, red meat), alcohol, sun exposure, environmental pollutants, infections, stress, obesity, and physical inactivity." The evidence indicates that of all cancer-related deaths, almost 25–30% are due to tobacco, as many as 30–35% are linked to diet, about 15–20% are due to infections, and the remaining percentage are due to other factors like radiation, stress, physical activity, and environmental pollutants.[180] Therefore, cancer prevention requires smoking cessation, increased ingestion of fruits and vegetables, moderate use of alcohol, caloric restriction, exercise, avoidance of direct exposure to sunlight, minimal meat consumption, use of whole grains, and use of vaccinations." Dear Reader, it could not be clearer! Dr. Anand also suggests that in some circumstances, regular check-ups for particular risk factors might be useful. However, we need to mention that not all check-ups are valuable; some, as we have noted, are harmful.

Recently, Dr. Kuanrong Li and colleagues reported[181] how lifestyle choices influence one's chances of dying. They reviewed remaining life expectancy for 40-year-olds with and without particular lifestyle risks. Dr. Li reports that male non-smokers who:

1. Maintain a moderate weight.
2. Drink little or no alcohol.
3. Avoid red meat and processed meats.

are likely to live 17 years longer (!) than men who did not behave this way. Women could expect to live 14 years longer than women who had risk factors related to being overweight, smoking, alcohol and eating processed and red meats.

Many, many people can avoid the scourge of premature death by taking this advice.

Other modifiable risk factors include getting enough exercise, avoiding polluted environments and drinking clean water. It is a simple fact that people who avoid the risk factors for cancers are less likely to develop cancer, leading many experts agree that "**Cancer is a Preventable Disease that Requires Major Lifestyle Changes**"[182] and that other conditions fit within the same category, as well.

Exercise

Scientists from the USA have developed a formula that uses a simple treadmill stress test result to predict the risk of death in the following 10 years. They make their prediction of survival based on the maximal heart rate achieved during the exercise stress test. The studies published in the Mayo Clinic Proceedings should be an impetus for people to maintain fitness levels and for clinicians to encourage their patients to do that.

The "FIT Treadmill Score is easy to calculate and cost effective," said the study authors. "*We hope the score will become a mainstay in cardiologists and primary clinicians' offices as a meaningful way to illustrate risk among those who undergo cardiac stress testing and propel people with poor results to become more physically active*", said

180 Anand P, Kunnumakkara AB, Sundaram C, et al. Cancer is a Preventable Disease that Requires Major Lifestyle Changes. Pharmaceutical Research. 2008;25(9):2097-2116. doi:10.1007/s11095-008-9661-9. https://pubmed.ncbi.nlm.nih.gov/18626751/. Accessed Sept 8, 2023.

181 Kuanrong Li*, Anika Hüsing and Rudolf Kaaks, Lifestyle risk factors and residual life expectancy at age 40: a German cohort study, BMC Medicine 2014, 12:59 doi:10.1186/1741-7015-12-59. https://bmcmedicine.biomedcentral.com/articles/10.1186/1741-7015-12-59%20. Accessed Sept 8, 2023.

182 Anand, Pr., Kunnumakkara, A.B, Sundaram, C. et. Al., Cancer is a Preventable Disease that Requires Major Lifestyle Changes Pharm Res. 2008 Sep; 25(9): 2097–2116. Published online 2008 Jul 15. doi: 10.1007/s11095-008-9661-9. http://www.ncbi.nlm.nih.gov/pmc/articles/PMC2515569/. Accessed July 19, 2022.

senior author, Michael Blaha.[183] [184] Estimates of the maximum heart rate that people achieve during exercise predict life expectancy and fitness. A lower resting heart rate is also associated with better health and longer survival.[185] The ability to reach a higher heart rate during an exercise test is also a sign of better health. The good news is that regular exercise helps to improve these important markers.

We know that overweight and inactive people are more likely to become sick and that obesity measured by weight or estimated by belt size is a risk factor for sickness and deteriorating health. Excess weight is associated with increased mortality[186] [187] and morbidity (sickness)[188]. Obese people are more likely to have poorer health and a shorter life span.

For most people, moving more and eating less contributes substantially to health maintenance and improvement. Nevertheless, many children and adults are overweight or noticeably obese[189] and yet they ask doctors about hidden risk factors. The truth is that many risk factors are not hidden. Some worry, occasionally correctly, that weight gain is a sign of a hidden illness and just want to be sure. Many people would reduce their risk of illness if they could maintain a normal weight and engage in regular exercise. For others, especially people with recent rapid changes in weight, medical consultation is important in order to find out if the weight change signals an undetected illness.

Nutraceuticals

Many of us prefer simple solutions, even if they don't work. We seem to believe that drug and health food stores have the magic ingredients that will help improve and maintain health. Even people who eat well and exercise sometimes seek additional benefit by purchasing nutraceuticals. In response, companies have developed and marketed a large array of dietary supplements, including vitamins.

Pharmaceutical companies must clear many hurdles to receive approval for a new drug. The American Food and Drug Administration (FDA)[190] and corresponding organizations in other countries evaluate the safety of prescription medication. Drug manufacturers that have tested medications for safety and effectiveness apply for patent protection and usually market these drugs through physicians and pharmacies.

The nutraceuticals, on the other hand, are not subject to the same rigorous evaluation

183 Maximal Exercise Testing Variables and 10-Year Survival: Fitness Risk Score Derivation From the FIT Project Ahmed, Haitham M. et al. Mayo Clinic Proceedings, Volume 90, Issue 3, 346 – 355. https://pubmed.ncbi.nlm.nih.gov/25744114/. Accessed Sept 8, 2023.

184 High Exercise Capacity Attenuates the Risk of Early Mortality After a First Myocardial Infarction. Shaya, Gabriel E. et al. Mayo Clinic Proceedings, Volume 91, Issue 2, 129-139. https://pubmed.ncbi.nlm.nih.gov/26848000/. Accessed Sept 8, 2023.

185 Zhang D, Shen X, Qi X. Resting heart rate and all-cause and cardiovascular mortality in the general population: a meta-analysis. *CMAJ: Canadian Medical Association Journal.* 2016;188(3): E53-E63. doi:10.1503/cmaj.150535. https://www.ncbi.nlm.nih.gov/pmc/articles/PMC4754196/. Accessed July 19, 2022.

186 Samaras TT[1], Storms LH, Elrick H. Longevity, mortality and body weight. Ageing Res Rev. 2002 Sep;1(4):673-91. https://pdfs.semanticscholar.org/e397/a3316268d5cd203f6f880cffb071b9b1fad3.pdf. Accessed July 19, 2022.

187 Lorenzini A. How Much Should We Weigh for a Long and Healthy Life Span? The Need to Reconcile Caloric Restriction versus Longevity with Body Mass Index versus Mortality Data. Frontiers in Endocrinology. 2014; 5:121. doi:10.3389/fendo.2014.00121. https://www.ncbi.nlm.nih.gov/pmc/articles/PMC4115619/. Accessed July 19, 2022.

188 Abdelaal M, le Roux CW, Docherty NG. Morbidity and mortality associated with obesity. Annals of Translational Medicine. 2017;5(7):161. doi:10.21037/atm.2017.03.107. https://www.ncbi.nlm.nih.gov/pmc/articles/PMC5401682/. Accessed July 19, 2022.

189 Celia Rodd and Atul K. Sharma, Recent trends in the prevalence of overweight and obesity among Canadian children CMAJ 188: E313-E320. https://pubmed.ncbi.nlm.nih.gov/27160875/. Accessed Sept 8, 2023.

190 https://www.fda.gov/. U.S. Food and Drug Administration. Accessed July 19, 2022.

as prescription medications. Furthermore, there is often little evidence that they improve health, and some may do the opposite. Some nutraceuticals, for example Vitamin B12, are naturally occurring substances. Others are not. Patients use these agents to maintain health because they "believe" that taking supplements is helpful. The problem is correlating this belief with experimental evidence of effectiveness and of safety. Recognize that the term 'natural' is used propagandistically to put a positive spin on these substances. We must realize that anthrax and viruses, poisonous plants and rattlesnakes are 'natural' too.

The Cochrane Collaboration is an independent group that monitors research literature and systematically reviews research. They report[191] that Vitamin C and Echinacea don't help to fight colds but "that Zinc might". They also suggest that cranberries are useful for urinary tract infections. However, they note that there is no evidence supporting the idea that use of antioxidant supplements, such as "beta-carotene or Vitamins A, C or E", improve health or increase longevity. Realize that vitamin A is needed by the body but too much of it is poisonous – it causes a disease called 'hypervitaminosis A'. High levels of vitamin A are present, for example, in the livers of many arctic mammals, the eating of which has injured or killed arctic explorers.

Vitamins

The element carbon is essential to life. Organic compounds all contain carbon combined with other elements. Vitamins are a special set of organic compounds. They are essential, in very small amounts, for normal development and nutrition. Humans can make a small number of vitamins if they eat the food containing the components required to make these vitamins. In particular, humans can make Vitamins B3 and Vitamin D. With a little help from gut bacteria humans can also make Vitamin K, a vitamin that participates in the body's ability to develop blood clots to prevent runaway bleeding (hemorrhaging).

Vitamin B12, a nutraceutical, has therapeutic benefits for those who cannot absorb enough from their food or who do not eat sufficient amounts of B12-containing foods (like meat, fish, vegetables including spinach, mushrooms, asparagus and many others). If a supplement is taken beyond what the body needs, it is simply excreted in the urine. This is where the statement that many vitamins and other supplements are a means of increasing the dollar value of one's excretions.

Vitamin B12 in Particular

Vitamin B12 (sometimes mistakenly called 'folic acid' or 'folate', which is vitamin B9) plays an important role in blood production and neurological function. People who are deficient in Vitamin B12 or in folic acid have abnormal red blood cells – they are larger than normal ones and are called macrocytes (large cells). The symptoms of Vitamin B12 and folate deficiency include weakness and fatigue, pallor, bowel problems, nerve problems, including in some cases numbness and tingling, muscle weakness, visual problems and memory loss.

People develop low levels of Vitamin B12 if their diet is deficient in it or if they cannot absorb the vitamin because of a condition like pernicious anemia. Sources of B12 vitamin include fish, meat, poultry, eggs and milk, so vegetarians might be prone to B12 deficiency because the vitamin is not usually present in plant foods.

In people with pernicious anemia (low levels of normal red blood cells from decreased ability to absorb Vitamin B12), taking folic acid may mask the important symptoms (macrocytosis for example) of B12 deficiency. The problem is that folic acid will not prevent the progression of neurological problems related

191 http://canada.cochrane.org/news/where%E2%80%99s-evidence-top-ten-list-cochrane-reviews. Accessed July 19, 2022.

to B12 deficiency. Folic acid supplements are useful for people with folic acid deficiency but not if those supplements mask the signs of B12 shortage.

Most people absorb enough Vitamin B12 and folic acid. Pregnant women and their developing fetuses require more folic acid and B12 because these compounds are essential for the development of new cells. Consequently, physicians prescribe vitamin supplements to almost all pregnant women. Inadequate amounts of B12 and folic acid lead to newborns with neurological problems and neural tube (the part of the embryo from which the brain and spinal column develop) defects.

MENDAL BURNSTEIN ANECDOTE – VIT B12 PLACEBO

Vitamin B12 is a benign substance. When DZ started to practice, the senior doctor, Mendel Burnstein, had what seemed at the time to be an odd practice. If someone presented with symptoms of fatigue, low energy, or depression-like problems, he would do a complete investigation. If the investigation found nothing and the blood tests were normal, he would first suggest lifestyle (diet and exercise) interventions. If these were not effective, he would suggest they receive an intramuscular injection of Vitamin B12. He told them the shot was a Vitamin and that we didn't know how it worked, but that many people improved with an injection and that if it was effective, they could return when the effect of the injection wore off. (Current literature[192] suggests that about 40% of people improve with a placebo injection – not much different from the current reported 58% improvement rate with antidepressants.[193]

Most colleagues, at the time and now, prescribed antidepressant medication for those problems. We know that for mild to moderate depression, these drugs, which have possible side-effects, are not always effective. So, treating with a benign treatment (placebo) is preferable and, for those who don't respond, clinicians could next try a drug that may have side effects but is more likely to be effective.

Dr. Burnstein knew that unnecessary medication is harmful and chose instead to recommend benign treatments followed by more conventional and possibly harmful treatment if the benign treatment did not work.

BURNSTEIN - DRUGS ARE FOR PATIENTS

Dr. Burnstein really understood the harms that come from unnecessary medication. Early in his career DZ had a minor respiratory problem (that turned out to be benign and self-limited) and asked Dr. Burnstein if he should take the medicines usually recommended by most doctors. His reply, with his own unique inflection, was "David, drugs are for patients!" The implication was that for many drugs many doctors knew better than to take potentially harmful medication themselves. We expect that is a different perspective for most readers.

Recent evidence supports Dr. Burnstein's intuition, at least about medication for prolonged, unexplained fatigue or feelings of depression.

At best, antidepressants are useful only for the most serious cases and not for mild to moderate instances of depression.

Adding to the confusion is a recent study in the Journal of the American Medical Association[194] that reported "*Most US adults who screen positive for depression did not receive treatment for depression, whereas most who were treated did not screen positive.*" Weird, eh!

---

192 Arif Khan, Kaysee Fahl Mar, Jim Faucett, Shirin Khan Schilling, Walter A. Brown. Research Report: Has the rising placebo response impacted antidepressant clinical trial outcome? Data from the US Food and Drug Administration 1987-2013 World Psychiatry Volume 16, Issue 2. First published: 12 May 2017. https://onlinelibrary.wiley.com/doi/full/10.1002/wps.20421. Accessed July 19, 2022.

193 Karen Wagner, Antidepressants: Risk vs. Benefit in Depression, Psychiatric Times, August 1, 2012 Volume 29 Issue 8. https://www.psychiatrictimes.com/view/antidepressants-risk-vs-benefit-depression. Accessed Sept 8, 2023.

194 Olfson M, Blanco C, Marcus SC. Treatment of Adult Depression in the United States. JAMA Intern Med. 2016;176(10):1482–1491. doi:10.1001/jamainternmed.2016.5057. https://jamanetwork.com/journals/jamainternalmedicine/fullarticle/2546155. Accessed August 29, 2022.

Therapeutic Excess and Therapeutic Gap

The suggestion is that we live in a time when there is a **therapeutic excess** because many people receive drug prescriptions even though they do not fall into the category of people who might benefit. At the same time, however, there seems to be a **therapeutic gap** because people who might benefit do not receive the prescriptions they need.

Maintaining health means doing things that promote health and avoiding harmful activities, including the taking of unnecessary medication. It seems that it should be simple to maintain and improve health. Proper exercise and a well-balanced diet are simple things that we all can do. Community efforts to improve the environment and to avoid "food deserts" (areas where it is difficult for people to purchase nutritious food) also can help all of us in our quest for sustained good health.

VOLUME 1

Section 6

THE NATURE OF TREATMENT

DUMB MEDICAL JOKES

Q: *What do you call 2 orthopedic doctors reading an EKG?*
A: *A double blind study! (Orthopedist or orthopods deal with the bones and joints of the body and are not known for knowledge of the heart or its electrocardiographic signals – the EKG)*

Q: *What's the difference between a general practitioner and a specialist?*
A: *One treats what you have, the other thinks you have what he treats.*

Q: *What do you call a student that got C's all the way through med school?*
A: *Hopefully not your doctor. (The truth is that grades in med schools are not good indicators of the quality of their graduates. There is often too much 'Just In Case' learning and memorization).*

I told the doctor I broke my leg in two places. He told me to quit going to those places.

From https://www.quickfunnyjokes.com/doctor.html. Accessed Aug 3, 2022.

A Story: Carotid Endarterectomy: Yes, No, Maybe?

Peter, a prominent, active, busy, lawyer saw an optometrist for routine eye exam. The optometrist noticed a small cholesterol spot – a Hollenhorst plaque – on his retina. He saw his family doctor who worried that the cholesterol eye plaque originated from another artery. His doctor ordered tests on his carotid arteries – the arteries in the neck that carry blood to the brain – and found that one artery was completely, 100%, blocked. The other carotid artery was 80% blocked. Peter had no other symptoms, although he had risk factors including alcohol use and mild obesity.

Peter's doctor asked him "would you like to have blood vessel surgery, a stent to open the arteries and reduce the blockages". Peter quizzically asked: "why the hell are you asking me, I don't know how to treat blocked arteries". His doctor explained that some vascular surgeons think operating will reduce the risk of a stroke, while others believe the operations would pose unnecessary risk. When Peter learned that his choice of doctor would influence whether or not he had surgery, he decided to go with a conservative doc, one less likely to operate. Peter's own doctor had explained that, because Peter had no symptoms from the blocked arteries, he probably had collateral blood vessels (small blood vessels that go around the blockage and provide blood to the brain).

Peter asked how many people with blocked arteries in his city went on to have a stroke or die prematurely. Sadly, that information was unavailable. Nor could he learn how many people had postoperative complications or died within one or two months of the surgery.

Peter elected not to have surgery and has been doing fine. Several years later he noticed an article that said: "*Carotid endarterectomy (CEA) among asymptomatic patients involves a trade-off between a higher short-term perioperative risk in exchange for a lower long-term risk of stroke.*". The authors reported no statistical differences in fatal and non-fatal stroke, about 6% of people died over 5 years, between people who elected to have medical therapy (diet, exercise, cholesterol lowering drugs) and those who elected to have surgery. For people who are symptomatic (Peter had no symptoms) – having had ischemic episodes (transient changes indicating inadequate blood flow to their brains) or actual strokes (damage to the brain), surgical therapy seemed to produce better results.

The important lesson, when making treatment choices, is that doctors and patients must find out, if possible, how often the treatments produce benefit or harm, and what kinds of benefit or harms result. Sometimes, the answers aren't clear, and that is also important to understand.

Chapter 35: ——— Kinds of Treatment

KEYWORDS: Medication, Surgery, Physiotherapy, Lifestyle Changes, The Art of Medicine, Homeopathy

ABSTRACT: There are several categories of treatment, including medication, surgery, and lifestyle change. Although treatments differ, the methods used to demonstrate their effectiveness are the same. Some medications act as harmless placebos, while other medications create harm. Whenever patients are concerned, as they should be, about the benefits and risks of treatment, they should ask the prescriber about the basis for treatment and any possible alternatives.

Introduction

A 'treat' is usually something good. We give treats to our kids and, of course, they beat 'tricks' at Halloween. When a physician 'treats' someone, we assume or at least hope that's a good thing, as that is the intention.

Children are usually happy when they receive Halloween treats, especially candy. However, sometimes they just eat too much and are sad to wake up the next day with a stomach-ache. Medical treatments behave in the same way. Some promote happiness, others inadvertently make people sad.

A 'treatment' or 'therapy' is any intervention meant to relieve or correct problems, both physical and mental. In healthcare, therapy is defined broadly as any action meant to improve the function of any aspect of a person, the cells, organs, the body and the mind. Treatments are all aimed at improving individual comfort, the function of the body overall and of its parts and a person's lifespan.

Some treatments are designed to produce dramatic, possibly life-saving improvement in health. Others have more modest but nevertheless important goals. Patients and clinicians must think about the types of treatment and have some way of evaluating the chances that a treatment will help or harm.

Therapies that appear to be limited to the improvement of the function of a body part can also have a profound effect on the overall performance and health of the individual. For example, someone with a swollen and painful thumb-joint suffers not only discomfort but also a physical limitation that prevents doing certain things. An anti-inflammatory drug for joint pain might reduce the pain, yet a few people will unfortunately suffer from drug-induced gastrointestinal bleeding. Most treatments 'cut both ways' like this and must be applied carefully with the patient's full understanding of the proposed benefits and consent to undertake the risks from possible, serious and not so serious negative effects.

Throughout this book, we recognize that treatments designed for one body part are not successful if they lead to other physical or emotional problems. Hip-replacement surgery that successfully restores hip function is not a success if the patient suffers a stroke and has paralysis because of the surgery or the anesthetic. An antibiotic that successfully treats an infection but leads to a serious blood problem, is not a success.[195] Many have heard the saw: "the surgery was successful, but the patient died". That surgery benefitted no one!

We discuss the methods used to assess the benefits and harms[196] of treatment in another chapter. The purpose of this chapter is to outline the broad spectrum of categories of treatment that people often consider. They run from the very safe ones to those that pose high risk for the patient. The safest categories have lower risk of side effects, and patients might consider these before other more invasive and therefore less-safe options. The categories of treatment can serve as a way of ranking one's treatment options. Everybody has options and choices, like those illustrated in FIGURE 1.35.1.

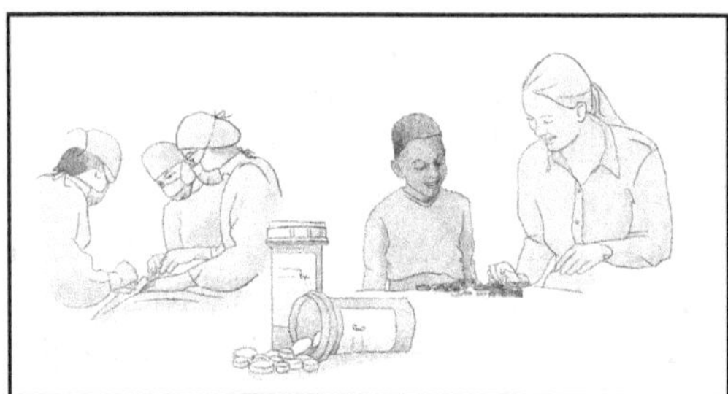

FIGURE 1.35.1: Patients have many options and must choose what's best for them

Treatment Options – Intrusiveness of Treatments

We can consider treatments based on how intrusive they are. There is often the focus on how 'invasive' treatments are, that is, if they involve cutting into the body. The real issue is their potential for harm, which can be on a spectrum spanning temporary mild discomfort to longer term levels of discomfort or significant pain. Treatments can also entail temporary, long-term or permanent infections, healing problems, damage to organs, functional disability and even death.

Surgery is often considered to be invasive because the surgeon uses instruments to enter the body. However, there are degrees of surgical invasiveness. Laparoscopic abdominal surgery is called 'minimally invasive' because the incision to enter the body is small. It is also called 'keyhole surgery'; the word 'laparoscopy' literally means 'to see into the body'. Other treatments are considered non-invasive because they do not penetrate the body. The problem is that we consider drugs as non-invasive, even though some also pose an equal or greater risk of serious harm. Diet and exercise are properly termed non-invasive.

Surgery, a clearly an invasive intervention, is almost always guaranteed to produce some immediate post-operative discomfort, including post-operative effects of the anesthetic. Medical interventions, which we could call 'microinvasive' – they enter the body via the mouth and the digestive system – might or might not be associated with decreases in comfort or function. So, they may be intrusive with the potential of the full range of harms. An antibiotic for pneumonia will often do its job without producing any adverse effects but sometimes it can cause problems.

The likelihood of benefit versus harm usually relates to the specifics of the treatment and not how invasive it is. For example, oral chemotherapy might pose a greater risk of immediate harm versus certain invasive surgeries, like an appendectomy (appendix removal). So, 'invasive' does not equate to 'harmful' even though surgery usually produces some immediate discomfort.

Medical Treatment Options

When we have a medical problem that does not immediately threaten life or limb, we often can consider the approach known as '**watchful waiting**' or '**tincture of time**'. This is the least

195 Chloramphenicol is the classic example of an effective antibiotic that caused about 1 in 25,000 people to suffer from aplastic anemia, a serious blood and sometimes deadly blood disorder.

196 Including Number Needed to Treat, Number Needed to Harm, Relative and Absolute Risk Reduction.

aggressive and least intrusive treatment. Many problems, like common colds, muscle sprains, minor cuts and burns or bad moods resolve on their own without intervention. Some clear up when we change our environment by removing allergens (for example, cats in the case of people allergic to cat hair) and pollutants in the air we breathe. Interventions like these, accompanied by encouragement to be patient and maybe some helpful guidance, such as getting additional rest or drinking more fluids, are among the most frequently used, safe and effective tools in the doctor's bag.

The next level of intervention is the use of '**talk therapies**', the more or less formal application of therapeutic conversations. Formal examples include Cognitive Behavioral Therapy and Psychodynamic. Therapy. An informal example is conversations with friends – we deal with matters like this in the Section 8 on Mental Health. These are important maneuvers when we are emotionally troubled or distraught, such as a consequence of a bad experience, a death or a rational or irrational fear of something happening.

Talk therapies comprise active listening, helpful enquiry, suggestions and advice, motivation and even recipes as to how to achieve calm, improve nutrition, lose weight, stop smoking, become more fit or avoid stress. There are even do-it-yourself possibilities, like improving relationships or seeking help from friends or trusted elders – not all talk therapies are delivered by a physician! Indeed, most helpful conversations are between people and their friends, relatives and co-workers. Mental health workers, such as psychologists and psychiatrists, label 'conversing' as 'therapy'. Rogerian therapy, for example, is attentive listening and showing understanding by questioning but without suggesting an intervention. From time to time, we all listen attentively to friends' problems without suggesting solutions.

People with more serious mental health problems like feeling deeply depressed, being unable to concentrate or rest, feeling hopeless and the like, may seek more formal interventions, called **psychotherapy** from professional therapists. They can perform interventions meant to improve mental well-being of people who have no detectable physical disease. They are also talk therapies, but more formal and structured in their nature, that help people to reframe how they perceive their situations, become better able to bear their personal challenges and alter their relationships. The interventions may include hypnosis, but mainly are conversations with mental health professionals, which we call psychotherapy and counselling. There are also behavior-altering therapies that use rewards and punishments or other techniques and environmental changes to encourage or discourage problematic behaviors. All are discussed in the Section on mental health.

Perhaps we should also include non-verbal interventions, such as massage, a facial or a stint in the spa, here as well. These are DIY-with-help.

Next, we need to mention **physiotherapy**, the purpose of which is to ease pain or improve function after an accident or physical strain. The same is true of occupational therapy (assistance and guidance in productive and creativity-engaging activities), which can be crucial for recovering function after a stroke, a head injury or other major bodily damage.

Then, often a big step up, are medicines – **pharmaceutical therapies** – that include drugs of many types. Some are designed to kill cancer cells (chemotherapy) that have major body-wide effects. Some target changing our metabolism (stimulants or drugs that calm), and some drugs replace substances (chemicals, vitamins, proteins or hormones) that the body is not absorbing or producing in adequate amounts. Examples of the latter include Vitamin B12 or thyroid hormone replacement therapy. There are also vaccines to prevent disease and antibiotics, antivirals, antifungals and immune system stimulants to cure or mitigate disease.

In the case of serious mental dysfunction, there are many drugs that may be used if less aggressive steps have failed. Some of these are quite powerful and may have unpleasant or dangerous side-effects.

Surgery

Some surgical treatments are dramatic and highly intrusive – think of a heart or lung transplant – while others are less so. In fact, some surgery might be termed 'micro-invasive' as it is usually quite focal, altering a single body part (e.g., the appendix) and only nearby structures, such as blood vessels. It can be that the risks and harms of surgery are not as great as those of some medical treatments, which can affect virtually every cell in the body.

Minor surgeries on the skin surface remove or 'biopsy' (obtain a sample for examination) various skin lesions, such as warts and worrisome or disfiguring growths. Going beyond the skin, surgeries become more aggressive and more likely to have unintended or long-lasting consequences. These more aggressive surgeries try to cure problems by invading body cavities and removing, repairing or otherwise changing things. Major surgery includes operations on internal organs in the abdomen, including the liver, spleen, bowels, kidneys, prostate, ovaries and uterus. Surgeries that invade the thorax (chest) to address problems of the lungs and heart can produce dramatic improvements in every dimension of health. Successful aggressive surgeries often improve comfort and function and prolong life in the long run, although patients usually experience short term and immediate post-operative pain and reduced function. Surgeries like these are made possible by special devices that breathe for the patient and support the function of the heart and by anesthetics that suppress consciousness and the experience of pain.

Today there are more and more 'minimally-invasive' surgical procedures that introduce surgical instruments and visualization equipment into the body through small incisions, rather than creating major openings. Even catheter-introduced tools can be used, one example being where a tube is introduced into a blood vessel to install a heart valve. It goes without saying that some brain surgery is more likely to produce unintended harm. The brain, on the other hand has no pain sensors and can be operated on with out major anesthesia. Similarly, people are astonished to learn that replacing the eye's cataract-obscured lens with a plastic one has very low complication rates and is associated with little discomfort and dramatic improvements in vision.

Today there is a vast palette of therapies. Indeed, the possibilities increase in type and number all the time. So, what's here ends up being a very incomplete catalogue of therapeutic interventions. Our intention, though, is to give an idea of the many types of intervention, the magnitude of their impact on the body and how they can influence physical and mental health. Other chapters describe the methods that researchers, clinicians and patients use to evaluate the likelihood that a treatment will be beneficial, harmful or a waste of time and money.

The Effectiveness of Treatments

In today's age of "fake news" and outright lying, it is important to recognize when claims for the effectiveness of an intervention are likely to be valid and when we are merely receivers of deceivers' marketing hype. Anyone who has tried to read the small print in drug and device ads will recognize the repeated warning that "these results are not typical of the results achieved by most people". This warning often accompanies advertising both for drugs that regulators have approved, as well as for unapproved drugs aimed at reducing weight, increasing libido, changing breast or penis size or helping to overcome depressed feelings. It is a jungle out there and predators seem to dominate.

Clearly, many drugs are worthwhile and provide almost miraculous benefits to many people. Yet, the comment "these results are not typical" must mean that the results are atypical for some and that not everyone is likely to benefit from the intervention. Paradoxically, if the results the ads depict are not typical it means that most people won't achieve the same result.

Knowing the questions to ask and how to find answers empowers all of us to participate in our own care and avoid the potential negative effects and costs of hyperbolic, unproven claims.

Alternative-Treatments

When clinicians, as is the case from time-to-time, do not have clear evidence to support this or that treatment for a particular patient, they rely on the 'Art of Medicine'. Medical artistry uses knowledge from scientific studies about the effectiveness of drugs, knowledge of human biology and experience to recommend a treatment that might not have been tested on a patient exactly like the person a doctor is treating. It is used when it is important to try something that might prevent or reverse suffering or dysfunction when no one has completed the necessary scientific studies that identify the most appropriate treatment. No intervention can be guaranteed to work. However, sometimes a therapeutic trial is worthwhile. Doing this is not a 'shot in the dark', as there is some possibility of good effects or at least of no bad consequences. It is a kind of 'thinking outside the box' and is one of the best demonstrations of the value of artistry in Medicine.

Clinicians are more likely to diverge regarding solutions when scientific evidence is lacking. The anecdote below describes the case of a man who had major blockages in his carotid arteries and how the problem was handled in the absence of strong evidence suggesting that surgical or medical treatment would be best.

THE ART OF MEDICINE AT WORK

An optometrist had told a 72-year-old, highly productive and thoughtful professional to see DZ, his family doctor, because the optometrist had asked the patient to pay for a picture of the retina and noticed the presence of a Hollenhorst plaque.

The optometrist explained that the picture helped to diagnose diabetes and high cholesterol (an ophthalmoscopic image of the retina is usually sufficient to diagnose diabetic retinopathy). The patient then said that he had high cholesterol. The optometrist reviewed the picture and noticed a Hollenhorst plaque, which is a cholesterol deposit or embolus that blocks one of the retinal arteries.. The optometrist was concerned that the patient was at higher risk of artery disease.

A Hollenhorst plaque (see FIGURE 1.35.2) is present in about 1.5% of men over 49 and its prevalence increases with age. Usually, the plaque originates from the carotid artery and is an indicator that cholesterol, which causes atherosclerotic plaques, may be partially or completely blocking the carotid artery or other blood vessels. The presence of Hollenhorst plaques is a stimulus for further investigation.[197]

On seeing the patient, DZ ordered appropriate investigations and confirmed that his patient had high cholesterol. Additional investigations showed that one carotid artery was completely blocked and another was 80% occluded. The patient was slightly obese but fully functional and brilliant at his work.

The challenge was to decide the best treatment to avoid a stroke or mental deterioration from the high cholesterol and blocked carotid arteries. The surgical treatment, one possibility, is performing a 'carotid endarterectomy', where the vascular surgeon attempts to remove the blockage. The other surgical intervention involves placing a stent, a device that holds the artery open, which is far less invasive. A non-invasive alternative, medication, treats the underlying condition (high cholesterol). In this case, the patient had

197 Kaufman EJ, Mahabadi N, Patel BC. Hollenhorst Plaque. [Updated 2019 Jun 23]. In: StatPearls [Internet]. Treasure Island (FL): StatPearls Publishing; 2019 Jan. Available from: https://pubmed.ncbi.nlm.nih.gov/29261979/. Accessed Sept 8, 2023.

full function, indicating that the carotid artery blockages were not causing harm. Some vascular experts recommend surgery, while others prefer medical treatment because there is little evidence showing that one or the other method is best.[198] *DZ sent his patient to a vascular expert who prefers less invasive intervention and 8-years later this patient is doing fine, taking cholesterol-lowering medication to reduce cholesterol and to reduce inflammation, and exercising more.*

Some experts were highly critical that treatment was not more aggressive. However, in this case, the treatment DZ and the vascular surgeon recommended represented the art of Medicine, considering the patient's values and what was known at the time. The fact that the patient's function was not impaired suggested that collateral circulation (other vascular pathways) was enabling his brain to get all the blood it needed. The alternative suggestion for aggressive surgery would also have been a recommendation based on medical art because there was no conclusive evidence one way or the other.

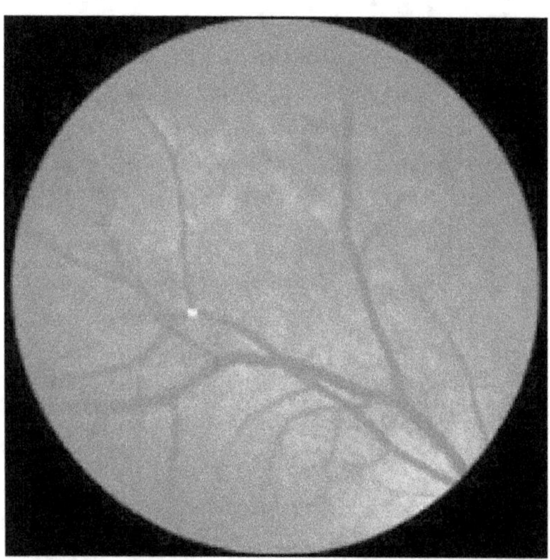

FIGURE 1.35.2: Picture of a Hollenhorst plaque

Art of Medicine versus Alternative Medicine (See FIGURES 1.35.3 and 1.35.4)

Another possible choice is the application of 'alternative medicine' treatments. However, these interventions rarely rely on accepted, peer-reviewed evaluation of the treatments' effectiveness and efficiency or even attempts to garner peer reviewed, statistically meaningful evidence. For example, homeopathic practitioners claim that dilute medicine (so dilute that there may not be a single molecule of the agent in the dose) is more potent than full-strength. However, there are no well-controlled trials supporting this contention and scientific theory in the areas of biochemistry, biology and pharmacology does not provide a rational basis for this claim. It has even been debunked by a team led by the Amazing Randi!.[199] The difference between "artistic medicine" and alternative medicine is that artistic medicine relies on the science of human biology and studies on patients similar, but not identical, to the one the doctor is treating. Chiropractic is another example of a 'medical' practice that often does not rely on scientific evidence (see link in the box below).

HOMEOPATHY

DZ had a patient who visited a physician who practiced conventional Medicine for which he charged government rates and he also charged market rates for homeopathic interventions. Oddly, he could bill patients high prices for unnecessary, non-peer reviewed, homeopathic care but lesser standard government rates for necessary conventional medical treatment. The patient had been persuaded to buy an expensive homeopathic remedy and was told that it would replenish itself, indeed become more potent – stronger – as he diluted it. DZ suggested he call the homeopath with feigned terror and report the bottle had fallen into the bathtub causing it to become

198 Salem MM, Alturki AY, Fusco MR, et al. Carotid artery stenting vs. carotid endarterectomy in the management of carotid artery stenosis: Lessons learned from randomized controlled trials. Surg Neurol Int. 2018; 9:85. Published 2018 Apr 16. doi:10.4103/sni.sni400_17. https://www.ncbi.nlm.nih.gov/pmc/articles/PMC5926211/. Accessed August 3, 2022.

199 The Memory of Water. Nature Magazine, https://www.nature.com/news/2004/041004/full/news041004-19.html. Accessed August 3, 2022.

so strong that the patient thought he was experiencing a severe side effect to the now very potent dilute nostrum.

When the treatments are demonstrably safe, alternative remedies are no worse (nor better) than a placebo. Homeopathy emerged as a discipline at a time when virtual poisons (such as mercury and arsenic) were used to treat disease. The homeopathic remedies at least did less harm. However, some alternative remedies may not be safe and may expose patients to the risk of harm without the opportunity of benefit. Furthermore, safe 'treatments' are not safe if they inhibit people from seeking appropriate, validated therapies that offer a real opportunity for benefit. Although we wish that our current medicines were more effective for some forms of cancer, there is clear evidence that many people do benefit. People who opt for unproven, placebo-like alternative remedies – these have included factitious remedies, extracts of peach pits[200], "psychic surgery"[201] and tea concoctions[202] – lose the opportunities for cure or control offered by conventional treatments.

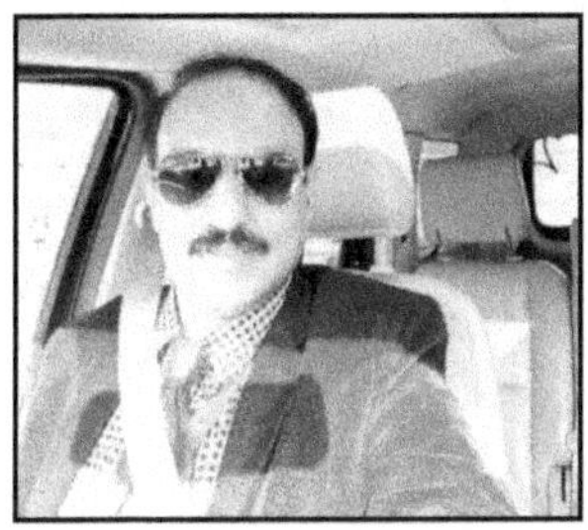

https://www.researchgate.net/post/Why_does_dilution_of_homoeopathic_medicines_enhance_their_potency_Is_this_not_against_scientific_phenomena. Accessed August 3, 2022.

I have been told by homoeopathic practitioners that dilution and potency of homoeopathic medicines are inversely proportional. This means the higher the dilution the more potent the medicine will...

FIGURE 1.35.3: Alternative medicine – homeopathy

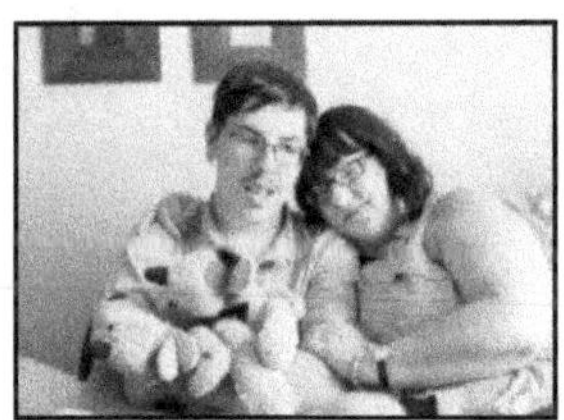

https://www.researchgate.net/post/Why-does-dilution-of-homoeopathic-medicines-enhance-their-potency-Is-this-not-against-scientific-phenomena. Accessed August 30, 2022.

Chiropractors at a crossroads: The fight for evidence-based treatment and a profession's reputation. For more than a decade, Ontario's regulator has been steered by 'vitalists' who promote...

FIGURE 1.35.4 Alternative medicine – chiropractic

200 https://www.cancer.gov/about-cancer/treatment/cam/patient/laetrile-pdq. Accessed August 3, 2022.
201 https://en.wikipedia.org/wiki/Psychic_surgery. Accessed August 29, 2022.
202 https://www.cancer.gov/about-cancer/treatment/cam/patient/essiac-pdq. Accessed August 3, 2022.

Chapter 36: Issues in Treatment - The Patient's Wager

KEYWORDS: Treatment, Purpose of Treatment, Evaluating Treatments, Effect of Treatment, Proxy Measures, Blood Pressure, Hypertension, Menopause, Hormone Replacement Therapy, HRT, Health System Mistakes

ABSTRACT: Treatments include a spectrum of interventions from psychotherapy, to drugs, to surgery. The essence of treatment is to help people feel better, do more and live longer. Health systems dedicate themselves to doing investigations that lead to interventions that measurably improve lives. Sometimes, however, success is not well-defined, and people must rely on proxy measures like a decrease in blood pressure. They may change the proxy, BP, but may not address the underlying cause or the interventions might cause unintended harm. The intervention to change one risk factor – hypertension – might itself be a risk factor for another problem – cancer. Clinicians' decisions must take advantage of good effects and avoid potential bad effects. Studies of mistakes suggest that too many people suffer because doctors prescribe the wrong drug or the patient takes it at the wrong times or dosage. We touch on hormone replacement to demonstrate how thinking about treatments evolves as new evidence accumulates, and how clinicians and patients can make artful choices.

Introduction

Treatment is any intervention intended to change the status quo. In health care, treatments include a spectrum of interventions from engaging a patient in psychotherapy, to using drugs, manipulating a body part or performing surgery. The essence of treatment and all clinical practice is to help people to feel better, do more and live longer. Health systems dedicate themselves to the ideal that their diverse, sometimes expensive, investigations will lead to interventions that measurably improve lives.

Understanding the selection and evaluation of treatments is necessary for everyone who participates in health care. After all, in agreeing to a treatment, patients are betting that the chance of benefit from a treatment will outweigh the risk of harm.

The goals of treatment are usually quite clear. Someone in pain expects to experience relief or reduction of pain. People with a dermatitis (inflamed skin) expect to receive a medication that reduces the redness, swelling and itching that come with the inflammation that is causing their discomfort. Patients with limited joint movement expect to be able to regain motion and have better function. People who have limited energy, whatever the cause, usually expect to be able to feel better and do more after treatment. Patients with enlarged lymph nodes from early Hodgkin's disease, but who have no pain and their usual level of energy, expect that treatment of the disease will eliminate Hodgkin's disease and prolong their lives. Sometimes, however, success is not well-defined, and people must rely on proxy measures of success such as a decrease in blood pressure.

REMINDER: THE PURPOSES OF TREATMENT ARE SOME OR ALL OF THE FOLLOWING:

- *To improve comfort.*
- *To improve function.*
- *To increase lifespan.*

In addition, people expect clinical visits to provide information about current health, any hidden disease and predictions about future health and what they can do to maintain optimum comfort, function and lifespan.

Proxy Measures

Proxy measures are indirect measures that provide information about our health and what we can expect. Proxy measures for health include waist circumference, walking speed, resting pulse and resting pulse rate. These measures relate to the overall health of an individual and contribute to predictions of future illness. Sometimes, instead of measuring directly whether a person feels better or can do more, clinicians use these proxy measures to estimate if an intervention has helped or harmed.

Sometimes proxy measures are useful; at other times they are misleading.

Proxies are common in our lives. We dye our graying hair. What we are actually doing is changing others' perception – and maybe our own feelings – of how gray hair, a natural consequence of aging, makes us look. The gray hair is a 'proxy', an external indicator of the process of aging. In reducing the manifestation, we are not altering the underlying process of aging, a deeper issue.

Occasionally, clinicians use 'proxy measures' to evaluate the effect of treatment. This means that they are assessing or measuring an effect that is really just associated with a deeper problem. A medical example of the use of a proxy is related to hypertension (high blood pressure). Studies tell us that people with high blood pressure are more likely to die from heart attacks or strokes, so clinicians monitor blood pressure (BP) and intervene to lower it if it is outside certain limits. They do this believing that lowering BP will prevent heart attacks and strokes, thereby extending healthy life. In the case of hypertension, drugs as well as lifestyle changes are possible interventions. If we use drugs to lower BP, we must realize that they are not all the same. Some drugs help people achieve lower BP but not necessarily to have longer or healthier lives.[203] They may change the proxy, BP, but may not address the underlying causal problem – perhaps vessel disease – or the drugs might cause other, unintended harm. Problems that can cause hypertension include the loss of resilience of arteries (some call 'hardening'), dietary sodium, certain hormones, rare tumors and so on. Often, the real cause is not detected, so called essential hypertension.

What can be of concern is that some anti-hypertension (BP-lowering) drugs reduce BP but may increase the risk of other conditions. For example, 'angiotensin converting enzyme inhibitors' (ACE Inhibitors) seem to cause an increased risk of lung cancer.[204] The important idea we are focussing on here is that the intervention to change one risk factor

---

203 Cooper-DeHoff RM, Gong Y, Handberg EM, et al. Tight Blood Pressure Control and Cardiovascular Outcomes Among Hypertensive Patients with Diabetes and Coronary Artery Disease. JAMA. 2010;304(1):61–68. doi:10.1001/jama.2010.884. https://jamanetwork.com/journals/jama/fullarticle/186169. Accessed August 3, 2022.

204 Hicks Blánaid M, Filion Kristian B, Yin Hui, Sakr Lama, Udell Jacob A, Azoulay Laurent et al. Angiotensin converting enzyme inhibitors and risk of lung cancer: population-based cohort study BMJ 2018; 363: k4209. https://www.bmj.com/content/363/bmj.k4209. Accessed August 3, 2022.

– hypertension – might itself be a risk factor for another problem – cancer. This illustrates that we must learn if, overall, the benefits of a treatment outweigh its harms.

Reducing the proxy (high BP) of deeper problems like vascular (blood vessel) or kidney disease, without addressing the underlying problem is not often a good thing. Sometimes, physicians make diligent and well-intentioned efforts to reduce a proxy like BP by using multiple medications without achieving their BP target. It can be that the underlying problem is unaffected by the treatment. The problem may only become obvious very late and it may be that only surgery can deal with it. This is the case with some adrenal (glands above the kidneys) tumors – pheochromocytoma. Treating the proxy can actually mask the real problem and delay appropriate care.

Purpose of Treatment

The only valid purpose of a treatment is to produce better health. Unfortunately, a treatment may also make people sicker. Clinicians must always have this in mind and must make decisions that take advantage of the good effects of interventions and avoid the potential bad effects. In other words, medications and other interventions can help a patient, injure a patient or even bring about death.

Patients and clinicians should have an idea of the frequency of the promised benefits, and the types and frequencies of unintended harms associated with treatments.

Studies of health system mistakes[205] suggest that too many people suffer because doctors prescribe the wrong drug or the patient took the right drug at the wrong times or dosage. It can even be a bit more complicated than that. For instance, it is common, especially in older people, that doctors – sometimes several different doctors – prescribe several medications. This even has a name: 'polypharmacy'. Each prescription might be appropriate for one of the patient's problems, but the combination of drugs could be harmful or deadly…they can interact (see FIGURE 1.36.1)!

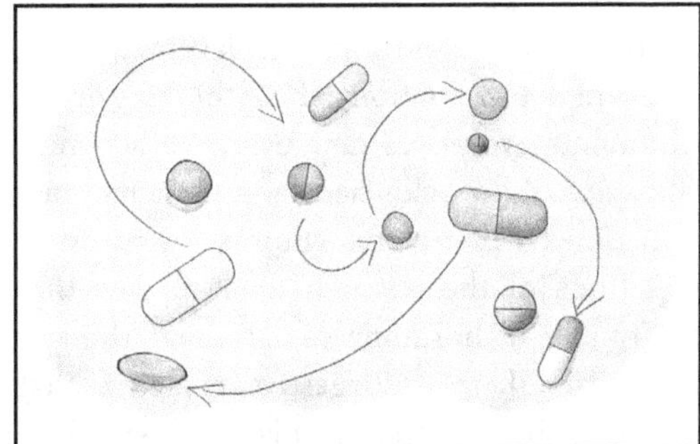

FIGURE 1.36.1: Pharmaceuticals, non-prescription drugs and supplements interact

Sometimes, drugs harm people because the state of medical knowledge is insufficient and what the drugs do to the body may not be fully understood. Sometimes, too, a medicine can be more like a shotgun birdshot load than a silver bullet, affecting multiple body systems and not all of them desirably. At other times, the doctor might not know enough about a patient and the patient's medical history, might not be familiar with recent research results regarding the condition or might have misunderstood the effects of the drug.

HORMONE REPLACEMENT THERAPY (HRT)

Prior to 2002 estrogen replacement therapy was accepted and recommended to reduce post-menopausal symptoms. Most practitioners believed they knew that estrogen replacement was appropriate. However, "In July 2002, researchers at the National Institutes of Health abruptly halted the nation's largest study on Hormone Replacement Therapy (HRT), because the study found that the long-term

205 Appendix 3, Baker and Norton Canadian Adverse Events Study https://www.cmaj.ca/content/cmaj/suppl/2007/05/15/170.11.1678.DC3/adverse-baker-online_appendix_3.pdf. Accessed Sept 8, 2023.

use of synthetic estrogen and synthetic progesterone drugs increase a women's risk of breast cancer by 26%, her risk of a heart attack by 29%, her risk of stroke by 41% and her risk of blood clots by 113%[206].

The history of hormone replacement is an excellent demonstration of how thinking about treatments evolves as new evidence accumulates, and of how clinicians and patients must sometimes make artful choices. New interpretations of the research data suggest that the timing of hormone replacement therapy is crucial. There is suggestive evidence that use early in menopause might be safe and comforting (e.g., by reducing hot flashes) while not increasing other diseases. Late use seems of little or not benefit and possibly harmful.[207] Many clinicians will recommend hormone replacement, after discussion, to women who have symptoms they find intolerable. Otherwise, they will not recommend it. Unfortunately, current knowledge does not enable clinicians to recommend non-medicinal measures to reduce menopausal symptoms or indicate why some women have symptoms that are more pronounced. Of course, proper diet and exercise help in reducing the chances of postmenopausal osteoporosis but the role of exercise to reduce "hot flashes" is inconclusive.[208]

206 Rossouw JE, Anderson GL, Prentice RL, et al. Risks and benefits of estrogen plus progestin in healthy postmenopausal women: principal results From the Women's Health Initiative randomized controlled trial. *JAMA*. 2002;288(3):321-333. https://pubmed.ncbi.nlm.nih.gov/12117397/. Accessed August 26, 2022

207 Clarkson, T.B.; Meléndez, G.C.; Appt, S.E., Timing hypothesis for postmenopausal hormone therapy: its origin, current status, and future, Menopause: The Journal of The North American Menopause Society: March 2013 - Volume 20 - Issue 3 - p 342-353 doi: 10.1097/gme.0b013e3182843aad. https://pubmed.ncbi.nlm.nih.gov/23435033/. Accessed Sept 8, 2023.

208 Mishra N, Mishra VN, Devanshi. Exercise beyond menopause: Dos and Don'ts. J Midlife Health. 2011;2(2):51-56. doi:10.4103/0976-7800.92524. https://www.ncbi.nlm.nih.gov/pmc/articles/PMC3296386/. Accessed August 3, 2022.

Chapter 37: ——— Treatment Benefit Vs Treatment Harm

KEYWORDS: Benefit, Harm, Risks and Benefits, The Patient's Wager

ABSTRACT: Recommended treatments always promise benefit. However, most occasionally produce unintended harms. Whenever patients accept treatments, they are accepting that the chances of overall benefit outweigh the chances of possibly serious harm.

Weighing the Benefits and Harms of Treatment

We all live in hope!

Related to health care, we and our doctors hope that every treatment offers only benefit. However, we now know that few treatments are risk-free. Some treatments, for example chemotherapies for cancer, offer the promise of important benefit, sometimes lifesaving, at the risk of short- (such as pain and hair loss) or long-term (such as later cancers or heart damage) harm. Other treatments, like over-the-counter elixirs for coughs and colds, promise minor benefit for some people and a small risk of serious harm for others. The truth is that the over-the-counters are usually not that helpful nor that harmful. When thinking about the idea of betting on OTC treatments, it's like playing the nickel slots!

Treatments might offer the chance of a large, small or absent benefit. Treatments might also be associated with a risk of serious, minor or non-existent harm. The fact is that the likelihood of experiencing benefit or harm from a drug varies for each patient and each drug and is determined by patient characteristics, such as genetic makeup, health status, organ function, weight and many other factors. Clinicians, patients and those who administer the care process should be knowledgeable about the chance of both the beneficial and adverse consequences of any intervention.

The gambles that patients are prepared to make about treatments reflect not only their knowledge but also their personal values. Chemotherapy for cancer is, again, a good example. It often offers an important chance for cure, which is a major benefit. However, many chemotherapeutic treatments lead to immediate side effects (harms) like those we mentioned. For most people, the promise of a longer life justifies the risk of temporary harm.

At the other end of the spectrum, consider Aspirin. It helps many. On the other hand, about 10% of people with chronic respiratory disease experience a worsening of their problem when they take Aspirin, some have bleeding in their stomachs and about 1 person in 1,000 suffers hives and itching from Aspirin.[209] Luckily, only a few suffer serious allergic reactions or death.

209 Gollapudi RR, Teirstein PS, Stevenson DD, Simon RA. Aspirin Sensitivity Implications for Patients with Coronary Artery Disease. JAMA. 2004;292(24):3017–3023. doi:10.1001/jama.292.24.3017. https://pubmed.ncbi.nlm.nih.gov/15613671/. Accessed Sept 8, 2023.

The Need for Information and the Effects of Its Absence

Choosing drugs and accepting a doctor's prescription would be simple if information about how many people a drug helps or harms were readily available. Usually, doctors are forced to estimate the chances of benefit or harm because the scientific evidence for or against a certain intervention is unavailable. When scientific evidence is available, doctors should inform patients about the chances of benefit or harm; when evidence is lacking, then at least guesstimating the range of potential health outcomes would seem appropriate.

In the absence of compelling evidence, doctors make artful recommendations based on their own knowledge, experience, values, beliefs, personal biases and predictions of what is most likely to work. It is simply not always possible to act scientifically in treating patients. Reality is that doctors choose treatments either based on medical science or, absent definitive evidence, they choose based on the art of Medicine and make decisions on what they think they know about the patient and the intervention and what they believe is important. Therefore, it's not surprising that, in the absence of definitive scientific evidence about what to do, different clinicians reach different conclusions.

According to the type of intervention and how complicated and risky it is, a varying degree of sophistication is required on the part of clinicians. Some non-intrusive interventions like verbal therapy or counselling sound easy but applying them effectively is a challenge as we discuss at greater depth in the chapters on mental health. In contrast, complicated intrusive procedures, like thoracic (chest) surgery, require sophisticated knowledge, skill and dexterity. In either case, there is always a risk that a patient may suffer untoward effects from any treatment. Even when excellent information is available and scientific choices are made, patients must accept the risk that the state of knowledge might not be adequate, that a mistake might occur or that one is just unlucky. Every treatment, scientific or artful, poses some risk.

Consequently, it is beneficial when non-clinicians, like patients and their families, participate in their care because they provide a second set of eyes and minds that help prevent mistakes or simply help make better choices for themselves. When patients ask about the chances of benefit or harm, clinicians must provide information either about the research or the rationale for treatment. This additional step sometimes leads clinicians to reconsider their recommendations and avoid a mishap or an intervention that won't fit with the person's values and preferences. Be aware that there are often caution signs, the message of FIGURE 1.37.1.

FIGURE 1.37.1: There are often warnings of possible errors

Medication Errors Can Lead to Disability, Dysfunction and Death

The classic Canadian Adverse Events study by Baker and Norton describes medical mistakes. Common mistakes they document include drug errors leading to disability, dysfunction and death. Patients may have received commonly used drugs they did not need or drugs that would be useful for someone else but wrong for them. Examples included people with problems such as renal (kidney) failure getting much worse because they received ordinary drugs, including Aspirin, ibuprofen and indomethacin.[210] Sometimes the cause was an administration or pharmacist error.

See further detail on errors at the end of this section.

ACCIDENTAL DIABETES PRESCRIPTION

One of DZ's patients was prescribed an antibiotic for an infection. She picked up the prescription and returned to the office the next day complaining that she craved sugary substances, even noting that she had put maple syrup on the ½ dozen sugar donuts she ate the night before. DZ called the pharmacist, who apologized and said that instead of filling a clearly written prescription for an antibiotic, she had dispensed a drug for diabetes. The person became hypoglycemic (low blood sugar) and her craving might have saved her life! Fortunately, her body detected possible harm from abnormally low sugar and she developed the urge for a sugar splurge.

The Patient's Wager

With what we already know about treatments, we can recognize that some are helpful, some harmful and some are a waste of money. Every day, people experience seemingly miracle cures from any number of conventional and unconventional treatments, including applying and then burying a potato to eliminate a wart.[211] Others only suffer from the side-effects of medications that were meant to cure. Still others spend money on things that are irrelevant because they have no effect.

Unfortunately, it is nearly impossible for any doctor to always prescribe the exact drug that each patient needs. Patients vary in how they or their disease react to treatment. Patients also differ in their preferences or expectations for outcomes and what they will accept as treatment. Although there is a promise of a future that will deliver 'personalized medicine' or 'precision medicine', we are not there yet. Today, the way we choose a drug, assign a dose and schedule its application leads many patients to get the wrong drug or more or less of the drug than they really need, even if the doctor is following established guidelines. Sometimes there are many guidelines, and the clinician requires a guideline as to which guideline to follow! The material on drug dosing and the dose-effect curve derived from research may determine why physicians often prescribe drugs in higher doses then is necessary.

Occasionally, patients must choose between different doctors' opinions about which treatment to accept. Few people reflect on what they should consider when faced with differing treatment choices. Sometimes, even when they know which questions to ask, the answers are not easy to find because many of the scientific papers, easily accessible to academic faculties, are hidden behind paywalls and they'd have to pay for access. We have touched on searching for information in Chapter 6.

Yet getting information to assist in decision-making is important. The fact is that whenever doctors suggest a diagnostic test or a medical treatment, they are proposing that the patient make a wager on the outcome. Another way of deciding what to bet on is to consider what happened to similar patients in the past. Patients could ask the doctor if, based on medical research, previous patients benefitted rather than suffered harm, what those benefits and harms were and how many were in each category.

All patients want doctors to share their values and to prescribe exactly what they prefer. To have such a doctor, patients must select one that fits with them. Some would prefer a doctor who treats aggressively. Other patients might prefer more cautious physicians.

210 CMAJ. 2004 May 25;170(11):1678-86. The Canadian Adverse Events Study: the incidence of adverse events among hospital patients in Canada. Baker GR[1], Norton PG, Flintoft V, Blais R, Brown A, Cox J, Etchells E, Ghali WA, Hébert P, Majumdar SR, O'Beirne M, Palacios-Derflingher L, Reid RJ, Sheps S, Tamblyn R. https://pubmed.ncbi.nlm.nih.gov/15159366/. Accessed Sept 8, 2023.

211 https://hillsborough-homesteading.com/old-wives-tales/. Accessed July 19, 2022.

Each style of practice benefits some people and harms others. The choosing of a doctor is tantamount to choosing an intervention…it may even be the most significant choice! We address the issues of aggressive versus cautious physicians elsewhere.

Chapter 38: —— Art and Science of Medicine

KEYWORDS: Art, Science, Polypharmacy, Treatment, Diabetes, Loose vs Tight Control Of Diabetes.

ABSTRACT: Medical practice is both an art and a science. Recommended treatments must meet the overall needs of patients and not merely address specific biomarkers. Deciding whether a person with diabetes should rigorously or less rigorously control blood sugar is one example of the dilemma that doctors and patients face. The art of Medicine refers to both how physicians deal with science unknowns, but also with the overall humanity with which they interact with and treat patients.

ART VERSUS SCIENCE

Clinicians use medical science when they adopt solutions that research shows are effective. Clinicians use intuition and their knowledge – the art of Medicine – when they recommend unproven solutions. Usually, clinicians have a reason for artful recommendations based on their perhaps imperfect understanding of Biology or on their prior clinical experiences. Many recommendations are based on the art of Medicine because trials may have not been completed on patients like the one the doctor is treating.

The Art of Treatment

Doctors recommend treatments based on "the art of Medicine" when patients need treatments and appropriate research studies are not available to provide statistical and scientific support for the interventions.

What people refer to as the 'art of Medicine' is the need for practitioners to recommend rational and probably useful but not-fully-validated treatments. When doctors recommend treatment based on pertinent scientific and statistical evidence, they are practicing 'Medical Science'. When scientific evidence is not available, doctors use information from their experience with previous patients and their knowledge of Biology, Biochemistry and Pharmacology to make a recommendation. The selection of the proper treatment also requires numeracy and sophistication in understanding the results of research. Regretfully, patients are not usually told which recommendations are based on art and which on science.

One problem with recommendations based on 'art' is that, without statistical support, it is difficult to choose between the recommendations of two thoughtful clinicians who offer different opinions about what is best. Medical publications recognize the wide variation in care when there is not a scientific consensus.[212] The lay press also recognizes that some recommendations are artful and that patients are not

212 Clara Westwell-Roper, Joanna M. Lubieniecka, Kelly L. Brown, et. Al., Clinical practice variation and need for pediatric-specific treatment guidelines among rheumatologists caring for children with ANCA-associated vasculitis: an international clinician survey, Pediatric Rheumatology volume 15, Article number: 61 (2017). https://www.ncbi.nlm.nih.gov/pubmed/28784150. Accessed July 19, 2022.

always told when recommendations are not based on proven science or that some artful recommendations might not even hold the promise of being effective.[213]

Most patients prefer to receive what doctors prefer to recommend, namely treatments based on research studies and scientifically known probabilities of benefits and harms. However, often doctors must deal with illnesses, aches and pains when there are no solutions that have strong research support. Some diseases may even be life threatening but lack a widely accepted and scientifically tested solution.

Fortunately, most patients indicate they feel comfortable receiving treatments based on the art of Medicine when there are no scientifically validated solutions.

Theoretical understanding of human illness and treatment requires sophisticated knowledge of a variety of medical sciences. Doctors with such knowledge can reasonably speculate and suggest innovative treatments. Sometimes, such suggestions might even be effective. It is important that we recognize, however, that they are place-fillers until scientists discover definitive approaches. It is equally important to encourage the collection of data linking artful recommendations to subsequent health in order to reveal objectively what works and what does not. FIGURE 1.38.1 illustrates these points.

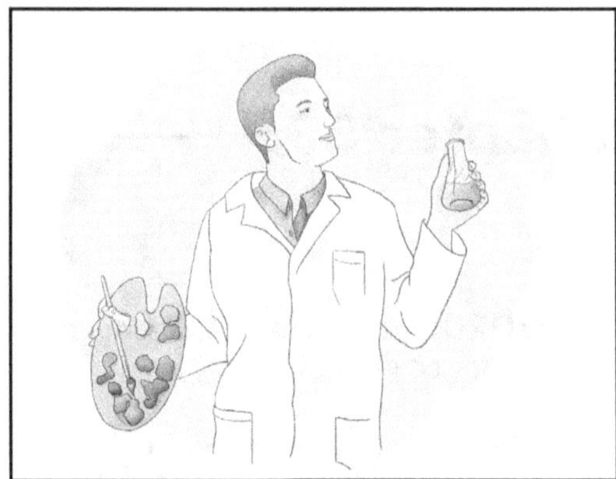

FIGURE 1.38.1: Physicians are both scientists and artists

The Science of Treatment[214]

Treatment may be merely an educated guess and a gamble, absent information about the characteristics of patients most likely to experience benefit or harm. Therefore, the lack of such information is only temporarily tolerable – something must be done about it. In order to get information about the helpfulness or harmfulness of a medication, it is crucial that we diligently search for it if it exists. However, it may be difficult to find or that we must work towards producing that information.

The effectiveness of care depends on formal studies of the results achieved when a meaningful number of people try a treatment. These studies are the 'clinical trials'[215] we have mentioned. Each trial of a medication produces information regarding the 'efficacy' of the drug. But we need to go even further, including natural experiments. Natural experiments are ones where researchers track the fate of large numbers of people who receive a treatment.

213 https://www.nytimes.com/2019/08/26/upshot/why-doctors-still-offer-treatments-that-may-not-help.html. Accessed July 19, 2022.

214 The diagram at the end of this document shows the evidence pyramid and indicates the types of information clinicians use when making choices and the scientific rigour of the method. We hope that predictive modeling techniques will enable people to capture information from clinical encounters to better learn which treatments are most likely to help particular people. https://www.google.com/search?q=medical+evidence+pyramid&client=firefox- Accessed July 19, 2022.

215 https://clinicaltrials.gov/ct2/about-studies/learn. Accessed July 19, 2022.

For example, in Vaccinology, researchers track the fate of people who receive yearly influenza vaccine and those who don't. It is beyond this book to discuss the details of the methods but be aware that such methods exist, and they allow us to determine how repeated flu immunization impacts people with different characteristics.

In medical research the **efficacy** of a drug indicates how well it works under ideal circumstances, that is, during a formal research project when it is under the careful observation of researchers and subject to careful management of the patient population. The **effectiveness** of a drug is how well the drug works in the real world with people in the general population. Doctors recommend treatments based on science when research studies at least demonstrate statistical indication that an intervention is efficacious. They hope the treatment will also be effective in the real world.

During clinical trials (efficacy studies) researchers monitor the effects of the test medication in the context of other agents the patient is using, and they attempt to control those. Researchers and participating clinicians together oversee the care process during the trial. This careful monitoring and review do not normally happen in everyday health care! So, a trial is a special testing situation and that needs to be taken into account when interpreting its results. To get to the level of understanding drug effectiveness, researchers must monitor patients after the trial ends. Pharmaceutical companies sometimes facilitate studies like this that are called 'post-market reviews', but objective researchers must participate if there is to be reasonable certainty that the review is 'arms length.'

If those effectiveness studies have been completed, doctors will have reasonable knowledge of a treatment's effectiveness. If not, they have at least a satisfactory basis for believe that the treatment will prove to be effective for their real-world patients.

We previously described another type of analysis that strengthens our belief in the results of trials. This involves looking at and combining the overall results of multiple trials on similar patients (a 'systematic review' or 'meta-analysis').[216] This latter analysis is often the strongest evidence on which physicians can base treatment decisions.

A scientific way to understand the effects of treatment is: (1) to determine the detailed characteristics of patients whom we wish to treat, (2) understand how the treatment might affect or be affected by each of these characteristics, (3) apply the treatment, and then (4) measure the effects of the treatment on those characteristics. Each characteristic or groups thereof can potentially be the subject of benefit or harm from the treatment. This makes it clear that, in a trial, the selection of patients with certain characteristics is crucial. In carrying out the trial, we establish the characteristics of patients most likely to achieve benefit or harm from a particular treatment. Studies like this are 'parametric studies.' In order to develop the information needed for science-based care, parametric studies that show convincing sta tistical indicators are essential. Ideally, when a doctor prescribes a drug or drugs for a patient, that patient and the drug(s) should be at least comparable to the patients and the drug(s) involved in the research trials.

Clinical Trials are Limited – Polypharmacy Rarely Evidence-Based

Unfortunately, some drug studies exclude large groups of ordinary people, for example

216 Uman LS. Systematic reviews and meta-analyses. J Can Acad Child Adolesc Psychiatry. 2011 Feb;20(1):57-9. PMID: 21286370; PMCID: PMC3024725. https://www.ncbi.nlm.nih.gov/pmc/articles/PMC3024725/. Accessed July 19, 2022.

women.[217] Another example is related to polypharmacy, defined as "patients taking many medications or using more drugs than clinically indicated"[218].

If there are types of patients that trials have not addressed or when patients are using drug combinations not tested, as is often the case with polypharmacy, doctors must subjectively use their experience and knowledge of the human body to assess the likely benefits and harms of treating them.

This situation is common. Over 60% of Canadian seniors take 5 or more medications and 30% of those over 85 are taking more than 10.[219] When doctors prescribe several drugs for a patient's various conditions, it is highly likely that the prescribing was artful and not based on science. What is interesting is that some clinicians are more likely to choose from a broader selection of drugs[220] or to prescribe more drugs[221]. Again, it seems that physician style often importantly influences prescribing.

Polypharmacy is an important matter. It makes it more likely that people will suffer because of mistakes both in how the drugs are taken and from adverse drug reactions. Multiple medications increase the chances of confusion, falls and hip fractures.[222] Physicians who deal with the elderly (geriatricians) are or should be aware of this and should take steps like asking the patient to bring in all medications and then consider if all are essential and appropriate in combination. Whenever a patient is taking many medications it is almost certain that studies are lacking on the effects of these combinations. It may just be that it was too difficult to create thoughtful research studies examining the effect of multiple drugs on a large group of patients or that there are simply too many combinations to test.

In thinking about this, we should also realize that the actions of drugs may be different for men and women, for people simultaneously taking or not taking certain drugs or for those drinking certain fruit juices or alcohol and those not.[223] A later chapter discusses the biology of some drug treatments and drug interactions.

Often doctors must use the art of Medicine to adjust treatments and dosages, trying to make them appropriate for the patient. However, most medical experts, including geriatricians, accept that, whenever possible, patients and clinicians should avoid polypharmacy. Easily said!

---

217 Holdcroft A. Gender bias in research: how does it affect evidence-based medicine? Journal of the Royal Society of Medicine. 2007;100(1):2-3. https://www.ncbi.nlm.nih.gov/pmc/articles/PMC1761670/. Accessed July 19, 2022.

218 Farrell B, Shamji S, Monahan A, French Merkley V. Reducing polypharmacy in the elderly: Cases to help you "rock the boat." Canadian Pharmacists Journal: CPJ. 2013;146(5):243-244. doi:10.1177/1715163513499530. https://www.ncbi.nlm.nih.gov/pmc/articles/PMC3785194/. Accessed July 19, 2022.

219 Farrell B, Shamji S, Monahan A, French Merkley V. Reducing polypharmacy in the elderly: Cases to help you "rock the boat." Canadian Pharmacists Journal: CPJ. 2013;146(5):243-244. doi:10.1177/1715163513499530. https://www.ncbi.nlm.nih.gov/pmc/articles/PMC3785194/. Accessed July 19, 2022.

220 Joyce GF, Carrera M, Goldman DP, Sood N. Physician Prescribing Behavior and Its Impact on Patient-Level Outcomes. The American journal of managed care. 2011;17(12): e462-e471. https://pubmed.ncbi.nlm.nih.gov/22216870/. Accessed Sept 8, 2023.

221 Alkhateeb, F., Khanfar, N.M, Clauson, K., Characteristics of Physicians Who Frequently See Pharmaceutical Sales Representatives Journal of Hospital Marketing & Public Relations 19(1):2-14 February 2009 DOI 10.1080/15390940802581374. https://pubmed.ncbi.nlm.nih.gov/19197653/. Accessed August 26, 2022

222 Härstedt M, Rogmark C, Sutton R, Melander O, Fedorowski A. Polypharmacy and adverse outcomes after hip fracture surgery. Journal of Orthopaedic Surgery and Research. 2016; 11:151. doi:10.1186/s13018-016-0486-7. https://www.ncbi.nlm.nih.gov/pmc/articles/PMC5122200/. Accessed July 19, 2022.

223 Bailey DG, Malcolm J, Arnold O, David Spence J. Grapefruit juice–drug interactions. British Journal of Clinical Pharmacology. 1998;46(2):101-110. doi:10.1046/j.1365-2125.1998.00764.x. https://pubmed.ncbi.nlm.nih.gov/9723817/. Accessed Sept 8, 2023.

Diabetes and the Art of Medicine

Diabetes is a condition where a patient does not produce enough insulin (most people with Type 1 diabetes) or where patients' bodies are resistant to the effect of insulin (patients with Type 2 diabetes). People with diabetes are more likely to suffer from a variety of problems including cardiovascular, kidney and liver disease. It is relatively easy to detect. An elevated blood glucose (sugar) level is its usual biomarker and there are often symptoms that warn of it. Physicians use injected insulin and various oral drugs to treat diabetes with the objective of reducing blood sugar to levels closer to normal.

Physicians understand the basic Physiology, Pharmacology and Biochemistry of diabetes, including the Krebs cycle. The Krebs cycle is a biochemical description of how the body processes energy. Although most medical students learn about it, very few practitioners can recall all the details about how insulin, a treatment for diabetes, works. This is true even though insulin is important in that it has a profound effect on how the body uses energy and diabetes is relatively common.

Insulin is an injected drug. There are also 'oral hypoglycemic' agents that reduce blood sugar and patients take by mouth. A controversy in diabetes, not yet resolved by science, is whether or not diabetic patients should aim to have a treated blood sugar that is very close to other people's normal blood sugar. That seems logical, doesn't it? Furthermore, there is no disagreement about the importance of treating very high blood sugar, which poses an immediate risk of serious complications. These morbid problems include ketoacidosis (where fat is metabolized too fast, producing fruity-smelling breath) that leads to coma and sometimes death. However, mildly elevated blood sugar levels do not pose an immediate risk. Nevertheless, many clinicians and researchers believe that even a modest chronic excess of blood sugar contributes to premature heart disease and organ failure. Surprisingly, this may not be correct, as recent clinical trials have revealed!

So, there are two positions. One, strong or tight blood sugar control, favors bringing the blood sugar as close to 'normal' as possible. The other holds that a slightly elevated blood sugar is acceptable. Those who argue for the less rigid approach believe that rigid control increases the chances of complications from low blood sugar. The tight control types believe that lower blood sugar reduces the risk of diabetic complications, including circulatory problems leading to limb damage and blindness. Deciding which position is correct, however, is not possible, as no one has yet completed a rigorous and persuasive study that resolves the disagreement. However, for type 2, non-insulin-dependent diabetes, it seems that tight control is probably worse than more casual control.[224] [225]

Those with a scientific understanding of diabetes can try to infer from the results of existing studies which treatment is most likely to help or harm a given patient. However, even sophisticated knowledge of Biology and Biochemistry may be insufficient for definitive judgement. Knowledge of sugar metabolism does not enable a clinician to predict if a patient will be better off if treated one way or the other. The only answer is careful monitoring of patient progress and adjustment of medication.

224 Newman, D., Medicine by the Numbers A Collaboration of The NNT.com and AFP Tight Glycemic Control for Type 2 Diabetes Mellitus (Over Five Years), Am Fam Physician. 2015 Jun 1;91(11): online. https://www.aafp.org/pubs/afp/issues/2015/0601/od2.html. Accessed Sept 8, 2023.

225 Rodríguez-Gutiérrez R., Montori VM Glycemic control for patients with type 2 diabetes mellitus: our evolving faith in the face of evidence. Circ Cardiovasc Qual Outcomes. 2016; 9: 504-512. https://pubmed.ncbi.nlm.nih.gov/27553599/. Accessed Sept 8, 2023.

LOOSE OR TIGHT CONTROL OF BLOOD SUGAR IN DIABETES

Researchers recognized that using hypoglycemic (sugar-lowering) agents may be harmful when clinicians make aggressive attempts to lower blood sugar. Aggressive therapy, aimed at bringing sugar as close as possible to normal levels, is associated with adverse events including decreased comfort, hypoglycemia (too low sugar levels that may cause patients to lose consciousness) and weight gain.[226]

People with a parametric understanding of diabetes may be able to determine the characteristics of people likely to be helped by various treatments including insulin or oral hypoglycemic agents. They will also adjust, over time, the amount of insulin based on the patient's weight and the changes in patient's blood sugar when insulin dosage is changed.

Most people with diabetes have the same reactions to drug treatments but a few have idiosyncratic responses. Clinicians with proper knowledge can suggest rational, likely helpful, treatments even when research does clearly indicate the dose or type of medication most patients must take for good results.

This research does not mean that, forevermore, tight glycemic control is inferior. As techniques for monitoring blood sugar improve and as scientists develop techniques for more precise drug administration (like implanted insulin pumps with sensors to monitor blood glucose), we might reasonably expect that the disadvantages of tight glucose control will disappear.

In the absence of a deep scientific understanding of the nature of a disease, researchers can only resolve some controversies by using statistical methods (that document numerically what happened when physicians treated many patients) to analyze results. That does not always work, though. For Type 2 diabetes, it seemed logical that tighter blood sugar control would be better. Yet trials showed that very tight blood sugar control isn't good. Statistical methods, showing numerically what worked and did not work during a trial, revealed that we still do not know the best course of care. Research made it clear that we need deeper knowledge of diabetes and its treatments. If there is a theoretical reason to deem that a treatment will work, but statistical analysis of the results of a trial do not demonstrate that, then the theory is either incorrect or requires refinement.

Because of the inherent ambiguity regarding treatment, the patient's choice of doctor often determines if the patient will be subject to tight or more casual blood sugar control.

CONTROL OF DIABETES

A diagram from NNT.COM indicates that, with tight control, one patient in 250 avoids a limb amputation, while 1 patient in 6 will require hospitalization at some time because of low blood sugar. Patients must be the ones to decide if a 1 in 250 chance of avoiding a limb amputation is worth the price of an increased risk of hospitalization. a hospitalization. Of course, it's never so simple because some patients prescribed tight control will not achieve it and others, to avoid the hazards of uncontrolled diabetes, will eat better and exercise more as a means of managing their diabetes.[227]

---

226 Moodahadu LS, Dhall R, Zargar AH, Bangera S, Ramani L, Katipally R. Tight Glycemic Control and Cardiovascular Effects in Type 2 Diabetic Patients. Heart Views: The Official Journal of the Gulf Heart Association. 2014;15(4):111-120. doi:10.4103/1995-705X.151084. https://pubmed.ncbi.nlm.nih.gov/25774253/. Accessed Sept 8, 2023.

227 Newman, D., Medicine by the Numbers A Collaboration of TheNNT.com and AFP Tight Glycemic Control for Type 2 Diabetes Mellitus (Over Five Years), Am Fam Physician. 2015 Jun 1;91(11): online. https://thennt.com/nnt/tight-glycemic-control-for-type-2-diabetes-over-5-years/. Accessed Sept 8, 2023.

Chapter 39: Evaluating Treatments – Number Needed to Treat and Number Needed to Harm

KEYWORDS: Number Needed to Harm, Number Needed to Treat, Benefits of Treatment, Harms of Treatment, The Patient's Wager, Sources of Information about Benefits and Harms, Treatment Error, Needless Treatment, Home Birth Controversy

ABSTRACT: Drugs help many people, but they also harm some. Clinical practice, including patient informed consent, requires an understanding of systematic methods to determine whether an intervention is more likely to help or harm. Examples in this chapter include issues of home birth, and some sources of information about the effectiveness or dangers of treatments.

Introduction

We have emphasized that treatment choices are almost always risky; treatments help some people and harm others. Further, the chances of benefit or harm are not often known. When they are known, two important measures are available. They are like the rating stars in advertising but provide more information and are not subjective. The measures are **Number Needed to Treat** (NNT) and **Number Needed to Harm** (NNH). The NNT answers the question: On average, how many people must be treated for one person to have benefitted? On the other hand, the NNH answers the question: On average, how many people must be treated for one person to have been harmed?

Imagine a roulette wheel with red and black numbers (FIGURE 1.39.1). The red numbers reflect the number of people who are harmed, the black numbers the number of people who are helped. The zeros reflect instances where treatment is neither helpful nor harmful, just a waste of money.

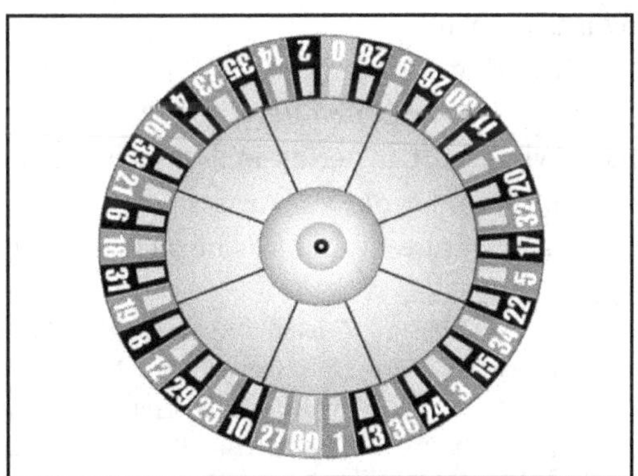

FIGURE 1.39.1: There is a chance of being helped or harmed

In roulette, there are 38 red, black and green numbers spread around the wheel. However, even the most ardent gambler would not bet on a roulette wheel where the numbers were hidden, and pay-out was based on a guess as to how many different numbers were on the wheel. Yet, just as in our blinded roulette, people don't normally know or ask about the chances of benefit or harm from treatments and only later do they discover if they won or lost at the treatment game. We can only hope that clinicians, administrators and researchers keep track of health outcomes, so they capture the information necessary to determine the chances of benefit or harm from treatments.

Consider, again, the treatment of hypertension. Physicians often prescribe medication to control mild hypertension for patients who have not had heart attacks or strokes. Their purpose is to reduce the risk of the patient having one. Antihypertension medication does reduce the chance of reoccurrence in people who have had a prior heart attack or stroke. However, doctors use these drugs commonly in people who have mild hypertension without a history of heart or stroke events. Physicians do this even though research evidence suggests that such treatment does not seem to reduce overall mortality or morbidity[228] in patients with mild hypertension. To no one's surprise, some people believe otherwise and feel that tight control of blood pressure is best, so they prescribe antihypertensives. Shades of diabetes management!

Measuring blood pressure seems simple but is a bit complicated because some people have 'white coat hypertension' – their blood pressure spontaneously increases when a professional measures it, but it is normal at other times. Assuming a person does really have mild hypertension and is prescribed a medicine, they should ask how confident the doctor is that the benefits outweigh the harms. Studies[229] [230] suggest that caution is appropriate and good financial sense suggests the same.

Again, the studies of patients who had not had a heart attack or stroke and who were taking antihypertension drugs for mild hypertension, showed the drugs prevented neither strokes nor heart attacks and didn't affect death rates. In the studies, patients taking antihypertensives and those taking placebos were equally likely to die. However, for every 12 people taking an antihypertensive drug, one stopped because of side effects. Some of those side effects were serious ones, including low pulse rate associated with fainting, fluid retention and swelling, electrolyte disturbances and associated disruption in normal cardiac rhythm (beating of the heart). [231] [232] Of course, it could be that eventually, as with many other conditions, researchers will discover drugs that do delay the usual illnesses of life, like heart attack, stroke or cancer. Until then it is important that efforts to reduce harm from one condition do not provoke other harms.

Medical Guidelines

NNT and NNH are incorporated into medical guidelines (see an example in FIGURE 1.39.2), which provide clinicians with information on when and how to treat a patient disorder.

228 Diao D, Wright JM, Cundiff DK, Gueyffier F. Pharmacotherapy for mild hypertension. Cochrane Database of Systematic Reviews 2012, Issue 8. Art. No.: CD006742. DOI: 10.1002/14651858.CD006742.pub2. Link to Cochrane Library. [PubMed]. https://pubmed.ncbi.nlm.nih.gov/22895954/. Accessed Sept 8, 2023.

229 http://www.thennt.com/nnt/anti-hypertensives-to-prevent-death-heart-attacks-and-strokes/. Accessed July 19, 2022 from the NNT.Com.

230 Diao D, Wright JM, Cundiff DK, Gueyffier F. Pharmacotherapy for mild hypertension. Cochrane Database of Syst Rev. 2012, Issue 8. Art. No.: CD006742. DOI: 10.1002/14651858.CD006742.pub2. https://pubmed.ncbi.nlm.nih.gov/22895954/. Accessed Sept 8, 2023.

231 http://www.thennt.com/nnt/anti-hypertensives-to-prevent-death-heart-attacks-and-strokes/. Accessed July 19, 2022 from the NNT.Com.

232 Diao D, Wright JM, Cundiff DK, Gueyffier F. Pharmacotherapy for mild hypertension. Cochrane Database of Syst Rev. 2012, Issue 8. Art. No.: CD006742. DOI: 10.1002/14651858.CD006742.pub2. https://pubmed.ncbi.nlm.nih.gov/22895954/ Accessed August 26, 2022., "AUTHORS' CONCLUSIONS:"Antihypertensive drugs used in the treatment of adults (primary prevention) with mild hypertension (systolic BP 140-159 mmHg and/or diastolic BP 90-99 mmHg) have not been shown to reduce mortality or morbidity in RCTs.

Guideline developers try to recommend standards of care based on research showing which treatments are effective and usually produce benefit while avoiding harm. These developers include the USA Agency for Healthcare Research and Quality[233] (AHRQ; https://www.ahrq.gov. Accessed August 3, 2022.) and the Canadian Medical Association[234]. The Agree Trust also facilitates the development, adoption and promotion of clinical practice guidelines, including guidelines for treatment.[235] (clinical practice guidelines list: http://www.agreetrust.org/. Accessed August 3, 2022).

When guidelines incorporating useful and proven treatments do not exist, as we outlined when discussing the art of Medicine, excellent clinicians use their knowledge of how the body and drugs work to choose solutions.

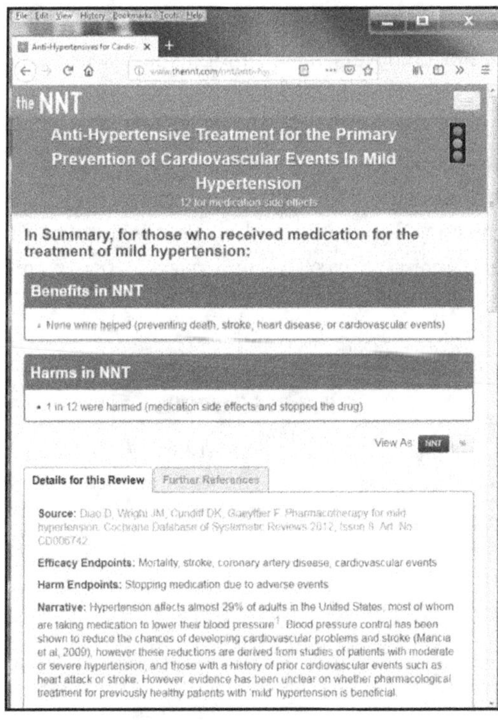

FIGURE 1.39.2: Example of NNT and NNH

Treatment Trade-offs

Patients expect drugs to improve comfort, function and/or life span. However, sometimes we make trade-offs. For example, people may accept immediate reductions in comfort and function if there is a reasonable potential for improvement in life expectancy. As we mentioned, they choose anticancer (chemotherapeutic) drugs to prolong life in the long term, though they often make people feel awful in the short-term.

Taking other drugs engenders similar considerations. If we are in pain, a doctor may prescribe narcotic analgesics but those may make us feel sleepy or become addicted. Antibiotics help cure infections, but some people experience serious harm from allergic reactions or a life-threatening infection, for example, C. difficile an antibiotic-resistant infection of the colon.

Pretty well every treatment involves a trade-off. This is like any wager. If we bet $1,000 in a lottery for a house, we might get a house cheaply, but we more likely will lose the money, as there is only a small chance of winning. It would be better to put the money toward a down payment and to eventually buy the house – then the money becomes a valued asset, not a wager. The message is that there are no sure things in treatment, only bets... some better than others.

Stakeholders

Stakeholders are people who have an interest in some process or outcome. They are participants.

In health care, the stakeholders include patients, families, care providers, health services administrators and insurers. They all need

233 https://www.guideline.gov/. Accessed July 19, 2022. National Guideline Clearing House, Agency for Healthcare Research and Quality.

234 CPG Infobase: Clinical Practice Guidelines Canadian Medical Association. https://joulecma.ca/cpg/homepage. Access to this URL will be cut off December 2023. Accessed Sept 8, 2023.

235 http://www.agreetrust.org/where-can-i-find-a-practice-guidelines/. Accessed July 19, 2022. The Agree Trust is a consortium of academics, clinicians and researchers mainly supported by the Canadian Institutes of Health Research.

information about the benefits and harms of treatment in order to give or receive informed consent, to decide how to deliver, accept or pay for care and to decide which treatments to insure. Lawyers also need information about the expected benefits and harms of treatment to know if an adverse event experienced by a client was unpredictable or represented the prescriber's poor judgement or failure to treat. Even journalists who report on new treatments must understand the measures that are necessary to decide that an intervention or innovation is worthwhile and to report it to their audiences.

Health informaticians, working with patients, researchers and clinicians, collect, store, analyze and interpret information about the effectiveness of treatments. They do this by integrating information systems into the care process to track the treatment outcomes of patients. They are also important resources to help other stakeholders achieve their goals. Informaticians' work is to produce reliable information to support treatment choices. Unfortunately, as we have mentioned, sometimes it is difficult, costly or just plain impossible to get important information. Worse still, some Internet searches lead people to promotional material or unfounded opinion, rather than reliable scientific evidence.

Some health systems, for example Kaiser Permanente in California, make good use of predictive modeling methods linking healthcare activities and results. Not all organizations are so dedicated.

Where to Get Information about Benefits and Harms

Several organizations provide credible, well-researched information about the benefits and harms of drugs, including Bandolier[236], the University of British Columbia Therapeutics Initiative[237] and the Cochrane Collaboration[238]. Medline, provided by the National Institutes of Health in the United States, is also an important source[239], as is NICE, the National Institute of Health and Care Excellence[240], in the UK Each of these organizations evaluates knowledge about drugs and other treatments and makes it available in ways that are easy to understand. Unfortunately, some publishers only release research information to paying subscribers or to people who purchase individual articles. The practice of hiding research behind paywalls becomes especially galling when taxpayers have funded the research. In the United States, Canada and Britain, government agencies support many forms of medical research and it seems odd that the publishers can demand money for the information they produce. Indeed, some believe it is outrageous and many efforts are underway to try to put it right!

SOME EVIDENCE-BASED MEDICINE RESOURCES

- *A guide created by the University of Illinois at Chicago's Library of the Health Sciences at Peoria. Please feel free to contact them with any questions at lib-pref@uic.edu. Accessed Aug 3, 2022.*
- *http://researchguides.uic.edu/c.php?g=252338&p=3963341. Accessed Aug 3, 2022.*
- *Dartmouth Medical Libraries: http://www.dartmouth.edu/~library/biomed/*

236 http://www.bandolier.org.uk/. Accessed July 19, 2022.

237 http://www.ti.ubc.ca/TherapeuticsLetter. Accessed July 19, 2022.

238 http://www.cochrane.org/. Accessed July 19, 2022.

239 https://www.nih.gov/. Accessed July 19, 2022. U.S. Department of Health and Human Services, National Institutes of Health, Turning Discovery into Health.

240 https://www.nice.org.uk/. Accessed July 19, 2022.

guides/research/ebm-az-list.html?mswitch-redir=classic. Accessed Aug 3, 2022.

- *University of Oxford Centre for Evidence Based Medicine: http://www.cebm.net/category/ebm-resources/. Accessed Aug 3, 2022.*
- *McMaster University Centres for Evidence-Based Practice: The 6S pyramid. Characterizes the kind of evidence available at each site note: http://hsl.mcmaster.libguides.com/ebm. Accessed Aug 3, 2022.*
- *The NNT: http://www.thennt.com/. Accessed Aug 3, 2022.*
- *Agree Enterprise Web Site promoted by CIHR for development and implementation of practice guidelines including treatment: http://www.agreetrust.org/. Accessed July 19, 2022.*

Treatment Errors

As we mentioned, the classic study by Baker and Norton, The Canadian Adverse Events study, described medical mistakes. Common mistakes (we address this in depth later) included drug errors leading to disability, death and dysfunction.[241] In the modern world, it is reasonable to expect that automated prompting systems would present information about benefits and harms to clinicians when they prescribe drugs. This should include cautions when liver or kidney function studies indicate the patient is likely to have difficulty with drug metabolism (breakdown in the body) and is more likely to suffer complications from treatment.

Understanding the NNT and NNH…and a Little Sarcasm

In order to prescribe drugs at a dose ample for most people, the standard doses are, by default, higher than they need to be for many. The possible adverse effects of drugs relate to the drug and the dosage, so many people are exposed to unnecessary risk of harm. Pharmaceutical companies suggest higher drug doses than should be effective for 95% of the population. However, many people would respond well at lower doses, incurring lower risk of undesirable adverse reactions. Unfortunately, we just don't know who is who. Again, the problem is the lack of information. We can see here why we look toward a future of Personalized or Precision Medicine, which promises the ability to determine the unique characteristics of each patient and to 'tune' the drug, dosage and duration thereto.

We have pointed out that the standard terms to describe the usefulness of medicines are 'Number Needed to Treat' (NNT) and 'Number Needed to Harm' (NNH). These numbers give us some idea of the probable positive value and negative impacts of a medication.

To look at this in a way that may make the issue even more glaringly, a summary article by Drs. Brophy and Bogaty in the journal Lancet reports that systematic nitrate (example, nitroglycerine, a drug to increase blood circulation to the heart muscle) use after a heart attack helps one person in 250. In other words, though one person will benefit, 249 people will not! The Number Needed to Treat Needlessly is 249/250! In other words, 99.6% of people will experience needless treatment for, on average, one to benefit.

Beta blockers are another example. Doctors prescribe beta blockers (e.g., atenolol or propranolol) to many patients with heart failure after a heart attack. In this case, 1 person in 33 benefits, so the Number Needed to Treat Needlessly is 32 of 33. Most people, 97%, receiving beta blockers for heart failure after a heart attack are treated needlessly because they do not benefit. Drs. Bogaty and Brophy coined their own somewhat sarcastic term "Index of Therapeutic Impotence" to describe the

241 The Canadian Adverse Events Study: the incidence of adverse events among hospital patients in Canada. Baker GR[1], Norton PG, Flintoft V, Blais R, Brown A, Cox J, Etchells E, Ghali. WA, Hébert P, Majumdar SR, O'Beirne M, Palacios-Derflingher L, Reid RJ, Sheps S,Tamblyn R., CMAJ. 2004 May 25;170(11):1678-86. https://pubmed.ncbi.nlm.nih.gov/15159366/. Accessed Sept 8, 2023.

proportion of people who do not benefit. Think of how many would be spared side effects and cost if we knew who that one person in 33 or 250 is who would, in fact, benefit! Eventually, we hope, research and data mining efforts will help to identify the characteristics of people most likely to benefit or be harmed.

In summary, treatment choices pose conflicts between the goals of improving comfort, improving function and increasing lifespan. It is important, but difficult, to choose among treatments. Sometimes the chances of benefit and harm are not clear. Sometimes people value different outcomes. Sometimes the chance of a life-preserving benefit makes it acceptable and worthwhile to risk the chance of adverse events.

Home Birth Controversy – Another Numbers Problem

Headlines about home birth in the New York Times and from the Canadian Broadcasting Corporation reflect the dilemmas all of us face.

The issue of home birth illustrates the need for accurate information to enable informed choices. A New York Times headline reads "*As Home Births Grow in the US a New Study Examines the Risks*."[242] This report cites an article in the New England Journal of Medicine (NEJM) that emphasizes the increased, but small, risk associated with planned home births. Birth does have associated risks that include the need for maternal blood transfusions, perinatal (around birth) infant deaths and depressed 5-minute Apgar scores. The Apgar score indicates the medical condition of the baby immediately after birth. It allows the delivery staff to assess: APGAR – the baby's Appearance (skin color); Pulse (heart rate); Grimace response (reflexes); Activity (muscle tone) and Respiration (breathing rate and effort). The baby gets from 0 to 2 points for each, with an ideal total score being 10.

Statistics indicate that neonatal deaths both at home and in hospital are rare. However, the NEJM article suggests that home birth leads to one additional infant death per 1,000 obstetrical deliveries (NNH = 1/1000). The beneficial trade-off of home birth, according to the NEJM, is that women are less likely to have obstetrical procedures, such as caesarean sections (C-section: surgical delivery through the abdominal wall rather than via the vagina). About 25% of the women who delivered in-hospital <u>and were expected to have a normal delivery</u> (note that!) had a caesarean section, compared with only 5% of women who planned a home birth. Note that a caesarian can make a following birth more complicated and is a surgical procedure with possible complications.

If the information is accurate, women are faced with the choice of a small but real risk of neonatal death balanced against maternal comfort. But that is not the final word.

The Canadian Broadcasting Company (CBC) headline has a different emphasis. The CBC headline states "*Low-Risk Births Just as Safe at Home as in Hospital: McMaster Study*".[243] The CBC report, based on an article in the Canadian Medical Association Journal (CMAJ), commented that McMaster study *"found little difference in the incidence of stillbirth or neonatal death — 1.15 for every 1,000 babies in the home births and 0.94 [per thousand] in the hospital group"*. [slightly more that the NEJM study, emphasis ours]

Both reports show that the rate of obstetrical interventions, caesarean sections and

242 As Home Births Grow in the US a New Study Examines the Risks, Belluck, P., As Home Births Grow in the US, a New Study Examines the Risks, New York Times, Dec 30, 2015. https://www.nytimes.com/2015/12/31/health/as-home-births-grow-in-us-a-new-study-examines-the-risks.html. Accessed Sept 8, 2023.

243 The CBC headline states "Low-Risk Births Just as Safe at Home as in Hospital: McMaster Study". Low-risk births just as safe at home as in hospital: McMaster study Craggs, S., CBC News Posted December 21, 2015. https://www.cbc.ca/news/canada/hamilton/headlines/low-risk-births-just-as-safe-at-home-as-in-hospital-mcmaster-study-1.3374764. Accessed August 3, 2022.

maternal lacerations was lower in the home birth group! This is essentially just a difference in emphasis but might lead one to a different conclusion. Expectant mothers face conflicting choices regarding home versus hospital delivery. Both reports recognize that women who delivered at home are more likely to avoid surgical interventions. However, in both studies there is a slight increase in the neonatal death rate for parents who opt for home delivery. That is what mothers-to-be must consider and balance it against the benefits they perceive.

There are some caveats, however. The Canadian authors recognize that "*findings from the study should be generalized only to settings that provide similar support [to that of hospitals] for women choosing home birth*". Note also that the NEJM report was modified by the statement "*who were expected to have a normal delivery*". In other words, it is necessary to understand any predictable risks as well as the local context and local results. In fact, in some communities, the infrastructure exists to support home births and to address unexpected events that threaten the baby or mother. In other communities, these supports might not be available (especially in remote areas). The choice depends on the knowledge, skills, experience and results achieved locally. Unfortunately, most communities in the United States and Canada do not bother to collect important information about the results of care, hence that information is not available, making it difficult for mothers to reach a thoughtful conclusion.

Basic Science Informing the Art of Medicine

Often it is not possible to do statistical studies to learn how drugs will work on everyone. One reason is that it is impossible to study the many variants of contexts and behaviors. For example, few studies examine the effect of different diets on the effectiveness of any drug. Researchers rarely learn if people who drink grapefruit juice, orange juice or cranberry juice react differently to drugs, even though we know that there are effects of local customs and behavior on the effectiveness of drugs.

Researchers and patients were surprised when they first learned that drinking grapefruit juice affects the required dosage of certain drugs.[244] This means that conclusions about the effective dosage are different if studies include grapefruit juice drinkers. Local context is often important.

Patients, wagering that a particular treatment will only be helpful can reassure themselves by asking about the expected results of treatment. How many people have lived longer with treatment? How many people have experienced improved function? How many people have been able to do more after treatment? How many people were more or less comfortable? How many people experienced harm? Often, though, specific studies have not been completed and clinicians must make inferences about what might be the best drug or drug dose for this patient.

Lack of information is a general problem. Not only women considering home birth lack the precise information they need to know the exact chances that a treatment will be helpful or harmful. All of us are in that situation. Perhaps by participating in our own care, we can influence this. Our questions can potentially induce change in health systems and push them to monitor the results of care. If we can do this, reliable information to support treatment choices will become accessible to anyone who seeks it and asks the right questions.

But life must go on even absent information. Lacking information, clinicians and patients must rely on conjectures and inferences about the benefits and harms of care.

244 Dahan, A., Altman, H. Food–drug interaction: grapefruit juice augments drug bioavailability—mechanism, extent and relevance. Eur J Clin Nutr 58, 1–9 (2004). https://pubmed.ncbi.nlm.nih.gov/14679360/. Accessed August 4, 2022.

Chapter 40: ——— Treatment Issues

KEYWORDS: Eldercare, Cautious and Aggressive Physicians, Therapeutic Excess, Therapeutic Gap

ABSTRACT: Physicians vary in how they interpret the medical literature or patient findings. Often, conscientious physicians offer different solutions for the same problem. Some are aggressive, preferring to make sure that no one who could benefit from treatment misses out. Others are cautious, preferring to reduce the risk that someone might be harmed by an adverse drug reaction. Treating Seniors, the challenge of eldercare, depicts some of the challenges.

The Challenge of Eldercare

As we age, we often face challenges from our bodies. There is both normal deterioration – especially if we place less emphasis on fitness or we suffer the accumulated effects of choices we made in our youth when we were immortal…or thought that. There is also senescence at the cellular and organ levels, i.e., our cells and body parts have 'Best By' dates. The overall impact of this – though some manage to delay it until the very end by good choices – is often multiple-organ disease or what are called 'co-morbidities'. Regarding the latter, we have mentioned that diabetes is often accompanied by cardiovascular and kidney problems. It can also be that mental decline can affect the patient's ability to remember to take medications and to avoid overdosing. So, treating the elderly is a medical challenge, especially as the intervention that helps one problem can worsen another.

The comeuppance is[245]: *"Elderly patients are frequent users of health services and medicines. Research, however, has identified problems in the effective use of medicines in this population. Adverse drug reactions are implicated in 5-17% of hospital admissions. Elderly people are also less likely to receive treatments indicated by guidelines including treatment for heart attacks – myocardial infarction. In addition, discrepancies with medicines prescribed in the hospital occur after discharge so patients do not receive the medicines they need, or overdose because they do not recognize that medicines prescribed in hospital are similar to the ones they were taking at home."* [246]

Patients expect doctors to use specialized knowledge, skill and experience to solve problems. They also expect most doctors to offer similar solutions to the same problem. There is the reality, though, that different doctors may give different advice for the same problem because sometimes, even for common problems, they harbor different opinions about the best approach. This is especially evident in Psychiatry where different professionals will apply diverse labels and suggest different treatments for the same person. Unfortunately, in

245 Spinewine A, Swine C, Dhillon S, et al. Appropriateness of use of medicines in elderly inpatients: qualitative study. BMJ. 2005;331(7522):935. doi:10.1136/bmj.38551.410012.06. https://www.ncbi.nlm.nih.gov/pmc/articles/PMC1261188/. Accessed August 3, 2022.

246 A. Spinewine, C. Swine, S. Dhillon, B. D. Franklin, P. M. Tulkens, L. Wilmotte, and V. Lorant Appropriateness of use of medicines in elderly inpatients: qualitative study. BMJ Oct 2005; 331: 935; https://www.nytimes.com/2015/12/31/health/as-home-births-grow-in-us-a-new-study-examines-the-risks.html. Accessed Sept. 8, 2023.

the absence of rigorous science, clinicians must rely on what they know in order to formulate artful recommendations.

Occasionally, differences in opinion arise because doctors differ as to which outcomes they value most. Sometimes, though, differences arise because doctors have a different understanding of how best to evaluate the effects of treatment.[247]

The patient's dilemma is to know which questions to ask to improve the chances of getting appropriate treatment and of receiving recommendations consistent with values and preferences. Patients who ask questions are encouraging their clinicians to find and communicate clear and patient-specific answers.

Drugs are useful only if they are helpful. It should be clear that we need to ask about the number of people who must take the drug for one of them to benefit (the NNT) and the number of people who must take the drug for one to experience harm (the NNH). Of course, it is also important to know the extent of the proposed benefits and possible harms. People who are invested participants in health care should ask these questions both to help clinicians choose among possible treatments and to help themselves decide to accept, eliminate from further consideration or reject a clinician's recommendations. However, we can only work with pharmacists and physicians if we understand the basic principles of medical treatment, including how drugs and dosage are decided.

Today, we can find out at least some of what is known about the potential benefits and harms of treatment. Increasingly, Health Informatics experts are capturing the information necessary for decisions but there is much yet they need to do. Several organizations do provide credible, well-researched information about the effects of drugs, as cited in this book. Each of these organizations evaluates and promulgates information about drugs and makes it available in ways that are easy to understand.

Cautious and Aggressive Physicians

We have mentioned that choosing a physician may be tantamount to selecting a treatment! Physicians are not all the same, harboring different attitudes towards patients' problems and their treatment. We will name physicians as 'Aggressive' who tend to treat everyone whom they believe might benefit from treatment, but also to treat some who might not. The patients getting unnecessary care are exposed to possible adverse effects of treatment, with no opportunity to benefit. Also, aggressive physicians may be more likely to prescribe more invasive or intrusive solutions. The option of cautious versus aggressive intervention is illustrated in FIGURE 1.40.1.

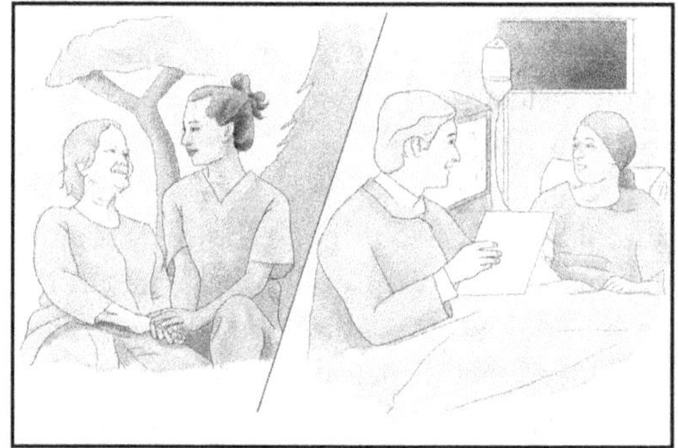

Figure 1.40.1: Cautious vs aggressive intervention

We would call physicians 'Cautious' if they avoid unnecessary or 'shot in the dark' treatments but who harm some of their patients who might benefit from tests or treatment because they suffer for longer than necessary or miss getting worthwhile treatments.

247 Johnston, B.C., Alonso-Coello, P., Friedrich, J.O., et. Al., Do Clinicians Understand the Size of Treatment Effects? A Randomized Survey Across 8 Countries, CMAJ. 2016 Jan 5;188(1):25-32. doi: 10.1503/cmaj.150430. Epub 2015 Oct 26. https://www.cmaj.ca/content/cmaj/188/1/25.full.pdf. Accessed July 19, 2022.

A good example is when more aggressive physicians use antihypertension medication to treat patients who have mild hypertension, while more cautious physicians may advise patients to adopt and maintain a healthier lifestyle to address the same problem. Physician beliefs, knowledge and even biases influence their recommendations. Patients who enquire about the benefits and harms of treatment are, at the least, prompting their doctors to do some further thinking and maybe to obtain the latest evidence. They are also telling their physicians that they have skin in this game and want a say!

If a physician makes a more aggressive proposal, asking questions about the potential upsides and downsides of the contemplated action can be quite important. Being careful can be important because a finding like an elevated blood pressure might be spurious. Some patients perceived to have mild hypertension may be victims of the way the clinician measured BP. They may have exhibited a high pressure in single measurement in the office, but repeated testing would have shown that their blood pressure was normal.

Physicians are human. Many medical decisions reflect, in addition to the physicians' knowledge and typical *modus operandi*, the physicians' personal tastes, rather than a scientific consensus. Even for common problems, for example treatments of sore throats in children, physicians show wide variations in the advice they give.

Therapeutic Excess and Therapeutic Gap

As we have indicated, some doctors (the aggressive ones) decide to prescribe drugs – or other interventions – whenever a condition might possibly benefit. The cautious ones, on the other hand, when faced with uncertainty, try to avoid prescribing, thereby reducing the likelihood of drug-induced harm. Of course, doctors usually try to prescribe the appropriate drug for the patient. The same applies to other interventions, like surgery.

This means that aggressive prescribers are more likely to overprescribe for some patients. This therapeutic excess leads to unnecessary and sometimes harmful complications. Unfortunately, some people who would recover without treatment also receive drugs that can cause complications.

Cautious prescribers are, as we have pointed out, more likely to under-prescribe. They do avoid the harms of unnecessary medication but some patients who would benefit from a prescription suffer or die needlessly because they do not get the treatment they need. Cautious prescribers produce a therapeutic gap because some people who would benefit do not receive it.

Therapeutic excess and the therapeutic gap must be considered in the context of litigation. Doctors who make or are thought to have made mistakes are prone to being sued. The risks for lawsuits are different for aggressive versus cautious prescribers. Aggressive prescribers harm some people because of medication side effects. Patients can elect to sue them for the harm the treatment caused. However, many people are aware that medicines may harm some people and might assume that the medication side effect was inevitable and do not sue. Patients of cautious prescribers can suffer harm because they don't receive a drug that might have helped them. Patients are more likely to be upset and to sue when they believe the doctors failed to act. There is no safe ground.

Consider a specific situation: the parent whose child has an earache and a very mild fever. Suppose the doctor did prescribe an antibiotic. If the child dies from an adverse, peculiar, rare and unexpected allergy to the antibiotic, the family might feel it was inevitable and the child needed it. It can also be that they decide that, in retrospect, the antibiotic was unnecessary – so they sue. On the other hand, if the doctor did not prescribe the antibiotic and the child dies from the rare complications of an infection, such as meningitis or mastoiditis, the parent might feel the doctor was negligent and did not do everything possible – so they sue. The appropriate expression that encapsulates both of these situations is: "You're damned if you do and you're damned if you don't!"

As the legal community becomes more aggressive and the courts more liberal, the possible outcomes of litigation will change. In any event, the success or failure of a defense might depend more on the sophistication of the lawyers and the medical experts they call than on the doctor's action or inaction. In some jurisdictions the legal standard is "common medical practice." If there are many local physicians with poor prescribing habits, the doctor is less likely to be found culpable.[248]

It is interesting that pharmaceutical companies, doctors and patients are aligned when drug companies try to reduce the therapeutic gap. Unfortunately, aggressive pursuit of reduction of the therapeutic gap may lead to a therapeutic excess. Everyone who needs a drug receives it, but some people who don't need it also get it and they can be injured. Again, we enter that state of damnation!

248 Moffett P, Moore G. The Standard of Care: Legal History and Definitions: The Bad and Good News. Western Journal of Emergency Medicine. 2011;12(1):109-112. https://pubmed.ncbi.nlm.nih.gov/21691483/. Accessed Sept. 8, 2023.

Chapter 41: Examples of Common Treatment Quandaries

KEYWORDS: Chris Cates' Diagram, Treatment Quandaries, Sore Throat, Otalgia (Sore Ear), Sleep Disturbance

ABSTRACT: Common conditions often illustrate the nature of treatment quandaries. When should doctors treat patients with medications, and which treatments should they prescribe for sore throats, sore ears, or sleep disturbances? Dr. Chris Cates has developed a methodology, illustrated, that visually depicts the chances that an intervention will help or harm.

Introduction

Choosing how to treat different people with different problems is seldom trivial. There are many factors that influence the choice including the nature of the illness, the nature of the person and the person's reaction to the illness, the spectrum of possible interventions and even the values and habits of the clinician. There is always a thought process, not the least important thought being how to avoid harming the patient.

Sore Throat

Sore throats are tricky, but there is a tendency to be quick on the draw. About 50% of doctors write prescriptions for antibiotics before they are certain the patient with a sore throat has a bacterial infection. Many doctors don't bother to get a throat swab to confirm if a bacterium was the cause.[249] If a virus caused the infection, an antibiotic would have no beneficial effect. Other doctors suggest waiting to see if the throat gets better before prescribing. Few of either group of physicians will be able to detail how many people they are likely to benefit or harm when they prescribe an antibiotic. This is even though commonly used antibiotics can cause both major and minor health problems.[250] Minor harms from antibiotics include diarrhea and allergic rashes; major ones, though rare, can include deadly allergic (anaphylactic) reactions or persistent bowel problems. It is important to recognize that the organisms growing in our bowels play important parts in our overall health. Killing them is not good news.

The strategy most doctors use, representing the art of Medicine, is to prescribe antibiotics if the symptoms are more significant, especially if

249 Science, M., Bitnum, A., McIsaac, W., Commentary: Identifying and treating group A Streptococcal pharyngitis in children CMAJ January 6, 2015 vol. 187 no. 1 First published December 15, 2014, doi: 10.1503/cmaj.141532. http://www.cmaj.ca/content/187/1/13.full; http://www.cmaj.ca/content/170/11/1678.full. Accessed Sept. 8, 2023.

250 Gillies, M., Ranakusuma, A., Hoffman, T., et. al. Common harms from amoxicillin: a systematic review and meta-analysis of randomized placebo-controlled trials for any indication CMAJ January 6, 2015 187: E21-E31; published ahead of print November 17, 2014, doi:10.1503/cmaj.140848. https://pubmed.ncbi.nlm.nih.gov/25404399/. Accessed Sept. 8, 2023.

fever is present or if there is a discharge around the tonsils (even though a viral infection can do this). The 'line' separating antibiotic versus non-antibiotic intervention is actually a fuzzy band.

Ear Pain or Infection in Children

Then there are earaches, and the parents are often right there. The chance of a child getting an antibiotic prescription for an earache depends as much on the parents' choice of physician as on their child's clinical condition.[251]

Most children (80-85%) with an acute ear infection feel better within 2 or 3 days without treatment and very few develop complications such as mastoiditis or meningitis – and antibiotic use does not seem to prevent these complications. Few children (about 1 child in 10; NNT = 10) benefit from antibiotic treatment. Reality is that most children taking antibiotics for ear infections would have gotten better just as quickly without the drugs. However, if 11 children are treated with antibiotics, one will have diarrhea, vomiting, abdominal pain or a rash[252] (NNH = ~10).

Some physicians adopt a strategy of giving parents a prescription for an antibiotic but tell them to wait a few days before administering it. If the child gets better, they have avoided unnecessary treatment and the risk of drug-induced complications. If the child is one of the few who needs an antibiotic, the child may face one or two days of suffering that might have been prevented, but then gets the needed treatment. This approach covers all bases. In short, most children with infected ears get better with or without antibiotics and most children, even those taking unnecessary antibiotics, do not suffer harm. Because the treatment choice relates to the style and values of the individual physician, patients who ask about and become aware of the potential benefits and harms of treatment can help in the choice by voicing their own values.

Dr. Chris Cates developed an elegant way to describe the possibilities, benefits and harms of treatment with antibiotics for acute ear infection causing pain.[253] Cates' diagrams (See FIGURE 1.41.1). (http://www.nntonline.net/visualrx/examples/.) are clear visual depictions of the potential benefits and harms of antibiotic treatment and are a useful resource for clinicians and patients.

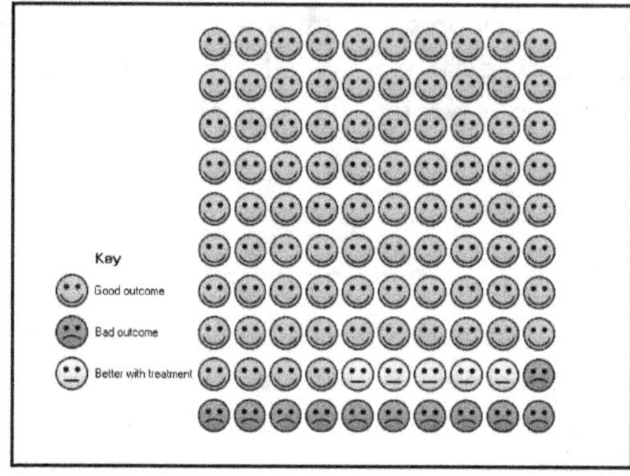

FIGURE 1.41.1: Cates plot of pain, 2-3 days in children given antibiotics vs placebo for earache

Sleep Disturbance (Insomnia)

Falling asleep and getting a good night's rest can be challenging, especially for the elderly. Many people use medications for sleep even though the chance of harm is often greater than the opportunity for benefit. For older people, 13 people must take a sleeping medication (sedative hypnotic) for one person to benefit from improved sleep. However, for every 6 people taking a sedative hypnotic one will be

251 Worrall G. Acute earache. Canadian Family Physician. 2011;57(9):1019-1021. https://www.cfp.ca/content/57/9/1019. Accessed Sept. 8, 2023.

252 http://www.ncbi.nlm.nih.gov/pmc/articles/PMC3173423/. Worrall G. Acute earache. Canadian Family Physician. 2011;57(9):1019-1021. Accessed August 3, 2022.

253 http://www.nntonline.net/visualrx/examples/. Accessed July 19, 2022. Dr. Chris Cates' EBM Web Site. Diagram with permission of Dr. Cates.

harmed because they suffer from drowsiness, fatigue, headache, nightmares or gastrointestinal disturbances. In some cases, the medications can even be addictive.

There are many varieties of sleep-inducing drugs. These include nonbenzodiazepine receptor agonists (e.g., zopiclone, zaleplon), benzodiazepine receptor agonists (triazolam, etizolam), the selective melatonin receptor agonist (ramelteon) and sedating antidepressants (doxepin).

The benzodiazepine family of drugs (e.g., Valium, Xanax) is popular for the treatment of insomnia. People taking benzodiazepines (sedative hypnotics) are 5 times more likely to suffer from impaired thinking and daytime sleepiness and are at least twice as likely of having a serious fall or hip fracture. Hypnotics are high on the list of drugs that are often prescribed inappropriately for seniors. About 25% of seniors take benzodiazepines from time-to-time and about 10% take them daily.[254 255] This means that tens of millions of people in the United States are users! That's a lot!

What is interesting is that many people sleep better after taking a benign placebo. In other words, many of those who report better sleep after taking a sleeping pill would also report better sleep with a safer pill not containing an active medical agent. Sometimes placebos appear to be effective even when the patient knows the pill is an inert placebo tablet.[256]

Most sedative hypnotic medications are prescription medicines. However, some drugs, for example antihistamines such as Benadryl, are available over-the-counter (OTC). These prescription and non-prescription sleep aids are associated with increased drowsiness or 'hangover' the following day and 'rebound insomnia' the following nights. Rebound insomnia occurs when the body depends on sleep-inducing medication and the drugs eventually become ineffective. If continued, the dose must be increased to get the effect, or the patient will not be able to sleep without using a drug. This seems to be a kind of addiction!

Some over-the-counter supplements, benign in very small doses, are marketed as sleep and relaxation remedies. These include the herb Valerian, 5 HTP, Melatonin, Magnesium and Theanine – an amino acid found in green tea[257]. Today, it is possible in some jurisdictions to buy derivatives of the Cannabis plant (Marijuana) legally to use for sleep and relaxation. The clinical testing of marijuana derivatives is not complete, so people remain in the dark about their best use.

What is surprising is that physicians do not recommend benign medicine or placebo as the first choice. If they did, many people would obtain benefit without the risk of side effects. If benign treatments fail, the doctor could recommend more active, but potentially harmful, medicine as a follow up treatment.

Unfortunately, many physicians are not familiar with the literature on Number Needed to Treat and even some experts recommend potentially harmful drugs when more benign substances would work. At a recent Continuing Medical Education (CME) event DZ attended,

254 Jacqueline M. McMillan, MD, Elizabeth Aitken, BSc MLIS, Jayna M. Holroyd-Leduc, MD Management of insomnia and long-term use of sedative-hypnotic drugs in older patients. CMAJ November 19, 2013 vol. 185 no. 17 First published September 23, 2013, doi: 10.1503/cmaj.130025. http://www.cmaj.ca/content/185/17/1499.full?sid=1b456efe-1c96-4446-8fac-a7fdc04a37fd. Accessed July 19, 2022.

255 Jacqueline M. McMillan, MD, Elizabeth Aitken, BSc MLIS, Jayna M. Holroyd-Leduc, MD Management of insomnia and long-term use of sedative-hypnotic drugs in older patients.
CMAJ November 19, 2013 vol. 185 no. 17 First published September 23, 2013, doi: 10.1503/cmaj.130025 http://www.cmaj.ca/content/185/17/1499.full?sid=1b456efe-1c96-4446-8fac-a7fdc04a37fd. Accessed July 19, 2022.

256 Kaptchuk TJ, Friedlander E, Kelley JM, Sanchez MN, Kokkotou E, et al. (2010) Placebos without Deception: A Randomized Controlled Trial in Irritable Bowel Syndrome. PLoS ONE 5(12): e15591. doi: 10.1371/journal.pone 0015591. http://journals.plos.org/plosone/article?id=10.1371/journal.pone.0015591. Accessed August 4, 2022.

257 http://www.thebetterhealthstore.com/Newsletter/030510_Top-5-Sleep-Supplements_08.html. The Better Health Store. Accessed July 19, 2022.

a reputed expert who recommended sleeping medication was not able to report on the benefits and harms (NNT and NNH) of the concoctions he suggested. For many people – especially those over 60 – the benefits of sedating drugs may not justify "*the increased risk, particularly if the patient has additional risk factors for cognitive or psychomotor adverse events*"[258].

258 Glass J, Lanctôt KL, Herrmann N, Sproule BA, Busto UE. Sedative hypnotics in older people with insomnia: meta-analysis of risks and benefits. BMJ: British Medical Journal. 2005;331(7526):1169. doi:10.1136/bmj.38623.768588.47. http://www.ncbi.nlm.nih.gov/pmc/articles/PMC1285093/. Accessed August 3, 2022.

Chapter 42: About the Body and Drugs

KEYWORDS: Pharmacokinetics, Drug Metabolism, Prodrugs, Pharmacodynamics, Drug Detoxification

ABSTRACT: Drugs exert their influence by acting at the cellular level. Understanding how drugs work can help avoid problems that can occur when drug metabolism is altered either by other drugs that patient may be taking, by diet, or by problems with an organ that helps break down and eliminate the drug.

Introduction

What happens when I take a pill, have an injection or receive an anesthetic? Where does it go and what does it do?

Scientists who study and develop theories and practice regarding pharmaceuticals are called 'pharmacologists'. In a certain sense, they are where the rubber hits the road, where drugs and their effects are understood and our education about them starts. On the other hand, pharmacists are those who package and sell medications developed by pharmacologists.

There are two important topics addressed by pharmacologists that are worthy of a basic understanding: Pharmacokinetics and Pharmacodynamics. FIGURE 1.42.1. summarizes these.

Drugs' Impacts on the Body are determined by:

The Patient's Pharmacokinetics: *how the patient's body absorbs, distributes throughout the body, breaks down and excretes drugs and their breakdown products*

and

The Patient's Pharmacodynamics: *what the patient's various receptors (enabling chemicals to 'communicate' with cells), ion channels (pathways for chemicals to get into cells), enzymes (chemicals that interact with drugs) and immune system mechanisms (the body's response to any 'invader') are and what they can do.*

FIGURE 1.42.1: Pharmacokinetics and pharmacodynamics

Pharmacokinetics

Pharmacokinetics is the area of pharmacological research and experiment that addresses how drugs get into the body, move about within it and get out of the body.

The Merck manual defines pharmacokinetics as describing "what the body does to a drug…the movement of drug into, through, and out of the body (and) the time course of its absorption, bioavailability, distribution, metabolism, and excretion."[259]

The general objective is to get drugs to receptors on cells or get them into cells. Receptors are chemical sites on the surface of a cell that allow external agencies to communicate and interact with the cell. A good example would be how insulin interacts with cellular receptors making the cells better able to use sugar (glucose) in the bloodstream. Another objective is to eventually eliminate the drug and the drug's by-products (metabolites) to avoid possible harms from too much of a pharmaceutical.

What Happens to Drugs in the Body?

If we pop a pill, the chemicals in the pill are broken down in our stomach and intestines and transported across the walls of these organs into the bloodstream.

One can immediately see an issue: the possibility of the stomach or the intestine breaking the drug down or possibly even making it ineffective by deactivating it. This can be a big issue with certain protein supplements, which are supposed to affect some part of the body, like the brain. If the content of the pill is a protein (a chain of amino acids), it will be broken down into separate amino acids by the gastrointestinal system, so the original protein no longer exists…very big molecules cannot transit the intestinal wall. Therefore, only the amino acids are available to affect the brain rather than whole proteins…but food might deliver those same amino acids. It is highly improbable that the body will reassemble these amino acids into a protein like the original. This will have about the same probability as a dropped and shattered cup reassembling!

If we assume, though, that an antibiotic or analgesic (pain reliever) survives the transit into the bloodstream, then there is another possible problem. Whatever it is, it will circulate to the entire body, going everywhere. This can mean that a chemical, like a chemotherapeutic agent, can affect a cancerous tumor but it will also affect every other cell in the body. This is familiar because these agents cause hair loss or changes in the intestine and this is off target from its intended destination.

Once the drug is in the bloodstream, it will be absorbed into different components of the body, with fat being an important one. Fat can absorb a drug, reducing the amount available for other tissues, but then can release it back into the bloodstream gradually. Fat is particularly important with many anesthetics, delaying recovery – what we call 'waking up'.

The different tissues in the body that take up drugs are generically called "compartments" and different drugs will be absorbed by different ones. Predicting the amount of a drug that will be in the bloodstream at any time is dependent on the amount of drug put in (its concentration in the blood), its uptake by different compartments, its release rate from these compartments, its breakdown in certain organs (e.g., the liver) and how fast it is removed from the body, e.g., by the kidneys. Sometimes physicians give a 'loading dose' of a medication to take into account its absorption into different compartments and making sure that the concentration in the blood quickly reaches the desired level.

Regarding the breakdown and removal of a drug from the body, various organs, such as the

259 https://www.merckmanuals.com/professional/clinical-pharmacology/pharmacokinetics/overview-of-pharmacokinetics. Accessed July 19, 2022.

liver and kidneys, do it chemically. The kidneys excrete many drugs. Some drugs (called 'pro-drugs') are only effective when an organ, such as the liver, has changed them, i.e., created metabolites. Examples of prodrugs include aspirin, psilocybin, irinotecan, codeine, heroin, L-dopa, and various antiviral nucleosides.

WHY PRODRUGS?

The need to design and produce a prodrug is often related to issues including (1) bioavailability, such as poor aqueous solubility (e.g., corticosteroids), (2) poor absorption/permeability (e.g., ampicillin), (3) high first pass extraction (refers to the drug being removed by an organ essentially as soon as it makes one pass through the body, e.g., propranolol), (4) instability (e.g., short half-life – how long it takes for half of the drug to disappear – such as dopamine), (5) poor site specificity (i.e., that the site of action of an active drug is rather nonspecific such as anticancer agents), (6) incomplete absorption (epinephrine), (7) unfavorable organoleptic – i.e., we can sense or feel the effects of the drug – properties (chloramphenicol), (8) pharmaceutical formulation difficulties, and (9) other adverse effects or toxicities.

(Wu, Kuei-Meng, A New Classification of Prodrugs: Regulatory Perspectives, Pharmaceuticals (Basel). 2009 Dec; 2(3): 77–81., Published online 2009 Oct 14. doi: 10.3390/ph2030077). A New Classification of Prodrugs: Regulatory Perspectives - PubMed (nih.gov)

If a person's liver, for example, is not functioning properly it can fail to break a drug down or not break it down fast enough. When that happens, the drug will increase in concentration in the bloodstream if the person continues taking the medication. This increase of the concentration can continue until it reaches a toxic level, potentially damaging other organs. The same can be true if the kidneys fail to excrete the drug.

Summary of Pharmacokinetics

In summary, scientists must study every drug to determine how to put it into the body so that it gets to the bloodstream in the desired form. Some drugs are injected because, otherwise, they would be broken down in the gastrointestinal system. However, they may also be injected so that the concentration of the drug reaches an effective level quickly.

Pharmacologists also must study to see how the drug goes into and comes out of the various compartments we've described. This can be quite complicated and involve some serious mathematics (think: systems of differential equations). Finally, pharmacologists must understand how ultimately to get rid of the drug from the body and to be able to plan proper dosages that take into account the under- or over- functioning of various organs.

Pharmacodynamics

Pharmacodynamics is the other part of the picture. Pharmacodynamics is, according to the Merck manual, "the branch of Pharmacology concerned with the effects of drugs and the mechanism of their action." In other words, it tells us how drugs work and what they do in and to the body.[260]

This area can be quite complicated, as it requires the understanding of how chemicals affect cells and what cells do in response, that is, what happens in them. A simple understanding of these effects of some drugs can be had by imagining that cells have little locks on their surface. Chemicals, such as proteins, serve as keys to these locks. The locks are called receptors and proteins attach to or insert into these receptors. When this happens, the receptor causes a chemical change inside the cell. It's like it has received a message, like "work harder!" and passes this to the cell's machinery inside. There are many different kinds of receptors

260 https://www.merckmanuals.com/en-ca/professional/clinical-pharmacology/pharmacodynamics/overview-of-pharmacodynamics. Accessed July 19, 2022.

that have different effects internal to the cell. Sometimes, chemicals are simply absorbed through the cell wall directly into the cell, stimulating the cell or possibly even killing it.

Drugs can be thought of as keys that unlock receptors and change the cell in some desirable way. For example, insulin tells the cell, through receptors, to process glucose.

Every different drug has specific effects on cells. The important thing to remember is that if the cell has a specific receptor, the drug will affect it, even if we don't want it to affect that cell type, for example in the heart. The various ways in which drugs can affect cells is manifold and is beyond what we can address in this book. However, it is worthy of note that today many pharmacologists use computer systems to design the shape of drug molecules so that they will interact with cellular receptors. It is quite accurate to say that these are "designer proteins" and they "unlock" cells to have desired effects on them.

In Summary

You now have a basic understanding of how drugs are processed by the body, excreted by it and how they affect the performance of cells in the body. There really isn't much magic involved, but there is a great deal of detailed study of the characteristics of chemical compounds, like proteins, the investigation of how the body deals with them and determination of the effects that they have. Pharmacology has absorbed (no pun intended!) biochemists, biophysicists, computer scientists, mathematicians and many other types of scientists for decades and will continue to do so into the future. There are even scientists who are creating incredibly detailed mathematical models of the inner processes of cells that attempt to imitate their every function and to be able to study what actually happens at a molecular level. It is one of the most interesting areas of biological science!

Chapter 43: The Peril of Ignoring Evidence - The Opioid Epidemic

KEYWORDS: Opioid Epidemic, Evidence, Harm Reduction, Access to Fake Drugs, Drug Addiction, Mind Altering Drugs, Control of Drugs, Health Policy

ABSTRACT: Policymakers, like clinicians, must define the purposes of policy, the evidence for the expected benefits of policy and how someone will measure the impacts of the policy. Evidence suggests that some policy, like that intended to reduce harm from opioid use, might have the paradoxical effect of increasing harm. Also, policies can help to maintain high prices for illicit drugs, thereby increasing the incentives for street vendors to sell them.

We face important questions:

Is the goal to reduce prescribing or to reduce harm?

Is the war on drugs a war on people?

Should addicts have access to safe drugs?

Introduction

The response of regulators, law enforcement agencies and clinicians to the opioid epidemic is one example of the implementation of expensive policies based on intuition, rather than on evidence![261 262]

People take drugs not only to cure illnesses but also to feel better. Doctors prescribe mood-altering drugs, including antidepressants (e.g., Paxil), amphetamines (for example, Ritalin), relaxants (like diazepam or Valium[tm]) and analgesics (pain relievers, including codeine and morphine). Street vendors also sell

261 Facing the Opioid Epidemic (FOE): Assessing and Responding to Prescription and Illicit Opioid Use and Misuse in 5 New England States, Stopka, T.J., Beletsky, L., Kreiner, et. Al., Power Point presentation. http://www.pdmpassist.org/pdf/PPTs/26C_Stopka_Young_Opioid_Use.pdf. Accessed November 5, 2017.

262 Finley, E.P., Garcia, A., Rosen, K., et. Al., Evaluating the impact of prescription drug monitoring program implementation: a scoping review, BMC Health Services ResearchBMC series – open, inclusive and trusted201717:420. https://doi.org/10.1186/s12913-017-2354-5; https://bmchealthservres.biomedcentral.com/articles/10.1186/s12913-017-2354-5. Accessed Sept. 8, 2023.

mood-altering drugs, including marijuana, amphetamines, analgesics – codeine and morphine, again – and sedatives (calming and sleep-inducing drugs). Now provincial governments in Canada have increased their approval and even marketing of mood-altering agents to include marijuana as well as alcohol.

Both prescription and non-prescription mood-altering (also called 'psychoactive') medications expose people to the risk of addiction and side effects. Drugs can make a person feel better but sleepy (a side effect). A drug prescribed by a physician may be no safer than the same one sold by a street vendor, though, unfortunately, street drugs often are fraudulent or adulterated, making them more dangerous. The hope is that physicians will prescribe only quality medications to people where the chances of benefit substantially outweigh the harmful side effects. Unfortunately, clinicians sometimes prescribe the wrong drug, for the wrong reasons, at the wrong dosage or for longer than is appropriate. And there are fraudulent drugs that sometimes slip into the healthcare system and there have been examples of pharmacists adulterating drugs.

Mood altering drugs are a particularly challenging case, as these are meant to help people to feel better. Consequently, people are more likely to become addicted because they crave the good feelings produced by the drug. In the case of some drugs, the body adapts when they are taken regularly. When these drugs are withdrawn, people can experience severe discomfort. The time until addiction can be as short as one to two weeks; in the case of some antidepressants, 5 or 6 weeks.

Examples of the effects of withdrawal include:

- Tremor when withdrawing from chronic heavy drinking.
- Panic attacks, tremor, nausea, confusion, nervousness and anxiety when withdrawing from antidepressants.
- Restlessness, muscle aches, abdominal cramping and rapid heart rate when withdrawing from opioids.

Oxycodone (OxyContin is the brand name of time-release oxycodone), both a prescription and a street drug, is highly addictive and easily available on the street. Researchers suggest that the overprescribing of this drug by physicians is a major cause of the opioid addiction crisis.[263] Of course, as mentioned, street vendors may sell any drug, including opioids, relaxants and amphetamines, which helps people to feel better. Antidepressants are inexpensive and widely available by prescription and are one class of "feel good" drug that does not seem to have a corresponding street market.

Oxycodone teaches us many lessons, including that many clinicians are as susceptible to marketing as patients. Drug companies are like that too because often drug ads in medical journals are similar to those in popular magazines. Also, clinicians in some jurisdictions have little time for independent research and rely on pharma to provide information, even though drug companies are self-interested and profit from selling the drugs they market. Purdue pharma had reports in 1997 that Oxycodone seemed attractive to street vendors and was addictive. A way to deal with this is if patients, when accepting drug prescriptions, ask about the chances of benefit and the chances of harm. The settlement regarding the Oxycodone case is highlighted in FIGURE 1.43.1.

263 https://www.bmj.com/content/359/bmj.j4792. Makary Martin A, Overton Heidi N, Wang Peiqi. Overprescribing is major contributor to opioid crisis BMJ 2017; 359: j4792. Accessed July 19, 2022.

Purdue Pharma aggressively promoted Oxycodone to clinicians even though they knew the drug was highly addictive and had become a valuable street drug.

Justice Department Announces Global Resolution of Criminal and Civil Investigations with Opioid Manufacturer Purdue Pharma and Civil Settlement with Members of the Sackler Family - U.S. DoJ: https://www.justice.gov/opa/pr/justice-department-announces-global-resolution-criminal-and-civil-investigations-opioid

The history of OxyContin, told through unsealed Purdue documents:

https://www.statnews.com/2019/12/03/oxycontin-history-told-through-purdue-pharma-documents/

Nov. 30, 1999: "A sales representative emailed Dr. J. David Haddox, a Purdue executive, about the growing concern among physicians about news reports of the diversion and abuse of OxyContin, including people extracting the oxycodone in the tablet for "mainlining" illegally.

Sales Rep: "While many salespeople have sold controlled release opioids as having less abuse potential, the current situation has put us in an awkward situation I feel like we have a credibility issue with our product. Many physicians now think, OxyContin is obviously the street drug all the drug addicts are seeking."

Origins of an Epidemic: Purdue Pharma Knew Its Opioids Were Widely Abused (Published 2018) - The New York Times. https://www.nytimes.com/2018/05/29/health/purdue-opioids-oxycontin.html

FIGURE 1.43.1: Related to Oxycodone settlement

The lay press also recognizes research showing that, when doctors prescribe antidepressant drugs, some patients may become addicted and have serious difficulty with withdrawal problems.[264] This is exacerbated by the fact that, although there is little research supporting long-term use of antidepressant medication, some doctors prescribe antidepressants for many years and do not try to help patients withdraw. This is particularly important, as abrupt withdrawal often causes a reactive depression, as well as some reactions like those associated with opioids. Moreover, for some groups of patients, the risk of harm from antidepressant medication far outweighs the chance of benefit, especially for people who feel mild or moderate – not severe – depression.[265 266]

However, it is important to recognize that many patients, even those who might not meet the criteria for antidepressant drugs, report feeling better on taking them, in the same way that many report improvements with benign placebos. A part of the art of Medicine is helping patients understand the possible harms of medications so they can weigh the harms against the benefits and make an informed choice. Sometimes there is insufficient scientific evidence supporting a treatment and clinicians must propose artful, rather than scientific, solutions. Of course, the issue is that different physician "artists" might propose different solutions, and the preferences and biases of the clinician, rather any real scientific evidence, might determine what the patient receives.

One purpose of drug legislation and regulation is to promote health and to reduce the incidence of side effects and human difficulties posed by drug addiction. Efforts to reduce access to prescription and non-prescription addictive drugs to reduce their harmful effects

264 New York Times, April 7 2018, Many People Taking Antidepressants Discover They Cannot Quit. https://www.nytimes.com/2018/04/07/health/antidepressants-withdrawal-prozac-cymbalta.html. Accessed Sept. 8, 2023.

265 Gøtzsche P. Depression Severity and Effect of Antidepressant Medications. JAMA. 2010;303(16):1596–1599. doi:10.1001/jama.2010.506. https://jamanetwork.com/journals/jama/article-abstract/185744?redirect=true. Accessed July 19, 2022.

266 Kok RM, Reynolds CF. Management of Depression in Older Adults A Review. JAMA. 2017;317(20):2114–2122. doi:10.1001/jama.2017.5706. https://jamanetwork.com/journals/jama/article-abstract/2627976. Accessed July 19, 2022.

is a good thing. However, this must be balanced against the possible increase in human suffering if people needing the drug are not able to get its benefits. Another complementary approach is to help addicted people to reduce or eliminate their drug use but that is very difficult.

Some people function very well and contribute to their communities despite being dependent on anti-depressants or analgesics. For some, the efforts to discontinue 'addictive' drugs produces immediate incapacity and social disruption. Further, it is virtually impossible for certain people to discontinue the drugs without immediate harm. This means that many will seek drugs from whoever and wherever they can get them. Restriction of access to drugs that forces people to deal with street vendors is often a recipe for disaster! We need to remember that most drugs (often with dangerous additives like Fentanyl and actual poisons) are available at the 'drug store at the corner' if the corner drug store is off-limits. Therefore, in some circumstances, it is better for credentialed prescribers to continue prescribing these medications and monitoring the patient. This may seem, at face value, to be inappropriate but it may be better than deprivation, with its concomitant social dysfunction and drug dealers. The challenge is to recognize and help people with addiction to discontinue – or continue under safe circumstances – the drugs without imposing additional harm. Drug addiction itself is not a crime but in many cases carries a death sentence! It is worth reading about Uruguay's or Portugal's strategies of legalizing the use of drugs (not the pushing) to see what a better solution might be than North America's great and endless Drug War.[267]

A Lot of Drug Policy is Based on Intuition – Not Evidence

The recent response of regulators, law enforcement agencies and clinicians to the opioid epidemic is one example of what we have mentioned is the implementation of expensive policies based on intuition and not evidence.[268] [269] [270]

The National Institute on Drug Abuse[271] reports that: "every day, more than 90 Americans die after overdosing on opioids."[272] There is widespread agreement that the problem is important, but controversy surrounds all solutions. Controversy arises when no one can agree on which information to collect or when people fail to collect and analyze available information that would help decide between conflicting opinions. Sometimes such studies are even proscribed (e.g., related

267 United Nations Office on Drugs and Crime (UNODC), "World Drug Report 2009," (Vienna: United Nations Office on Drugs and Crime, 2009), 2. https://www.unodc.org/unodc/en/data-and-analysis/WDR-2009.html. Accessed August 26, 2022

268 Beletsky, Leo et.al. Today's fentanyl crisis: Prohibition's Iron Law, Revisited International Journal of Drug Policy, Volume 46, Pages 156–159 http://www.ijdp.org/article/S0955-3959(17)30154-8/fulltext. Accessed Sept. 8, 2023.

269 United Nations Office on Drugs and Crime (UNODC), "World Drug Report 2009," (Vienna: United Nations Office on Drugs and Crime, 2009), 2.

270 Finley, E.P., Garcia, A., Rosen, K., et. Al., Evaluating the impact of prescription drug monitoring program implementation: a scoping review, BMC Health Services. https://pubmed.ncbi.nlm.nih.gov/28633638/. Accessed Sept. 8, 2023.

271 National Institute on Drug Abuse, June 2017. https://www.drugabuse.gov/drugs-abuse/opioids/opioid-crisis#one. Accessed November 6, 2017.

272 United Nations Office on Drugs and Crime (UNODC), "World Drug Report 2009," (Vienna: United Nations Office on Drugs and Crime, 2009 United Nations Office on Drugs and Crime (UNODC), "World Drug Report 2009," (Vienna: United Nations Office on Drugs and Crime, 2009 Rudd RA, Seth P, David F, Scholl L. Increases in Drug and Opioid-Involved Overdose Deaths — United States, 2010–2015. MMWR Morb Mortal Wkly Rep. 2016;65. doi:10.15585/mmwr.mm655051e1. https://www.ncbi.nlm.nih.gov/pubmed/28033313. Accessed Aug 3, 2022.

to marijuana)[273]. Valid and relevant information can enable us to resolve policy disputes through intelligent consideration. Without enough information, proponents of one or another policy rely on hypothetical argument or, worse, biased opinions.

Sometimes the solutions just seed further problems. For example, many blame the addiction problem on aggressive marketing by pharmaceutical companies that promoted opioid pain medication as nonaddictive. Consequently, physicians were liberal in prescribing these drugs and many people became addicted. Subsequently, street vendors learned how to obtain these drugs by prescription from physicians so they could sell them. This effectively diverted these legally prescribed drugs to street purchasers.[274] [275] Of course, many street drugs are also manufactured by underground and illegal laboratories. These illegal drugs may be – and often are – contaminated or of unknown strength, making death a common 'side effect'.

Controlled substance prescription monitoring programs might succeed at reducing access to physician prescribed drugs but fail to reduce overall drug use or deaths from drug overdose. These programs have come about because many clinicians, administrators and law enforcement officials believe that one way to stop the opioid epidemic in North America is to make it more difficult for credentialed prescribers (physicians) to prescribe them. Partly this belief (a painful result of poor logic) comes from the observation that American states with larger sales of prescribed opioid pain relievers experienced more deaths from drug overdose. Consequently, in many jurisdictions, governments legislated the monitoring of controlled substance prescriptions, especially related to opioids. The result has been increased workloads for clinicians and for pharmacists who dispense opioids, with little impact except to increase the business of street vendors.[276] The increased workload associated with these programs disincents prescribing narcotics or even engaging with patients who might be addicted. So, many patients with real medical problems suffer without relief.

Unfortunately, street vendors never offer counselling and the drugs they sell are unregulated. Consequently, to emphasize an earlier point, the street drugs people get are often not the ones they thought they had purchased. When licensed physicians will not engage with people who seek certain drugs, people feel forced to look for other suppliers and may turn to street vendors. As prescription-monitoring programs make more aggressive efforts to reduce misuse of prescription drugs, people can get fewer physician-prescribed medications. Instead, they purchase pharmaceuticals of unknown quality from completely unregulated street vendors. Wow! What progress!

Ergo, deaths from heroin and fentanyl overdoses rise. Thoughtful regulators should (but often do not) study, monitor and report how reducing access to prescription drugs influences drug use, deaths and sickness from both prescription and street drugs. Without those reports, it is not possible to know if policies are

---

273 United Nations Office on Drugs and Crime (UNODC), "World Drug Report 2009," (Vienna: United Nations Office on Drugs and Crime, 2009. https://www.popsci.com/science/article/2013-04/why-its-so-hard-scientists-study-pot/. Accessed Aug 3, 2022.

274 Canadian Medical Protective Association: Preventing the Misuse of Opiods. June 2015.https://www.cmpa-acpm.ca/en/advice-publications/browse-articles/2015/preventing-the-misuse-of-opioids. Accessed August 3, 2022.

275 Hahn KL. Strategies to Prevent Opioid Misuse, Abuse, and Diversion That May Also Reduce the Associated Costs. American Health & Drug Benefits. 2011;4(2):107-114. https://www.ncbi.nlm.nih.gov/pmc/articles/PMC4106581/. Accessed Sept. 8, 2023.

276 Beletsky, Leo et.al. Today's fentanyl crisis: Prohibition's Iron Law, Revisited International Journal of Drug Policy, August 2017 Volume 46, Pages 156–159. http://www.ijdp.org/article/S0955-3959(17)30154-8/fulltext. Accessed Sept. 8, 2023.

good or bad for people. It is a simple reality that prescription-monitoring programs do further harm to addicted people by driving them from credentialed clinicians into the arms of street vendors and their especially harmful drugs.[277]

Persuasive arguments in favor of prescription-monitoring programs should be based on formal evidence that they reduce the overall use of inappropriate medication and that the harms, including deaths from drug overdoses, decrease. Unfortunately, in many communities, deaths from overdoses of street drugs seem to show an increase following the introduction of prescription-monitoring programs.[278] Addressing this issue based on evidence would involve monitoring not only health system prescribing but surveying street drug selling and usage, as well as deaths and overdose treatment and resuscitation delivered by hospitals and emergency response programs. Clearly a major challenge. Without evidence, though, we can never make adjust to the realities!

These programs exemplify how governments often introduce health policy without thoughtfully considering the evidence of the effects of interventions.

Information to Inform Health Policy

Regulators must have information to study and determine the impacts of health policy and changes to it. Health services administrators must organize systems to capture information from the process of care so the public and regulators have worthwhile data that enables them to evaluate interventions. Because clinicians collect that kind of information about individual patients, they are the natural information resource for decision-enabling facts. Collaboration between physicians and administrators is essential to realizing the hope that actual clinical information and evidence from the 'mine face', so to speak, will inform health policy. We must start to create and promulgate 'evidence-based policy'! Community access to effective and efficient care demands that communities recruit healthcare experts[279] to work with clinicians to collect and analyze clinical information to inform health services management, evaluation and regulation so that appropriate analysis advances excellent care.

Most jurisdictions in the United States and Canada do not use modern information system techniques to link healthcare activities to changes in health so they can determine the value of health interventions. This avails partly because of ineptitude and partly because of the failure to see the societal value of capturing and mining clinical data. Fortunately, the information necessary for performance measurement and management is usually the same as the routine information that clinicians must collect to care for patients.[280] It just needs to be accessed and analyzed.

277 Beletsky, Leo et.al. Today's fentanyl crisis: Prohibition's Iron Law, Revisited International Journal of Drug Policy, August 2017 Volume 46, Pages 156–159. http://www.ijdp.org/article/S0955-3959(17)30154-8/fulltext. Accessed Sept. 8, 2023.

278 Fink DS, Schleimer JP, Sarvet A, et al. Association Between Prescription Drug Monitoring Programs and Nonfatal and Fatal Drug Overdoses: A Systematic Review. Ann Intern Med. [Epub ahead of print 8 May 2018] 168:783–790. doi: 10.7326/M17-3074. https://annals.org/aim/article-abstract/2680723/association-between-prescription-drug-monitoring-programs-nonfatal-fatal-drug-overdoses. Accessed July 19, 2022.

279 Clinicians including physicians, nurses, pharmacists, dentists, physiotherapists, occupational health experts, health services administrators and regulators.

280 In addition to the routine information collected at the time of care some studies also survey patients and communities for additional information about health and health status and link this information to the information collected by clinicians.

Summary

Every single day, clinicians capture the information necessary to assess health system performance. At every visit, doctors make assessments of patients' health (their comfort, function, the results of laboratory tests, and estimates of life expectancy). That information is captured and present in the medical record.

More sophisticated and ubiquitous health information systems can aggregate information from many clinicians to develop more refined, statistically validated, estimates of the health benefits or harms that follow when many similar patients receive treatments.

THE PROBLEM WITH RELYING ON EXPERIENCE

Pharmaceutical companies have been extremely generous in providing drug samples to busy clinicians. The idea is that the clinician would try the drug on a patient and that those patients would do well because of the drug, recover on their own, or experience neither benefit nor harm following drug treatment.

If the doctor gives the patient the drug and the treatment is a success, the pharmaceutical company representative can enthusiastically emphasize the excellent result.

If the patient who received a sample is worse off after treatment the drug representative could, appropriately, remark that the sample was too small to reach a conclusion and that larger trials had been completed indicating the drug is effective.

Chapter 44: Medical Errors

KEYWORDS: Medical Errors, Standards, Options, Guidelines, Harm Reduction, Avoidable Adverse Events, Non-Avoidable Adverse Events, Identifying Adverse Events from Administrative Data, Patient Participation

ABSTRACT: Clinicians, like all of us, sometimes make mistakes leading to adverse outcomes. However, not all adverse outcomes are preventable. Adverse outcomes resulting from the failure to comply with standards for care or systematic processes are almost always avoidable. Whenever patients or groups of patients have adverse outcomes, efforts should be made to learn if those outcomes were preventable and thereby show how we can improve future patient care.

Introduction

"Patient Loses Leg to Surgical Error!" Read all about it!

Medical errors are frequent news items. A clinician injures (or worse) someone by wrongly prescribing a drug or surgically removing a healthy limb. Clearly, not good! Definitely a medical error! However, is it a 'medical error', or a brilliant insight if an apparently incorrect or contraindicated intervention solves a patient's problem? What the doctor did was not what many would recommend but it seemed to work. Well, that is not all that uncommon! Think of all the times the wrong cause of a problem is 'diagnosed', the patient treated for the wrong cause, and the problem goes away because the drug worked on the patient's problem or the problem resolved itself. It's an error to think that an 'error' means the same thing to all of us, so we have to clear up some confusion.

SOME DEFINITIONS: STANDARDS, GUIDELINES AND OPTIONS

Standards are things that must be done in the specific circumstance. For example, stopping bleeding from a severed artery or treating airway obstruction. Guidelines apply in most instances. For example, we usually treat people with low levels of thyroid hormone; however, if they are clinically well, we might not. Options for care occur when there are many possible choices that are regarded as appropriate. For example, treatment of prostate cancers or enlarged prostate.[281]

Researchers have recognized that they can cause confusion if they use terms like 'medical error,' 'medical mistake' or 'medical misadventure'. These are attempts to characterize doing the wrong thing. It is far clearer to, instead, characterize the results. Hence, we will use their term 'adverse medical events' or just 'adverse events': actions that result in outcomes that are undesirable regardless of the cause. Adverse Events are "*unintended injuries or complications resulting in death, disability or prolonged hospital*

281 2009 Eddy DM. Designing a Practice Policy: Standards, Guidelines, and Options. JAMA. 1990;263(22):3077–3084. doi:10.1001/jama.1990.03440220105041. https://jamanetwork.com/journals/jama/article-abstract/382154. Accessed Aug 3, 2022.

stay that arise from healthcare management."[282] This would include, for example, a patient who has an allergic reaction to penicillin, who had never had penicillin previously and where it would have been impossible to anticipate the allergic reaction. Worse is a 'preventable adverse event', sometimes just characterized as a mistake, which is when a person who had a previous reaction to penicillin has an allergic reaction. In that case, the result was foreseeable.

An information system that prompted clinicians when they were prescribing inappropriate medication would reduce some of these adverse events. It would also help prevent mistakes if clinicians diligently searched for evidence of previous allergic reactions to drugs before prescribing them. Sometimes, though, relevant information, e.g., on a previous reaction is buried in an old chart and it's not clear if the clinician could have been expected to foresee the adverse result.

Avoiding Harm from Health System Mistakes

Maybe it is surprising, but not all health care is good care. There may be mistakes or errors in diagnosis, treatment and follow-up. The clinician may come to the wrong conclusion as to the cause of a patient's problem and apply a treatment appropriate to that incorrect cause. This may injure the patient or delay finding and treating the actual cause. Even knowing the actual cause, the clinician can intervene inappropriately. After intervening, the clinician may fail to follow up with the patient, which may result in injury or drug complications. Surgeons can do the same sort of thing by performing the wrong surgical procedure or by damaging a body part during surgery. These missteps plague patients with avoidable discomfort, disability and death. Consequently, to avoid repeated adverse events, it is essential that health organizations implement objective methods to detect and report on both good and bad results in general and on any harms that occur because of blunders – better characterized as 'adverse events' – especially preventable ones.

An article published in the Canadian Medical Association Journal (CMAJ) in 2004, estimated that between 9,250 and 23,750 deaths occurred because of preventable adverse events – preventable mistakes.[283] Regretfully, it is surprising that in 2020 no Canadian hospital can report if we make more, fewer or about the same number of mistakes as originally reported. Fifteen years have passed (at publication time) and no Canadian hospital informs people about having better or worse performance than before. In fact, many clinicians and health services administrators believe adverse events are becoming more common.

Part of the problem is that the information we need to learn about adverse events is not available. Canadian and American hospitals do not report adverse event rates in consistent and systematic ways. Both the U.S. Institute of Medicine (IOM) report "To Err is Human"[284] and the Canadian "Adverse Events Study"[285]

282 Ross Baker, Peter G. Norton, Virginia Flintoft, Canadian Adverse Events Study CMAJ Oct 2004, 171 (8) 834-834-a; DOI: 10.1503/cmaj.1041120. https://www.cmaj.ca/content/171/8/834.2. Accessed August 3, 2022.

283 Baker GR[1], Norton PG, Flintoft V, Blais R, Brown A, Cox J, Etchells E, Ghali WA, Hébert P, Majumdar SR, O'Beirne M, Palacios-Derflingher L, Reid RJ, Sheps S, Tamblyn R., The Canadian Adverse Events Study: the incidence of adverse events among hospital patients in Canada. CMAJ. 2004 May 25;170(11):1678-86. https://pubmed.ncbi.nlm.nih.gov/15159366/. Accessed Sept. 8, 2023.

284 Institute of Medicine. 2000. To Err Is Human: Building a Safer Health System. Washington, DC: The National Academies Press. https://doi.org/10.17226/9728. https://www.nap.edu/catalog/9728/to-err-is-human-building-a-safer-health-system. Accessed July 19, 2022.

285 Baker GR, Norton PG, Flintoft V, Blais R, Brown A, Cox J, et al. The Canadian Adverse Events Study: the incidence of adverse events among hospital patients in Canada. CMAJ 2004;170(11):1678-86. http://www.cmaj.ca/content/170/11/1678. Accessed July 19, 2022.

described methods to detect and reduce adverse events in order to make health care less of a risk factor for illness. It is a crime that they have not been implemented!

Governments normally regulate industry to improve product authenticity, consistency and safety. Canadian hospitals are different because we (somewhat irrationally) expect governments, as the owners and funders of hospitals, to regulate themselves. Good luck! If the government, as regulator, payor and evaluator, finds problems, it would have to slap its own wrist. Moreover, governments, as administrators, must pay to fix the problems they find in their role as regulator and evaluator. That is a real disincentive!

Canadian Reporting Versus U.S. Reporting

Canadian federal and provincial governments have not insisted that health organizations capture information and report on whether or not patients are in the appropriate setting for care or what the outcomes of care are. They also do not systematically capture information about preventable and nonpreventable adverse events, despite the Baker and Norton study showing that these measures can be captured in a meaningful way. Therefore, Canadians have little information about preventable adverse events, with the result that no one knows if the incidence of preventable mistakes has been increasing, decreasing or has remained the same.

Contrast that with the fact that, in the United States, the Pennsylvania Health Care Cost Containment Council[286] has required that every health organization measure and report on severity-adjusted costs and outcomes. There is no such mandate for Canadian hospitals to do likewise.

MATERIAL FROM USA

https://www.cnbc.com/2018/02/22/medical-errors-third-leading-cause-of-death-in-america.html. CNBC Feb 2018. Accessed August 3, 2022.

https://www.ncbi.nlm.nih.gov/books/NBK499956/. Rodziewicz TL, Houseman B, Hipskind JE. Medical Error Reduction and Prevention. [Updated 2022 May 1]. Accessed August 3, 2022.

The relatively recent major studies of Adverse events in hospital are included in FIGURE 1.44.1.

RECENT MAJOR ADVERSE EVENTS STUDIES

U.S. Institute of Medicine: To Err is Human: Building a Safer Health System (2000):

https://pubmed.ncbi.nlm.nih.gov/25077248/

The Canadian Adverse Events Study (2004): the incidence of adverse events among hospital patients in Canada:

https://www.cmaj.ca/content/170/11/1678/tab-related-content

FIGURE 1.44.1: US/CDN hospital adverse events studies

Kinds of Adverse Events and Their Causes

Patients can experience a variety of adverse events, some preventable, some not. These include damage, injury or loss of a body part, poisoning, infection, allergic reaction (anaphylaxis), bleeding, arrhythmia or circulation stoppage, loss of brain functions (memory, cognition, motor function), burns and inappropriate radiation exposure, various psychosocial dysfunctions (fear, terror, PTSD) and increased risk of follow-on medical problems,

286 http://www.phc4.org. Pennsylvanian Health Care Cost Containment Council. Accessed July 19, 2022.

such as an untreated problem or immune system damage.

Avoidable causes of these events can include:

- The administering of the wrong drug, or a drug at the wrong dosage, or administered for the wrong duration to treat a specific problem.
- Surgically intervening using the wrong procedure, or on the wrong body part, or with the wrong supporting interventions, such as pharmaceuticals, other chemicals and blood products, or anesthesia agents.
- Performing inappropriate tests that entail false positives and false negatives.
- Manipulating or examining the body using inappropriate techniques or machines (e.g., neck manipulation causing a carotid tear, radiation burns from the Therac-25[287]).
- Giving inappropriate advice or counsel, for example, in a psychiatric encounter or failing to intervene when a person is a clear danger to self or other.

Patients surrender, to some degree, their control of their bodies and minds to clinicians and are thereby exposed to clinicians' ventures and misadventures, any of which can help or harm. Patients can help reduce the chances of mistakes by asking questions and helping the clinician know about any medical factors or current drugs that might influence the value of an intervention.

Why Adverse Events are Not Reported

It is difficult to get information about health system mistakes because most clinicians, administrators, and governments exhibit unfamiliarity with the methods they could use to detect adverse events. Typically, hospitals ask clinicians and other workers to self-report mistakes and near-mistakes (sometimes called 'near-misses'). However, if you are not aware you have made a mistake, you have nothing to report. And, if no one is watching, even if you knew you made a mistake, you might not be forthcoming. Such is the human condition.

Every day, North American hospitals discharge thousands of patients. Statistics tell us that quite a few of them have experienced errors of various types. Unfortunately, it may be that most hospital efforts to find mistakes are unworkable or unproductive. They fail because they ask people to recognize and self-report their mistakes. They do not routinely measure clinical outcomes and consequently lack data that would alert them to situations and processes that were more likely to be error prone. When there is a poor patient outcome, it might or might not have been preventable. The belief is that the clinician who makes a mistake will recognize that the adverse outcome was preventable and would report it. However, the clinician might believe the adverse outcome was an inevitable result of the disease and not the result of an error or omission. A patient who has pneumonia together with unrecognized kidney disease, for instance, might be treated for the pneumonia and die of the kidney disease, while the clinician remains unaware of the mistakenly overlooked condition.

To be fair, patients can have poor outcomes absent any mistakes. It might be that clinicians who make an error might truly believe the poor outcome was inevitable even with the best care.

287 Leveson, N.G., Turner, C.S., An Investigation of the Therac-25 Accidents, from Computer 26,7 July 1993 Pg 18-41. https://web.stanford.edu/class/cs240/old/sp2014/readings/therac-25.pdf. Accessed August 26, 2022

That being said, the reality is that there was a mistake! We know that some poor outcomes are preventable – the Canadian study estimates that about 30% might be.[288]

One way to screen for systematic mistakes (those that occur regularly) is to learn which groups of patients in an organization are most likely to have unexpectedly poor health outcomes. People enter hospital with a set of characteristics. Some are very sick – they might have anemia (lack of healthy red blood cells), low levels of blood oxygen, poor kidney function, poor heart function, or a combination of disorders of any bodily systems. We expect, in general, that patients who are very sick will have worse results compared with patients who are less sick on admission. Groups of patients whose results are worse than expected are more likely to be suffering because of systematic mistakes.[289]

SOME CANADIAN STATISTICS ON ADVERSE EVENTS

For 51.4% of the AEs (Adverse Events), the service most responsible for the delivery of care was Surgery; for 45.0%, it was Medicine and for 3.6% it was another service (e.g., Dentistry, Physical Therapy, Podiatry). The most common types of AEs were related to surgical procedures and the next most common were associated with drug- or fluid-related events. In the Medicine service, AEs resulting from errors of omission (the failure to carry out necessary diagnosis or treatment) were more common than those resulting from errors of commission (57.1% v. 42.9%). In the Surgery service, the frequency of these errors was assessed as being roughly equal (50.8% v. 49.2%).

Some AEs are the unavoidable consequences of health care, such as an unanticipated allergic reaction to an antibiotic. However, 37%–51% of AEs have been judged in retrospect to have been potentially preventable.

http://www.cmaj.ca/content/170/11/1678. Accessed July 19, 2022.

Identifying Adverse Events

Finding and documenting adverse events requires organizations to develop, promulgate, implement and enforce formal and continuously applied policy supported by suitable information systems to screen for poor outcomes of individual patients and to determine if the poor outcomes were preventable or if they were likely inevitable. Success also requires training to recognize mistakes, even when harm did not occur, and to learn from 'near misses' (a mistake that was averted before it affected a patient). Organizations like the FAA (Federal Aeronautics Administration) have a far more systematic approach to detecting and reporting errors but are still far from perfect. The point is that there are models in other industries.

The somewhat haphazard approaches health organizations do use have a low sensitivity (they do not detect errors not recognized and reported by the offender) and are open to coverups. Unsophisticated systems also have a low specificity (they have a lot of false alarms). They sometimes suggest that a department is error prone because its results differ from other organizations treating people with similar diagnoses. However, it can be that subsequent analysis finds no objective evidence of systematic error. They are just statistical outliers or clinicians are treating patients who are very sick. Inept error-finding methods can doom hospitals to expensive retrospective reviews.[290] These reviews are seldom complete and often

288 Baker GR, Norton PG, Flintoft V, Blais R, Brown A, Cox J, et al. The Canadian Adverse Events Study: the incidence of adverse events among hospital patients in Canada. CMAJ 2004;170(11):1678-86. http://www.cmaj.ca/content/170/11/1678. Accessed July 19, 2022.

289 Developing regression equations using patient lab values is one way to develop expectations. Ken Rockwood at Dalhousie with other researchers have developed frailty measures that provide some indication of the health outcomes possible with treatment.

290 Screening methods that rely on reporting by staff risk being too sensitive- suggesting mistakes when there were none. They also risk having a high specificity and missing mistakes when a mistake occurred (see section on testing).

inaccurate. After the fact, crucial information may be unobtainable, having been lost or deliberately hidden or altered.[291] However, modern information systems have features that track changes and corrections in the record.

How to Detect Preventable Adverse Outcomes See FIGURE 1.44.2 for examples)

Finding significant preventable adverse outcomes in health care is easier when there is commitment and dedication to the goal of quality improvement.

It is most crucial that we identify adverse outcomes when they result in unnecessary and preventable discomfort, disability or death. This does not mean organizations should ignore lesser mistakes, as these can indicate that a risk of harm lurks in the future and can eventually emerge. Whenever they are detected, mistakes can provide an opportunity to learn which procedures and processes are most likely to be error-prone and may give early indication of potential pitfalls that need attention. When showing someone how to drive a car, for example, one doesn't wait for a crash to occur but notices the failure to do a shoulder-check. That is a lesser mistake that can predict the propensity for a big and costly mistake, a collision. In health care, for an analgesic medication like acetaminophen, a mistake in timing is unimportant. However, for other medications like digitalis or insulin, a timing mistake might be serious. Learning from minor mistakes or near mistakes could help prevent other more serious errors.

e-Appendix 3: Brief description of clinical details of adverse events occurring in 255 patients, by corresponding maximum degree of preventability*

Case	Description of adverse event†
Virtually certain evidence of preventability	
1	Acute on chronic renal failure caused by NSAIDs
2	Acute renal failure with hyperkalemia and intractable constipation with large-bowel obstruction ending in death. Lack of effect of enemas recorded in nurses' notes and results of bowel radiograph not acted upon
3	Admission because of severe anemia. The anemia had been documented in previous admission but not investigated fully, which resulted in delayed diagnosis of colorectal carcinoma
4	Delirium caused by benzodiazepines given to patient with hepatic encephalopathy
5	*Clostridium difficile* colitis following antibiotic therapy. Patient did not receive sufficient volume expansion, which led to acute renal failure and death
6	Cardiac valve replacement. Three days before discharge nurse noted wound was red, inflamed and painful, but no treatment or medical note. Nontherapeutic international normalized ratio (INR) on discharge. Readmitted at 2 weeks with a wound infection, echogenic mass on prosthetic valve and possible infective endocarditis
7	Chronic renal failure in patient taking sotalol and given increasing doses of digoxin, which led to increased QT interval, digoxin toxicity, heart block and worsening renal failure
8	Delayed diagnosis of rectal cancer in patient with long-standing rectal symptoms
9	Delayed diagnosis of uterine cancer in patient with vaginal bleeding for over a year
10	Delayed treatment of digoxin toxicity in patient with acute renal failure, diarrhea and dementia

FIGURE 1.44.2: A selection of the major preventable errors from the CDN study[292]

291 Published by Canadian Medical Protective Association. October 2009 and accurate at the time of their publication. https://www.cmpa-acpm.ca/en/advice-publications/browse-articles/2009/the-medical-record-a-legal-document-can-it-be-corrected. Accessed August 3, 2022.

292 The Canadian Adverse Events Study: the incidence of adverse events among hospital patients in Canada, Appendix 3. 2004. https://www.cmaj.ca/content/170/11/1678/tab-related-content. Accessed August 31, 2022.

There are steps necessary to screen for and identify unexpected poor results that are linked to preventable mistakes. However, we must recognize that many methods used traditionally to detect, attempt to correct and to prevent adverse events have been found lacking.

It is easy to imagine why this is the case. For instance, there is no mechanism that can detect harm to a patient before the error is made (although it may be possible to predict the risk of harm). Of course, the bad effect on the patient may also be delayed. Then there is the tendency of humans to ignore their mistakes and hope they will go away, especially if there are no witnesses. Of course, there is also the good old capacity we have for denial. "It wasn't I!" Logically, however, at least the following must be in the recipe:

1. Develop and promulgate policy that focuses on the identification of potential errors and the prevention, detection and correction of errors.
2. Create an environment of blameless or anonymous reporting.
3. Teach safety awareness, the effects of errors, the opportunities for errors and prevention techniques.
4. Inculcate a philosophy of carefulness, self-critiquing and error reporting in all staff.
5. Based on experience and thoughtful analysis, identify clinical situations and interventions that have an associated likelihood of engendering errors. Focus attention on the high-probability ones initially and proceed to lesser ones when possible.
6. Define bounds of acceptable patient status (an envelope) for error-prone conditions, situations and interventions. Be especially wary when a patient is not 'in the envelope.'
7. Measure and document every patient's health status before, during and after treatment, alarming when the patient's condition departs from the pre-defined envelope.
8. Use systems to manage procedures and document divergences. This has been called 'workflow management' and is largely in the future.

We must counsel, however, that the devil (actually, a whole hoard thereof) is in the details and that this is a challenging domain.

FORMAL ERROR DETECTION METHODOLOGY

The following represents the essence of a method to detect medical errors:

1. *We must derive estimates of life expectancy by use of predictive modeling and other techniques to learn which variables (comfort, function, laboratory results and demographic factors) contribute to expected life and sickness.*
2. *We must categorize patients for likelihood of survival and other health outcomes using the information from the Cox survival tables, including measures of comfort, function, life expectancy and demographic variables, including age.*
    - *The people most likely to survive seek health care but do not have major abnormalities. They might have an ache or pain or gait disturbance, but important measures of health are normal, including blood tests and x-rays.*
    - *People who are less likely to survive have some abnormal values.*
    - *People least likely to survive have major abnormalities in important measures. Respiratory rates might be abnormally high or low, pulse rates and blood pressures might be far from the norm, they might exhibit cyanosis (a blueish tinge suggesting lack of oxygen) or extreme pallor of their complexion or their nail beds (paleness from marked decrease in hemoglobin, the substance in the blood that carries oxygen).*

3. ***Examine the health results for people in each category.***
    - *If large numbers of low severity patients have poor results it suggests that either:*
        - *Investigations have been incomplete. Examples include laboratory investigations not completed or ignored. The consequences of not recording an abnormal laboratory finding could be that the patient appears to have lower severity. For example, if the patient has kidney failure but tests for kidney function have not been ordered, the person would fit into a category of patient that is more likely to survive.*
        - *Or care that is inappropriate.*
4. ***Identify those with unexpectedly poor outcomes and search for the causes of these outcomes.***

The benefit of this approach is that it detects groups of patients with poor results even if the clinicians do not recognize the problem.

Specific Examples of Health System Mistakes

Baker and Norton[293] reported the kinds of preventable adverse events that happen in our hospitals. The important word is 'PREVENTABLE'. Hospitals could implement procedures to avoid mistakes and the harms from mistakes, but they have been reluctant to pay for and implement either failsafe processes to prevent mistakes or information systems that would detect mistakes before (or even after) they cause harm.

The following are some of the types of definitely preventable and harmful mistakes reported by Baker and Norton:[294]

1. **People were harmed when doctors prescribed a drug that the medical literature suggested would make their condition worse. Examples include**:
    a. Someone with kidney failure was given a non-steroidal anti-inflammatory drug (ibuprofen is one example).
    b. Another patient with brain problems caused by liver disease was given diazepam (Valium is an example).

   These are preventable because a capable information system could prompt the clinician prescribing a drug when laboratory tests have shown the person has a condition that contraindicates the drug.

2. **People were harmed when clinical staff did not pay attention to abnormal blood results (like anemia). The result was a delayed diagnosis of colorectal cancer.**

   Capable information systems could reduce this kind of error by prompting the clinician to investigate whenever patients have abnormal blood results. The doctor could ignore the prompt if the problem is already known.

3. **People were harmed when problems were ignored.**
    a. One patient had long-standing rectal symptoms from a rectal cancer.
    b. It took over a year to diagnose uterine cancer in a patient with a long history of vaginal bleeding.

293 Baker GR, Norton PG, Flintoft V, Blais R, Brown A, Cox J, Etchells E, Ghali WA, Hébert P, Majumdar SR, O'Beirne M, Palacios-Derflingher L, Reid RJ, Sheps S, Tamblyn R. The Canadian Adverse Events Study: the incidence of adverse events among hospital patients in Canada. CMAJ. 2004 May 25;170(11):1678-86. https://pubmed.ncbi.nlm.nih.gov/15159366/. Accessed Sept. 8, 2023.

294 Baker GR, Norton PG, Flintoft V, Blais R, Brown A, Cox J, Etchells E, Ghali WA, Hébert P, Majumdar SR, O'Beirne M, Palacios-Derflingher L, Reid RJ, Sheps S, Tamblyn R. The Canadian Adverse Events Study: the incidence of adverse events among hospital patients in Canada. CMAJ. 2004 May 25;170(11):1678-86. See Appendix 3 for a list of the mistakes. https://pubmed.ncbi.nlm.nih.gov/15159366/. Accessed Sept. 8, 2023.

Prompting systems could remind patients and physicians that certain problems require investigation and an explanation.

4. **People were harmed when doctors did not complete indicated investigations of signs and symptoms.**
   a. One patient had rectal bleeding and numerous visits without clinicians asking for or performing a colonoscopy (a test to visualize the lower bowel).
   b. One patient had several admissions for falls and received drug therapy without complete investigation.

   Prompting systems could note important signs and symptoms and remind patients and physicians to investigate them.

The complete list of adverse events is available as part of Appendix 3 of the Canadian Adverse Events Study-Baker and Norton, 2004.

Health informaticians are the experts who organize and implement prompting systems to ensure that doctors do not ignore important information of any kind, including the potential for drug-drug and drug-patient (allergic, for example) interactions. This is one of the most cogent reasons for deploying information system in the first place.

What Patients Can do to Protect-Themselves

The errors reported by The Canadian Adverse Events study occurred in hospitals, but similar errors occur in other settings. People can help their doctors provide appropriate and safe care by being active participants and asking questions about problems, abnormal laboratory results and proposed treatments. When doctors say they have investigated all the possible causes for a problem, people should ask how many of the possible causes the doctors considered and why none were judged to be the cause. The same goes for proposed treatments. Many medical conditions are possible causes of most problems – aches, pains and disabilities. If they ask their doctors for the list of possible causes for and treatments of a problem, it is more likely that the doctor will consider all factors.

If patients' problems do not appear to have an explanation, they should persist in asking questions:

- Ask what the doctor thinks is going on.
- Ask if the doctor ordered all the appropriate investigations that could reveal the problem's important possible causes.
- When considering treatment, ask how likely it is that the treatment will be of benefit and what the alternatives are.
- Also, ask how likely the treatment is to cause harm and what the possible harms are.
- When patients receive a prescription, they should ask the doctor and the pharmacist if the prescription is likely to interfere with any other medications they might be taking and be sure they have brought those up.
- They must not forget to ask about side effects and what should be done if there are any.
- They should ask if anything might interfere with the beneficial effects of the prescription, like taking it with or without food or drink.
- They should read the descriptive material with the prescription so that they learn, for example, if grapefruit juice or anything else could interfere with it.

Every day people derive almost miraculous benefits from modern medicine. So, they are among those who enjoy the benefits and avoid the harms that occasionally result, they should become active participants in their care.

REMINDER: HEALTH SYSTEM AND GOVERNMENT SPENDING ON THE DETERMINANTS OF HEALTH

In Canada, about half of all government spending is on treatment of people who see doctors and other health professionals because they are sick or think they might be sick. The other half is on public sector activities that influence the overall health of the population. These latter activities, which are determinants of health, are largely paid for by government. They include social assistance, education, nutrition programs, public housing, disease prevention and promotion, Public Health and safety agencies that address drug, chemical, work, air, water and food safety.

Public Health experts use the health information, which doctors get from individual patients, to assess the health of populations and to learn if changes in public policy influenced population health. In addition to the clinical and administrative information collected at the point of care, governments and other public health groups also do periodic surveys of their citizens to learn about their health and to link patient health to the individuals' contexts, such as where they live, what they eat and how they behave. The overall health of populations, measured by community health surveys and medical visits, is largely influenced by these and by factors such as socioeconomic status and environmental pollution.

VOLUME 1

Section 7

THE CHALLENGE OF TESTING

SECOND AUTHOR'S WEIRD SENSE OF HUMOR

- *An FBI program for relocating dumb criminals: Witless Protection Program.*
- *People who are unreliable from the day they were born: Post Natal Drips.*
- *Will taking a Zinc supplement daily galvanize a person to action?*
- *Most needed instrument in today's misinformation milieu: a Truth Decay Detector.*
- *A Nordic car that run on salt water: The Fjord.*
- *Becoming more like this book's authors: Going Over to the Dork Side.*
- *(For the math inclined) Can Go Home the Same Way We Go to Work: Travel Commutes!*
- *Politics sounds just like Public Health: Delusion is the Solution.*
- *She wanted the job, but it required standing before the Hiring Squad.*
- *(For Physics buffs) Electrons are Repulsive!*
- *(For authors) All writers kern for more space.*
- *(For Political Science types) Problems getting people out to vote: Electoral Disfunction.*
- *(For military personnel) His wife declared Marital Law!*
- *(For statisticians) Sign: "The Bureau of Statistics Will Probably Close."*
- *(For chemists) Masked chemist's friend: Chemo-sabe.*
- *(For veterinarians) Device to cause horse to get larger: bronco-dilator.*
- *(For syringe haters) Exercising Parenteral Discretion.*

Ok. Ok. Sorry about that!

Dr. Sam and His Screening: Should He Have Known Better?

Surgeon Sam, the 63-year-old head of the surgery department at a large teaching hospital, hired Dr. Mike a talented new G.I. surgeon (a surgeon who deals with the digestive tract). Apart from being a talented administrator and surgeon, Dr. Sam was unusual because his dad, a fire fighter, died in a firetruck-automobile collision when responding to a prankish, but deadly, false alarm.

Dr. Sam showed his confidence in his new hire, Dr. Mike, by asking him to do his screening colonoscopy – a visual inspection of the lower bowel meant to detect early signs of cancer using a flexible tube with a video camera. Unfortunately, for both doctors, Dr. Sam experienced a bowel perforation, a rare complication of that exam, the first one Dr. Mike had done at his new hospital. Fortunately for Dr. Mike, he went on to have a successful career. The Chief of Surgery and the other hospital clinicians knew that fate sometimes deals rare, but not statistically unexpected, events. A recent report noted that for every 225 colonoscopies, one person suffers harm, including bowel perforation in 6 out of 10,000 colonoscopies and death in 3 of 100,000 colonoscopies.

According to the American Association of Family Physicians "*Colonoscopy is accurate in detecting adenomas but has no evidence of decreasing Colo-Rectal Cancer related mortality. Colonoscopy detects adenomas measuring 10 mm or larger with 89% to 98% sensitivity and 75% to 93% sensitivity for adenomas measuring at least 6 mm.*"

It seems that screening is successful for the early detection of lesions (adenomas) that can lead to colon cancer, but there is little evidence of decreased Colo-Rectal Cancer deaths in those who are screened. Nevertheless, many credentialed experts recommend regular colon cancer screening for everyone, including people who do not have risk factors (family history, for example) for colon cancer. Of course, anyone experiencing symptoms or signs such as severe constipation, abdominal pain, or rectal bleeding should have a colonoscopy to be sure they do not have cancer that requires treatment.

Chapter 45: Introduction to Testing and Screening

KEYWORDS: Screening, Case-Finding, Diagnosis, Public Health Screening, False Positive Test Results, False Negative Test Results, True Positive Test Results, True Positive Test Results, Test Sensitivity, Test Specificity, Positive Predictive Value, Negative Predictive Value, Reliability, Prevalence, Safe Screening for Disease Detection, False Alarms, Pretest Probability, Low Value Testing

ABSTRACT: Screening tests help clinicians find hidden disease. Case finding tests help clinicians to diagnose an existing problem. It is important to understand the characteristics of tests and the prevalence of disease, as discussed in this chapter, to avoid misinterpreting a test result.

Introduction

In patient care, performing tests – such as laboratory analysis of blood chemistry or radiological imaging of organs – is often a crucial step in formulating a definitive diagnosis. What may not be obvious is that the results of tests can be false alarms, indicating problems that can be highly consequential. These false alarms can frighten people, can engender harm from needless interventions and can divert important human and financial resources from necessary and important work to harmful or superfluous activity.

Finding diseases can be like finding needles in a haystack! Sometimes, a very small needle in a lot of haystacks.

If we reflect on the haystack analogy, success in finding a needle is more likely with very large needle and one small haystack. Diagnostic testing and screening involve identifying the haystacks and finding the needles, where the 'needles' are disease causes. Sometimes, also, the pieces of hay and the needles can be hard to distinguish visually. Ok, let's assume we have iron-rich needles and a very powerful magnet. FIGURE 1.45.1 brings this home.

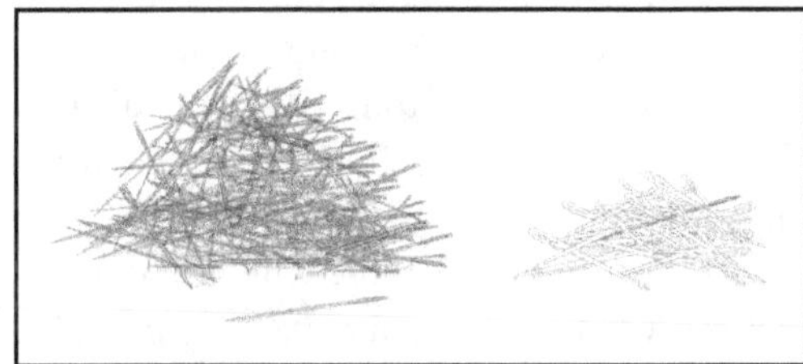

FIGURE 1.45.1: Finding a needle in a haystack or a pile of needles

Diagnostic testing and screening – the latter also defined as case-finding testing but we will use the word 'screening' here – are akin to the finding of needles in haystacks, and screening is the more problematic of the two as often the haystack is large, and the needles are few. Screening would only truly be useful if results were always positive for people with a condition and always negative for those without. Screening creates problems when it suggests a person has a disease when the person is disease-free or when it provides false reassurance to those who are sick.

Let's do it![295]

Why Patients Have Tests

People who feel sick see doctors because they want to feel better, be able to do more, live longer and maintain their health. Healthy people sometimes also worry that they might become sick, which would limit their activities and enjoyment. Most people are motivated to increase their 'health span' – the number of years they are and feel well and can be active – as well as their lifespan. Consequently, they ask for information about their health and what they can do to maintain and improve it.

Sometimes, medical interventions offer some promise of increased lifespan but cause immediate reductions in comfort and function – their health span. A good example is the treatment of some cancers. However, in all instances, patients must get the information they need to decide about treatment so they can make a personal decision. Testing those who feel sick makes good sense as it can help to discover what is wrong. We will call this 'diagnostic testing' or 'hypothesis confirming testing'.

On the other hand, those who visit doctors to learn what to do to maintain their health are hoping that a physical exam, questions from the doctor and laboratory testing will find hidden problems that will be resolved before they create serious harm. They believe that regular and comprehensive checkups are always good and that doctors can find impending problems before they are bothersome. This type of testing is to find a disease when there are no indicators that disease is present. It is called 'screening' and can be problematic when the problems from false positive tests outweigh the benefits of early detection. Furthermore, the evidence shows that the time and money spent on screening are often of little or no benefit.[296] [297] [298] [299] The Canadian Task Force on Preventive Health care[300] reports that "the traditional annual physical exam of asymptomatic adults is not supported by evidence of effectiveness and may result in harm." The task force further reports that "A systematic review of 14 randomized controlled trials (RCTs) indicated that these general checkups do not reduce total mortality, cardiovascular mortality, or cancer mortality". Instead, they recommend "a periodic (i.e., according to age, risk, and specific test intervals) preventive visit to provide preventive counseling and screening tests proven to be of benefit. Periodic preventive visits are particularly useful for people older than 65 years of age".

We will call screening 'case-finding' or 'discovering hidden disease' testing. Periodic screening tests for particular risk factors, for example, high blood pressure, anemia, blood sugar and other factors. Note that the choice of screening tests recommended by the task force

295 We are plagiarizing here. Gary Gilmore said this just before being executed by firing squad in the State of Utah on January 17, 1977. We trust that your experience in reading on will be more pleasant!

296 Hopkins Tanne J. Annual check-ups aren't needed, US study says. BMJ. 2007 Sep 29;335(7621):631. doi: 10.1136/bmj.39349.383194.DB. PMCID: PMC1995475. http://www.ncbi.nlm.nih.gov/pmc/articles/PMC1995475/. Accessed July 19, 2022.

297 Mehrotra A, Zaslavsky AM, Ayanian JZ. Preventive Health Examinations and Preventive Gynecological Examinations in the United States. Arch Intern Med.2007; 167(17):1876-1883. doi:10.1001/archinte.167.17.1876. http://archinte.jamanetwork.com/article.aspx?articleid=486857. Accessed August 4, 2022.

298 Roehr Bob. Routine screening for ovarian cancer harms more than it helps, says US authority BMJ 2012; 345: e6203. https://www.bmj.com/content/345/bmj.e6203. Accessed August 3, 2022.

299 Lin KW, Duane MR. Are some screening tests doing more harm than good? Am Fam Physician. 2007 Aug 1;76(3):351-2. PMID: 17708134. https://www.aafp.org/afp/2007/0801/p351.html. Accessed August 3, 2022.

300 Canadian task force on preventive healthcare. https://canadiantaskforce.ca/guidelines/periodic-preventive-health-visits/. Accessed August 3, 2022.

relates to the person's circumstances including age, family history and where they live.

Unfortunately, what physicians do is not always helpful. Something as simple as a checkup or undergoing a test for disease can be harmful. These harms are not obvious and include false reassurance that all is ok and consequent reduced vigilance. Patients, reassured by a checkup, are more likely to ignore new signs or symptoms that might indicate that there is a real problem, for example, serious heart disease.[301] Test results also can alarm people and cause anxiety (and more testing) by suggesting they have a disease when it's not there and further testing can produce false alarms as well needless and possibly harmful – or just unnecessary – treatments.

Information Gathering in the Doctor's Office

Doctors, in their clinical offices, learn about an individual's health by listening, asking questions, and examining patients. They can also get additional information through laboratory testing that examines and analyzes bodily substances including blood, urine, sweat, tears, saliva, mucous or even tissue samples. Even more can be gained from other types of testing, including imaging (using x-rays, magnetic resonance, radioactive tracers and ultrasound) and the electromagnetic signals that all humans generate. These signals include electrocardiograms (ECGs or EKGs) of the heart, electroencephalograms (EEGs) of the brain, electromyograms (EMGs) of the nerves and muscles and the galvanic skin response (GSR) to assess the body's response to stress.

Using all this information, doctors assess and estimate the patient's health status, make a diagnosis, prognosticate (try to predict what may happen) and determine if interventions might be helpful, harmful or unnecessary – or even unwise.

To do their jobs properly, doctors (as well as administrators, informaticians and others who define, manage, evaluate, opine on and decide on funding health facilities) must understand and apply the essential ideas related to testing and screening. They must do this because test quality, availability, applicability and the dependability of test results profoundly influence health care and health policy.

Also realize that, as we will elaborate on later, often we can test or screen ourselves. Sedentary lifestyle and overeating leading to obesity are risk factors we all know about. If people are sedentary, it is unlikely that they need a doctor to tell us that or to prescribe a regular walk or other exercise. It's already known! If one's waist size is too large, that is obvious to the person especially when shopping for clothes. Again, a doctor does not have to "diagnose" that you are overweight or obese.

There are good reasons to see a doctor, though. For instance, it might be that someone has a medical problem, and a doctor can determine that there is an underlying reason for weight changes, for example, thyroid disease. Simply eating too much fast food and not exercising can also explain it. To determine which of these is the problem, a doctor would enquire about eating and exercise habits and order laboratory tests to make sure only fast food and lack of exercise were the problems.

Most people have learned that overweight and inactive people are more likely to become sick and that obesity – indicated by weight or belt size – is a risk factor for

301 Marteau, T.M., Kinmonth. A.L., Thompson, S., The psychological impact of cardiovascular screening and intervention in primary care: a problem of false reassurance? British Family Heart Study Group. The British Journal of General Practice. 1996 Oct; 46(411)577. https://pubmed.ncbi.nlm.nih.gov/8945794/. Accessed Sept. 8, 2023.

sickness, deteriorating health and mortality.[302] [303] [304] Obesity portends poorer health, reduced quality of life and shorter life span.

For most people, being more active and eating appropriately contribute to health maintenance and improvement. Nevertheless, many adults and children are overweight or noticeably obese.[305] What is frustrating is that they ask their doctors about hidden risk factors, when the obvious is right in front of them: that bulge! Some do worry, occasionally correctly, that weight gain is a sign of a hidden illness and just want to be sure. For a few, especially those with recent rapid changes in weight, medical consultation is important.

Information from Public Health Screening

Some screening testing (case-finding or disease-discovering testing) is very useful and important, particularly for Public Health surveillance. The results of tests can inform governments and insurance companies about the prevalence (frequency) of the risk of diseases in each community. This was crucial during the COVID-19 pandemic. Health agencies tested many people, symptomatic or not, to learn the frequency of COVID in the community. Some tests were better than others in providing positive results for patients with COVID infection and negative for those without. However, no test was perfect.

Information about the health of communities (we call it the 'Humongous Body' in the chapter on Public Health) is essential to inform government policy related to economic development, sanitation, housing, education, air pollution and water pollution. Public Health experts gather data not only by collecting information from clinical offices (including reports of many communicable diseases) but also by conducting specialized screening in the community. The key idea is to get early information about the existence and spread of disease or other health problems in a region.

The Public Health Agency of Canada[306] describes the information they collect to help inform Public Health policy. Some of it comes from the unique information captured in regular community health surveys[307], while other information comes from clinicians' reports regarding communicable disease. Still other information comes from physician billing information – how many physicians billed for treating pulmonary problems, for example. This gives Public Health experts an indication of the health problems that plague communities, especially related to their social and other conditions. The information also helps to identify the communities that seem healthier or sicker than average and the conditions that

302 Samaras TT, Storms LH, Elrick H. Longevity, mortality and body weight. Ageing Res Rev. 2002 Sep;1(4):673-91. https://pdfs.semanticscholar.org/e397/a3316268d5cd203f6f880cffb071b9b1fad3.pdf. Accessed July 19, 2022.

303 Lorenzini A. How Much Should We Weigh for a Long and Healthy Life Span? The Need to Reconcile Caloric Restriction versus Longevity with Body Mass Index versus Mortality Data. Frontiers in Endocrinology. 2014; 5:121. https://www.ncbi.nlm.nih.gov/pmc/articles/PMC4115619/. Accessed July 19, 2022.

304 Abdelaal M, le Roux CW, Docherty NG. Morbidity and mortality associated with obesity. Annals of Translational Medicine. 2017;5(7):161. doi:10.21037/atm.2017.03.107. https://www.ncbi.nlm.nih.gov/pmc/articles/PMC5401682/. Accessed July 19, 2022.

305 C. Rodd, A.K. Sharma, Recent trends in the prevalence of overweight and obesity among Canadian children CMAJ September 20, 2016, 188: E313-E320; published ahead of print May 9, 2016, doi:10.1503/cmaj.150854. https://www.cmaj.ca/content/188/13/E313. August 3, 2022.

306 Public Health Agency Reports and Publications. https://www.canada.ca/en/public-health/services/reports-publications.html Accessed July 19, 2022.

307 Canadian Community Health Survey. https://www.canada.ca/en/health-canada/services/food-nutrition/food-nutrition-surveillance/health-nutrition-surveys/canadian-community-health-survey-cchs.html. Accessed July 19, 2022.

promote better or worse health.[308] Even what people search for on the Internet may provide a warning of a problem. Awareness of the frequency of diseases in communities, informs physicians and suggests for which diseases a physician should screen.

The Two Purposes of Testing – Diagnosis and Screening

There are two main types of tests, as we have mentioned, diagnostic tests and screening tests.

Physicians do **Diagnostic Tests**, or hypothesis-confirming tests, to explore the reasons or causes for a patient's problem(s). Physicians also use these to explore why there was an abnormal result from a screening test.

Searching for a cause when someone complains of discomfort or disability is not the same as screening. It should not be surprising that doctors are more likely to find problems when patients have complaints than when they are ordering tests for people who believe they are well. The complaint is at least some indication of a problem possibly being there. In other words, the existence of a complaint makes it more probable that a problem exists.

The other type of testing is **Screening Tests** – disease-discovering or case-finding tests. These are investigations physicians do to learn if people showing no symptoms or signs have hidden disease. Screening is what clinicians are doing when looking for concealed disease or risk factors in people who seem otherwise well. Testing for risk factors is more likely to be helpful when performed for people who might be at risk because of genetics, an exposure to a noxious or infectious agent or family history. Just looking for risk factors without a reason related to an individual's personal complaints or environment is screening. A good example of appropriate screening would be checking asymptomatic or seemingly healthy people in a town who might have been exposed to a chemical or pathogen (a virus, bacterium, etc.). Sometimes, also, a Public Health agency may usefully screen a population to document its health status. In addition, doctors may order screening tests for patients if requested to do so or out of curiosity about some concern.

As we mentioned, screening tests can be harmful. This can happen (1) if they provide false reassurance or (2) suggest the presence of a disease when none is there. They can also be helpful, on the other hand, if they discover treatable but hidden illnesses or risk factors that can set the stage for disease. So, they present us with a quandary. Who should we test and for what conditions? When are tests results more likely to be helpful? When are they more likely to mislead? To answer questions like this cogently, we must understand the characteristics of tests. This understanding will allow us to develop an approach to making decisions about whom to screen, when to screen and how to understand what test results mean.

Therefore, let's get our heads around the key characteristics of tests.

The Important Characteristics of Tests

The fly in the ointment is that, like smoke alarms, many medical tests can produce misleading results. A test result is misleading when it is a 'false positive' (FP) – 'positive' (P) means a person has a disease; 'false positive' means that the result is wrong, and the patient does not have the disease. It is also misleading when a test result is a 'false negative' (FN) – meaning it indicates not having the disease when the person does have the disease. These options are listed in FIGURE 1.45.2.

308 Physical activity, access to excellent food, affluence are well accepted qualities associated with better health.

	Test Result is Positive	Test Result is Negative
The person has the Disease	True Positive - TP	False Negative - FN
The person does NOT have the Disease	False Positive - FP	True Negative - TN

FIGURE 1.45.2: False and True Positives and Negatives

This means that:

> Some patients with a disease will have a positive test result, correctly indicating the person has the disease.`
  - This is a True Positive (TP) Result.

> Some patients with a disease will have a negative test result, wrongly indicating the person is ok.
  - This is a False Negative (FN) Result.

> Some patients without a disease will have a positive test result, wrongly indicating the person has the disease.
  - This is a False Positive (FP) Result.

> Some patients without the disease will have a negative test result, correctly indicating the person is ok.
  - This is a True Negative (TN) Result.

Worthwhile (accurate) tests give early warnings of conditions; this is most useful when the conditions are treatable. Worthwhile tests produce few false alarms (test results that are positive when a person does not have a condition) and few false negatives (test results that are negative when a person has a condition). We want to make it clear that very few tests are perfect, that is, almost every test produces some misleading results, positive test results for healthy people and negative test results for people with the disease. Perhaps the only exception, where every conclusion should be accepted as truth, is the evaluation of one's outfit by a spouse!

It is worth repeating: Screening tests – ones not a direct part of the confirmation of a diagnostic hypothesis – become controversial if they lead to further, unnecessary investigations, treatments or procedures that result from a false alarm.

Take for example a person, with no signs or symptoms of bowel disease, who has false positive (FP) result of a screening tests for blood in the stool. False positive results from stool tests occur for various reasons, including having taken an iron supplement, having eaten meat recently or having taken certain drugs, like colchicine used for gout. The consequence of a false positive result from a screening test can be additional unnecessary investigations, akin to chasing a phantasm, and sometimes these further investigations can cause harm. For instance, a person can get an injury to the lower bowel from an unnecessary colonoscopy. Researchers and clinicians recognize that over-testing can lead to serious harm.[309]

Everybody could benefit if they knew the characteristics of tests, but patients and even diagnosticians are often in the dark about them.

Characteristics of Tests

There are several key characteristics of tests: their **Specificity** and **Sensitivity**, the **Prevalence** of the disease and the **Predictive Value** of a test result.

A test that correctly identifies every sick person as sick will be 100% sensitive even if it misidentifies some healthy people as sick.

A test that correctly identifies every healthy person as healthy will be 100% specific even if it misidentifies some sick people as healthy.

309 H. Singh, J.A. Dickinson, G. Thériault, R. Grad, S. Groulx, B J. Wilson, O. Szafran and N.R. Bell, Overdiagnosis: causes and consequences in Primary Care Canadian Family Physician September 2018, 64 (9) 654-659. http://www.cfp.ca/content/64/9/654. Accessed July 19, 2022.

The **Prevalence** of a disease is the frequency of the condition in the population or the group of people who are tested. If on average, the disease is present in 1 of 1000 people in a region, the prevalence is 0.1% in that region.

Putting this information together is essential to understanding the **Predictive Value** of a positive test result or a negative test result.

Please note that there are many illustrative examples in the next chapter that will help make these clear.

SUMMARY OF THE IMPORTANT CHARACTERISTICS OF TESTS

- ***Sensitivity*** = *The proportion of people with the disease who receive a positive test result.*
- ***Specificity*** = *The proportion of people who do not have the disease who correctly receive a negative test result.*
- ***True Positive (TP)*** = *A positive test result indicating correctly that a patient has a disease.*
- ***False Positive (FP)*** = *A positive test result when the patient is disease-free.*
- ***True Negative (TN)*** = *A negative test result indicating correctly that the patient is disease-free.*
- ***False Negative (TN)*** = *A negative test result when the patient is sick with the disease.*
- ***Positive Predictive Value*** = *The proportion of people with a positive test result who have the disease.*
- ***Negative Predictive Value*** = *The proportion of people with a negative test result who are disease-free*
- ***Prevalence*** = *The proportion of people in a population who have the disease – a number necessary to determine the positive and negative predictive value of a test.*
- ***Reliability*** = *Is the test result the same when a lab repeats the test, or another laboratory does the test?*

Note 1: *Regarding the pre-test probability: The PTP is the chance that someone will have the disease in the region of interest. It is related to prevalence or the frequency of the condition in the community. Diabetes has a high prevalence and high PTP. Addison's disease has a low prevalence and low PTP. So, the likelihood that a positive test result is a true positive (TP) is higher for diabetes than for Addison's disease.*

Note 2: *The American Academy of Family Physicians publishes "Summary of Recommendations for Clinical Preventive Services"*[310] *including recommendations for routine screening tests at various ages, and the academy indicates the strength of evidence supporting their advice.*

Unfortunately, doctors sometimes suggest screening – remember that is looking for a problem that has not shown itself in the patient – based on their belief that screening will be helpful. They do this even when there is little or no research-based evidence demonstrating that people who submit to screening have longer or better lives and they do this despite evidence that some people experience harms from unnecessary screening.[311] However, there are other factors to consider, one being discovering a condition that it is possible to treat successfully with tolerable side effects on comfort and longevity. The other is when knowing the patient has a condition can enable longer maintenance of comfortable living (e.g., pain minimization or avoidance). In the case of some conditions, for example screening for thyroid cancer, testing increases the frequency of the detection of thyroid cancer, but early diagnosis does not seem to avert deaths from the

310 American Academy of Family Physicians, Summary of Recommendations for Clinical Preventive Services July 2017. http://www.aafp.org/dam/AAFP/documents/patient_care/clinical_recommendations/cps-recommendations.pdf. Accessed August 29, 2022.

311 Recommendations on screening for colorectal cancer in primary care Canadian Task Force on Preventive Health Care* CMAJ 2016. DOI:10.1503/cmaj.151125 "No RCTs have reported on the mortality benefit of screening, colonoscopy, computed tomographic colonography, barium enema, digital rectal examination or fecal DNA testing. Resources, test availability and patient preferences should be considered when choosing a screening test." http://www.cmaj.ca/content/early/2016/02/22/cmaj.151125.full.pdf. Accessed July 19, 2022.

disease.[312] In other words, the screening engenders anxiety and treatments that might not help!

Simple Screening and Safe Screening

Some kinds of screening tests are simple, non-invasive and safe.

It is easy and safe, for example, for patients to ask their doctors to check their blood pressure or for them to monitor their own blood pressure using commercially available blood pressure measurement devices. The same can be said about monitoring weight; a scale does that trick. In fact, the more often people do these things themselves, the more likely they are to notice if things start going awry and then to do something about it. Perhaps the only issue might be the downside of becoming too compulsive and of worrying about every excursion. Vital signs, like blood pressure, vary throughout the day.

Somewhat More Risky Screening

Other screening tests are a little more intrusive.

Many find it distasteful to collect a stool sample (a sample of one's feces) to send to a laboratory to check for non-obvious ('occult') blood, which can be a warning sign of cancer. This is an important consideration particularly if a person has a history of bowel problems or is concerned on having seen some blood with their feces. Testing for blood or bowel cancer isn't screening for people who have a history of problems, have darker stools or have red blood on their stool. If they are in a higher risk group, testing is more likely to be life preserving and reliable positive tests more likely to be true positives.

If the result of a test for blood in the stool is positive, doctors will recommend colonoscopy (the rectal insertion of an imaging device to view the inside of the colon). This is not screening, but rather is cause-finding – the blood needs to be explained. The next appropriate test would be colonoscopy. Unfortunately, colonoscopy is sometimes dangerous because of the risk, albeit low, of bowel perforation during the procedure. Colonoscopy is important, as it can detect early cancer, but should not be undertaken unnecessarily because some can experience a reasonably serious complication. Another minor risk is a reaction to the anesthetic, though that is extremely rare. Again, this is not screening as it is appropriately following up on the evidence of blood in the stool.

People should always consult a clinician to explore the causes of signs (blood in stool, for example) or symptoms (discomfort, e.g.) of what might be a disease. However, they should also learn the reason for a procedure and if it can reliably detect the problem. To ascertain this, they should inquire about how often the test finds something, and how often positive test results are true positives. Clinicians, administrators and researchers must track the fate (what happens to) of people who have the test whether the result is positive or negative and how often the resulting tests are helpful or harmful. Regretfully, this is rarely done and should be corrected.

To further understand the need to limit testing to people who are at risk for colon cancer, consider the following. At age 50-years, fewer than 1 person in 100 (1%) will develop bowel cancer over the following 10 years. At age 70-years, about 2 people in every 100 (2%) will develop

312 Kato, E., Niebuhr, D.W. Putting Evidence into Practice, Screening for Thyroid Cancer, Am Fam Physician. 2018 Mar 15;97(6):406-407. "The USPSTF recommends against screening for thyroid cancer in asymptomatic adults (D recommendation). The USPSTF found inadequate direct evidence on the benefits of screening but determined that the magnitude of the overall benefits of screening and treatment can be bounded as no greater than small, given the relative rarity of thyroid cancer, the apparent lack of difference in outcomes between treatment and surveillance (for the most common tumor types), and observational evidence showing no change in mortality over time after introduction of a mass screening program." https://www.aafp.org/afp/2018/0315/p406.html. Accessed July 19, 2022.

bowel cancer over the following 10 years.[313] These are small numbers! As people age from 70 to 80 or 80 to 90 there is an increase in the frequency of all medical problems and very few people live past age 90 regardless of whether they do or do not have cancer.[314] Recall what we wrote regarding the minimal benefit of screening on lifespan. We all must be realistic about longevity and be careful not to cause harm when we try to improve life expectancy.

Percent of U.S. Men Who Develop Colorectal Cancer over 10-, 20-, and 30-Year Intervals According to Their Current Age, 2003-2005			
Current Age	**10 Years**	**20 Years**	**30 Years**
30	0.06	0.29	0.96
40	0.23	0.92	2.29
50	0.71	2.14	4.06
60	1.55	3.64	5.06
70	2.51	4.22	N/A

Percent of U.S. Women Who Develop Colorectal Cancer over 10-, 20-, and 30-Year Intervals According to Their Current Age, 2003-2005			
Current Age	**10 Years**	**20 Years**	**30 Years**
30	0.06	0.26	0.78
40	0.20	0.72	1.74
50	0.54	1.58	3.16
60	1.10	2.76	4.29
70	1.88	3.61	N/A

FIGURE 1.45.3: Chances of colorectal cancer in short and long term at various ages[315]

The data in FIGURE 1.45.3 shows the chances of cancer at various stages of life for men and women and helps to inform choices about the appropriateness of screening. At younger ages, colon cancer isn't likely, so the risks of screening outweigh the potential benefits. For those older, screening is more likely to detect something that is treatable, and the increased chance of benefit outweighs the potential harms. For the most senior among us, e.g., people over 80, screening asymptomatic people is not likely to prolong life, because sadly we all die.

To make it clear: Screening – not diagnosis confirmation or cause-finding – for possible disease in older people who have normal comfort and function often produces more harm than benefit because there is little opportunity to improve life expectancy. Furthermore, many treatments – and some tests – reduce comfort and function and can cause serious problems. Even surgery or chemotherapy for cancer usually reduce comfort and function, while having little likelihood of increasing the lifespan of elderly people. Worse still, some treatments shorten their lives. Given that the goals of treatment are to improve comfort and function, screening a healthy 85-year-old person for colorectal cancer makes little or no sense if they were functioning well and are comfortable.

Another Example: Detecting Heart Disease

Heart disease is a complicated and important matter.

Let's say a person goes to a physician to be tested for heart disease just as a matter of a checkup – to make sure everything is ok.

313 Haggar FA, Boushey RP. Colorectal Cancer Epidemiology: Incidence, Mortality, Survival, and Risk Factors. Clinics in Colon and Rectal Surgery. 2009;22(4):191-197. doi:10.1055/s-0029-1242458. http://www.ncbi.nlm.nih.gov/pmc/articles/PMC2796096/. Accessed July 19, 2022.

314 Haggar FA, Boushey RP. Colorectal Cancer Epidemiology: Incidence, Mortality, Survival, and Risk Factors. Clinics in Colon and Rectal Surgery. 2009;22(4):191-197. doi:10.1055/s-0029-1242458. http://www.ncbi.nlm.nih.gov/pmc/articles/PMC2796096/. Accessed July 19, 2022.

315 Haggar FA, Boushey RP. Colorectal cancer epidemiology: incidence, mortality, survival, and risk factors. Clin Colon Rectal Surg. 2009 Nov;22(4):191-7. https://www.ncbi.nlm.nih.gov/pmc/articles/PMC2796096/. Accessed August 26, 2022.

The test results show no problem; they are negative for heart disease. That sounds like good news, but is it? A negative test result for heart disease is reassuring. But suppose it didn't detect disease that's actually there – it's a false negative (FN)! If so, one might ignore further symptoms that crop up. Sadly, some small heart blood vessel blockages, previously undetected during routine checkup, can lead to major heart damage, severe illness and possibly death. Counterintuitively, a recent reassuring check-up can make it more likely that someone will ignore an important new symptom.[316]

On the other side of the coin, some results from cardiac testing are false alarms – false positives (FP) – they falsely indicate a problem and can lead to additional, more intrusive testing and even treatment. And some remedies are more likely to harm than help. The classic George Bush cardiac stenting event, referred to previously, is one example. We repeat it here as it so well illustrates the issues.

GEORGE BUSH-CARDIAC STENT:

The classic example is the President George W. Bush cardiac stent story.[317] *President Bush was a physically fit 67-year-old avid cyclist, who had no symptoms. Shortly before the stent placement he had participated in a 30-mile bike ride in the heat of summer. He had "routine" testing including cardiac stress test and follow up. The follow up testing suggested he had a coronary artery blockage, and this was followed by an invasive procedure, namely the insertion of a cardiac stent.*[318] *The good news is that President Bush did not seem to be harmed by the procedure. The bad news is that President Bush had no opportunity to benefit because research since then has demonstrated that stenting asymptomatic blockages does not lead to increased survival. If someone isn't having discomfort to begin with, the procedure can only induce temporary discomfort without any opportunity of benefit.*[319] *Patients who have not had pain and who have a stent for an asymptomatic blockage do not live longer than similar people who do not have a stent. Moreover, those who receive the surgery are at immediate risk of complications from the surgical procedure itself.*

The crucial message in all of this is that testing is not perfect! The results of testing can be valid (True Positives or True Negatives) and tell you correctly that you definitely have a disease (TP) or that you definitely don't (TN). Regretfully, the results can be invalid (False Positives or False Negatives) and worry you (FP) or give you bogus reassurance (FN). The fact that tests are not perfect is what makes screening problematic.

Screening: False and Real-Alarms

Maybe we need some explanation, as many are surprised to learn that some people are harmed because of a screening test or medical check-up. Well, harm comes in many forms; some we have mentioned. Harm can occur if a test result frightens people. This happens unnecessarily when a test, which should really have been

316 Cristina Renzi, Katriina L Whitaker, Jane Wardle Over-reassurance and under-support after a 'false alarm': a systematic review of the impact on subsequent cancer symptom attribution and help seeking. BMJ Open 2015; 5:2 e007002 doi:10.1136/bmjopen-2014-007002. http://bmjopen.bmj.com/content/5/2/e007002.short. Accessed July 19, 2022.

317 Cardiovasc Revasc Med. 2013 Sep-Oct;14(5):251-2. Doi: 10.1016/j.carrev.2013.08.008. Waksman, R., To stent or not to stent: the President Bush stent controversy. PMID:24034861 DOI: 10.1016/j.carrev.2013.08.008. http://www.ncbi.nlm.nih.gov/pubmed/24034861. Accessed July 19, 2022.

318 A cardiac stent is a device inserted into a coronary artery meant to open the artery.

319 Boden WE, O'Rourke RA, Teo KK, Hartigan PM, Maron DJ, Kostuk WJ, Knudtson M, Dada M, Casperson P, Harris CL, Chaitman BR, Shaw L, Gosselin G, Nawaz S, Title LM, Gau G, Blaustein AS, Booth DC, Bates ER, Spertus JA, Berman DS, Mancini GB, Weintraub WS. Optimal medical therapy with or without PCI for stable coronary disease. N Engl J Med. 2007;356(15):1503–16. https://pubmed.ncbi.nlm.nih.gov/17387127/. Accessed Sept. 8, 2023.

reassuring, produces a false positive report, suggesting that a healthy person is sick. It can also ensue when doctors prescribe unnecessary treatments because they ignore the possibility of false alarms and believe that a positive test result always means the disease is present.

Doctors and patients must understand the 'predictive accuracy' of the test – how likely it is to be correct in light of the nature of the test and the prevalence of the disease in their community.

The 'prevalence' part may not be intuitive. It makes clear that a positive test result – again, all tests generate false positive results (FP) – for a rare condition is less likely to be valid (a TP) compared with a positive test for a common condition. Consider again the needle in a haystack and searching with your hands. If it's a very large haystack with few needles, you are more likely to feel hard pieces of straw and not find the needle. On the other hand, if it's a tiny haystack or there are many needles, you are more likely to find a needle.

We can understand that the issue of prevalence may cause a "what the heck?" reaction! All we can say is that the next chapter will convince you!

AN ALARMING EXAMPLE

A familiar example might help. Let's look at smoke alarms again... we all have experience with them.

Consider a smoke alarm that always goes off when there is smoke. It is 100% sensitive to smoke. The problem is that most smoke alarms also go off when someone is overheating the French fries or Uncle Steve is smoking a stinky stogie. They are quite sensitive at the job of detecting smoke – with or without a fire. In other words, they are not sufficiently specific to fires, which is what we are mostly worried about. As smoke on its own can be life-threatening, concern about the smoke itself is appropriate. The alarm is sensitive to smoke, if it is 100% sensitive to smoke, it will go off every time there's smoke, a possible indicator of a fire, even if there is not actual fire burning up the house. The problem is that ANY smoke sets it off.

On the other hand, a smoke alarm system that is 100% specific would only go off when there is smoke from an actual fire or from smoldering material likely to burst into flames or combust. An alarm that detects smoke AND very high temperature (maybe with an infrared sensor) – not Auntie Minnie's hot flash – would be more specific to fires. If this type of alarm is installed, it would have a much higher specificity to fires. In other words, if it went off, there was likely a fire. Most smoke alarms have low specificity to fires.

False alarms are the problem. Cooking French fries sets off the alarm – too sensitive, not highly specific to fires, False Positive for fire, false alarm, lots of noise and concern, not good... especially if it automatically called the fire hall. The same is true of an alarm NOT going off when it should. If there's a fire, we want the detector to be sufficiently specific, NOT give us a False Negative when it should have detected the problem and doesn't. A sensitive alarm that is not specific will alarm too often and people will learn to ignore it ignore it due to its many false positives. False negatives aren't good, either, as lives can be lost because of them.

A smoke alarm is really intended to inform us that there may be a source of a lot of deadly smoke or a fire somewhere.

Then there is the issue of prevalence. If an alarm goes off in a wooden building, especially one with lots of inflammable material, it is more likely to signal an actual fire than it would in a steel and concrete bunker. The basis for supporting burning must be there.

A medical parallel to the smoke alarm in the wooden building above would be to consider people in a rural pig farming community susceptible to a disease that their creatures carry. Suppose a doctor sees a patient from this rural community who has the troublesome symptoms of a rare disease that might not be present in an urban community. If the doctor orders a test and gets a result, the doctor must have information about the likelihood that the condition occurs in the person's community. If the result is positive, it is more likely to be correct (a TP) if the person raises pigs – the patient is more likely has the disease. On the other hand, if the doctor ordered the test for a patient in an urban community who didn't travel to a farm or eat pork, a positive result is likely incorrect (an FP). Of course, one might wonder why the doctor did that. Well, maybe the patient's symptoms rang a bell potentiated by a recent online education session – who knows, but such things happen!

The problem of developing tests for disease detection is similar to the problem of developing a smoke detector. Ideal smoke detectors would sound the alarm only when there is life-threatening smoke or a fire. They would ignore smog in the air or overcooking French fries. This is an excellent illustration! Even the best smoke alarm will raise a ruckus secondary to some kitchen events... even just plain bad cooking! There are no PERFECT smoke alarms! Also, Virginia, there are no perfect tests! Furthermore, even an imperfect smoke alarm is more likely to be warning of an actual fire in a basement piled high with cardboard boxes and old paint cans near the furnace than it is in the kitchen!

The better the test and the more likely the disease, the more likely a positive or negative result reflects reality, i.e., is a true positive (TP) or a true negative (TN)!

Especially in health care, false alarms (false positives or false negatives) are not merely annoying or scary. False alarms create danger because they affect how people behave. They frighten people, produce side effects from needless interventions and divert important human and financial resources from necessary and important work to harmful or superfluous activity.

CLINICAL ANECDOTE

Way back in the early 1960s, DC was inoculated with the new polio vaccine created by Jonas Salk. Public Health personnel did the vaccination in a mobile unit deployed to distribute the vaccine to large numbers of people rapidly – polio was endemic at the time. At the same encounter, the personnel screened people for blood pressure – actually a great idea. However, it was a scary experience for a somewhat young person.

A few weeks later, the Public Health agency sent DC a notice to see a physician as soon as possible. That was even more scary! The physician revealed that the screening had detected high blood pressure and a doctor needed to measure it again. Sure enough, the blood pressure was elevated! However, the physician said to lie there for a few minutes and then repeated the measurement. The diagnosis: "white coat syndrome" – blood pressure increased by the scary situation. The screening result was a false positive for high blood pressure. Whew!

Being Careful with Our Elderly

Screening is a particular enigma for older people. We all want to live longer but we want to be comfortable and not cut life short.

There are some facts here that must be considered. As we age, our body systems tend to become less resilient and adaptive. Treatments like radiation or chemotherapy that disrupt metabolism may be even more distressing compared to the same treatment given to a younger person. Elderly people must be careful and consider if an immediate loss of comfort and function is reasonable when it is unlikely that the treatment will increase life expectancy. They need to weigh immediate changes in health, comfort and function against the chances that the discomfort will be worthwhile because of the potential increase in lifespan.

Pretest Probability in the Context of Diseases of the Elderly

'Pretest probability' refers to the chance someone has a specific condition before we test. The pretest probability is higher for people with symptoms or from areas that have a high prevalence of the illness. They are more likely to have the disease.

Diabetes and COPD (chronic obstructive pulmonary – lung – disease) are relatively common illnesses. People who are thirsty and must wake up at night to urinate are more likely to have diabetes compared with a group of people who feel well and have no known problems. People who smoke or live in smog-polluted areas are more likely to develop COPD.

Let's look at diabetes first. The World Health Organization suggests that the prevalence of diabetes for all age groups worldwide is about 4%[320] (4 of 100 people have the disease). Screening a random population of humans scattered throughout the world you would expect to find diabetes 4% of the time. This means that our pretest probability of diabetes is 4%. However, some countries and communities have more diabetes than others.

In the United States, the prevalence of diabetes is greater than the average worldwide at about 10%[321]; in American seniors it is about 25%.[322] If we screen American seniors for diabetes, a positive test result is more likely to be a true positive (TP) result than the same test performed on a younger American or in some other part of the world. In Canada, the prevalence of diabetes is about 7%; in Canadian seniors it is also about 25%.[323]

Next, if we consider COPD, researchers at the University of Ottawa[324] tell us that someone over 45 who is coughing has a 0.4% (4 in 1000) chance of cancer. This means that for people with a cough, fewer than 1 person out of 250 will have cancer. Three out of 100 (3%) will have pneumonia and most patients with a cough will have a benign and self-limited viral illness. Lung cancer is not that common a cause of coughing!

On the other hand, a smoker has a higher pretest probability of having cancer compared with a non-smoker. An x-ray image suggesting cancer in an older smoker is more likely to be correct and not an artifact compared with a similar x-ray picture in a 23-year-old, non-smoking athlete with a cough. The young athlete is very unlikely to have cancer and it is probable that a seemingly abnormal x-ray image will turn out to be a false positive (FP). Of course, rare does not mean never, so it is necessary to follow up abnormal test results even when they are most likely a false alarm. This is an example of testing leading to more testing.

The key point we need to understand is that doctors use information about disease prevalence, the potential for harm from a missed diagnosis or from over-investigation and other factors like age to decide how aggressively to investigate a problem and how to interpret a test result and decide on treating.

The message: The presence of a positive test result suggests but does not guarantee that a person has a disease! It can be a true positive or a false positive.

The Imperfection of Testing

Clearly, a test would be perfect and most useful if it gave a positive result for everyone with a disease and a negative result for everyone who does not.

We will go back to sensitivity and specificity now.

320 Wild, S, Sicree, R, Roglic, G., et. Al., Global Prevalence of Diabetes: /Estimates for the year 2000 and projects for 2030. https://pubmed.ncbi.nlm.nih.gov/15111519/. Accessed August 3, 2022.

321 Diabetes Prevalence Worldwide and By Country. https://worldpopulationreview.com/country-rankings/diabetes-rates-by-country. Accessed Sept 8, 2023.

322 M. Sue Kirkman, Vanessa Jones Briscoe, Nathaniel Clark, Hermes Florez, Linda B. Haas, Jeffrey B. Halter, Elbert S. Huang, Mary T. Korytkowski, Medha N. Munshi, Peggy Soule Odegard, Richard E. Pratley, Carrie S. Swift; Diabetes in Older Adults. *Diabetes Care* 1 December 2012; 35 (12): 2650–2664. https://diabetesjournals.org/care/article/35/12/2650/38582/Diabetes-in-Older-Adults. Accessed August 26, 2022.

323 https://www.canada.ca/en/institutes-health-research/news/2021/08/government-of-canada-announces-new-investment-in-diabetes-research.html. Canadian Institutes of Health Research Government of Canada Announces New Investment in Diabetes Research, August 13 2021. Accessed Sept. 8, 2023.

324 Ponka D, Kirlew M. Top 10 differential diagnoses in family medicine: Cough. Canadian Family Physician. 2007;53(4):690-691. http://www.ncbi.nlm.nih.gov/pmc/articles/PMC1952600/. Accessed July 19, 2022.

SUMMARY OF SENSITIVITY AND SPECIFICITY

Sensitivity (AKA the true positive rate) of a test measures the proportion of people who actually have a disease who have a positive test result who are correctly identified as such.

Specificity (AKA the true negative rate) of a test measures the proportion of people not having the disease who are correctly identified as such.

Very few tests have a sensitivity of 100% or a specificity of 100% and even fewer have both!

This implies that some of the positive tests results will be misleading (FPs) and so will some of the negative results (FNs). Almost every test sometimes leads to the wrong conclusion for some of the people tested. The important thing is to know the chance or likelihood that a test result accurately depicts the presence or absence of a disease. This means we need to know the test's sensitivity and specificity!

It is also worth mentioning 'false alarm fatigue'.

If we get frequent false positives, we eventually begin to ignore true positives, and that is not good! Tests that produce a lot of false alarms are properly called 'low-value tests'. Not only can they lead to false alarm fatigue, they also often engender 'low-value care' that includes sequences of further pointless testing, often more invasive in nature, labelling, unnecessary treatment and even patient injury.

LOW VALUE TESTING

Low-value care, or healthcare services that do not improve patient outcomes or for which harms appear to outweigh the benefits, is estimated to cost the US healthcare system between $75.7 and $101.2 billion annually.[325] Campaigns like 'Choosing Wisely' have led to the publication of hundreds of recommendations to reduce low-value healthcare services; however, prior research has shown that low-value care continues to be frequent despite these recommendations, with substantial ordering variation observed across institutions and clinicians. In addition to direct patient harms and costs associated with low-value testing, abnormal results from these initial tests can initiate care cascades (i.e., subsequent testing or treatment). Care cascades can increase costs to the healthcare system while also raising the burden of care on patients, including greater patient inconvenience and costs, and even exposing them to harms associated with subsequent, potentially unnecessary healthcare services.

It is useful now to consider some examples.

325 Bouck Z, Calzavara AJ, Ivers NM, Kerr EA, Chu C, Ferguson J, Martin D, Tepper J, Austin PC, Cram P, Levinson W, Bhatia RS. Association of Low-Value Testing With Subsequent Health Care Use and Clinical Outcomes Among Low-risk Primary Care Outpatients Undergoing an Annual Health Examination. JAMA Intern Med. 2020 Jul 1 https://pubmed.ncbi.nlm.nih.gov/32511668/ Accessed Sept. 9, 2023

Chapter 46: Details of Test Characteristics

KEYWORDS: Sensitivity, Specificity, Prevalence, Positive Predictive Value, Negative Predictive Value, Screening Tests

ABSTRACT: Few tests produce only useful information. Misleading false positive (false alarms) or false negative (false reassurance) test results can harm patients. Some screening programs, especially ones where the prevalence (commonness) the of the condition in the community is high, might be useful. Other screening, where the prevalence of the condition in the community is low, are more likely to mislead. Doctors and patients must consider these factors in deciding when to screen.

Introduction

Material about testing is likely unfamiliar and somewhat challenging, so let's consider it further and use different words and examples. If it is too confusing, feel free to skip the details, but remember that testing is imperfect and results can be misleading (tell you that you are sick when you are not, or tell you you're ok when you are not).

For clarity: a 'test' is a measurement process for attempting to determine for a patient if something is wrong or that indicate nothing is wrong. A 'test result' is the report of the outcome of the measuring process that the patient and doctor receive.

The sensitivity, specificity and predictive value of tests depends on the local prevalence of illnesses and the quality of the laboratories doing the tests. Most Canadian and American laboratories have quality assurance mechanisms in place to help improve the sensitivity, specificity and predictive values. See, for example: https://pathology.ubc.ca/2022/12/01/michael-a-noble/. Dr. Michael Noble is an expert in laboratory quality management.

Restating Specificity and Sensitivity

The **specificity** of a test tells us the % of disease-free people who will receive a negative test result. For the disease-free people, it indicates "no", and affirms they don't have the disease. However, some people with the disease may get an erroneous negative result indicating they are disease-free. The people who have the disease and get a negative test result, may falsely believe they are disease-free, but they aren't.

AN AIDE MEMOIRE FOR SPECIFICITY

As a way of remembering this, consider your spouse, a person very well-known to you. Your spouse is a specific person with unique characteristics. It doesn't matter how big the crowd, you will be able to go through and eliminate (give a true negative result for) everyone in the crowd who is not your spouse, and you will be sure of that.

The **sensitivity** of a test describes the % of people who actually have a disease who receive a positive test result.

REMEMBERING SENSITIVITY

Another way of remembering what test sensitivity is about is to think about being 'sensitive'. If you are 100% sensitive to a spouse, you will recognize "the glare" or snappy word. However, in the real world of relationships – not testing – you may be oversensitive, and assume the person is upset when not. Of course, like tests, not all of us are 100% sensitive and sometime miss that affect!

The challenge in understanding the results of tests is that the specificity and sensitivity of tests together indicate the likelihood that a test result is correct! They co-exist – we can't interpret the results without knowing both.

This may seem like a pain in the brain, but it is worth it.

Some Examples of Situations

It is useful to consider some cases.

FIGURE 1.46.1: Assume everybody has the disease, indicated by 100 dark squares.

Case 1: Everybody to be Tested Has Measles (See FIGURE 1.46.1)

[Sensitivity > Indicates the probability (% chance) that someone with the disease will receive a positive test result.]

[Specificity > Indicates the probability (% chance) that someone without the disease will receive a negative test result is.]

[Nuance: a test that is positive for the disease might also indicate false positive results for someone who is healthy. A test that is negative for a disease might also be a false negative for someone who has the disease.]

The sensitivity of a test is a measure of how likely a person with the disease will receive a positive test result. In the situation where 100% of the population has the disease, e.g., measles, if a test were 100% sensitive and 100% specific, then everyone who has the disease will be correctly informed.

If we know for sure that all 100 people in a group have measles (as Table 1.46.1 illustrates), and you are one of them, every positive test result will be a true positive result. Your positive test result means that you do have measles.

Of course, this would not be the usual circumstance, as everyone in a group is unlikely to have measles. In the circumstance where there are people being tested who are measles-free, even if the test is 100% sensitive, not everyone for which the test is positive might have measles. The hypothetical 100% sensitive test does detect every person with measles, but it may indicate some people without measles have it! Some people will get mislabeled as having measles (i.e., there can still be false positives).

Case 2: We Do Not Know If the People we are Testing Have a disease

Let's start this time with a very rare disease in a large population and a not-quite-perfect test (see FIGURE 1.46.2). This is more like the following:

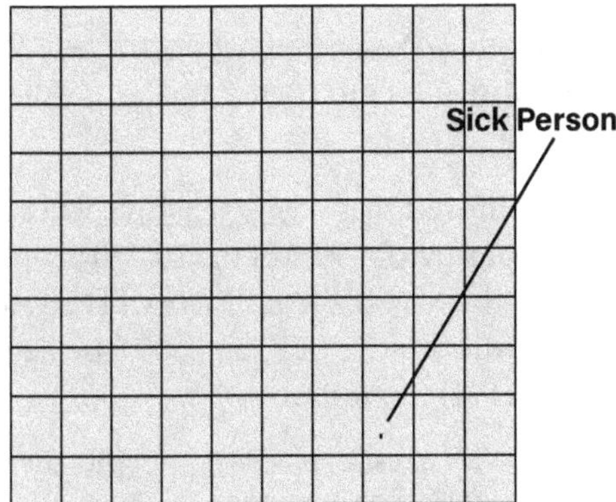

FIGURE 1.46.2: Assume almost nobody has the disease. The 100 dark squares each indicate 1000 (100,000 total) well people and the one black dot ('.') indicates the sick person..

Note: the black dot is in the 2nd row from the bottom, 3rd square from the right.

> *[Sensitivity > Indicates the probability (% chance) that someone with the disease will receive a positive test result.]*
>
> *[Specificity > Indicates the probability (% chance) that someone without the disease will receive a negative test result is.]*
>
> [Nuance: a test that is positive for the disease might also indicate false positive results for someone who is healthy. A test that is negative for a disease might also be a false negative for someone who has the disease.]

Suppose that one person in 100,000 has a rare disease and the test has 100% sensitivity. The test will identify that diseased person by giving a positive test result. However, it might also suggest that some people without the disease are ill. (Unless the test has 100% specificity as well.) Therefore, in order to identify everyone who is disease-free, further testing will be required to corroborate any positive test results.

If the test, on the other hand, has a specificity of 94%, then 94% of people who are disease-free will receive a true (correct) negative test result. However, it will also incorrectly identify – give false positive test results – for 6% of those tested, incorrectly suggesting that they have the disease. So, there will be 6,001 positive results, with only one being correctly positive. Consequently, 6,000 of those who are disease-free will have a test result claiming they have the disease. Therefore, the chance that you have the disease (the predictive value of the test) is 1/6,001 or about one-hundredth of 1% (0.00017%). Most of the positive test results would be false positives!

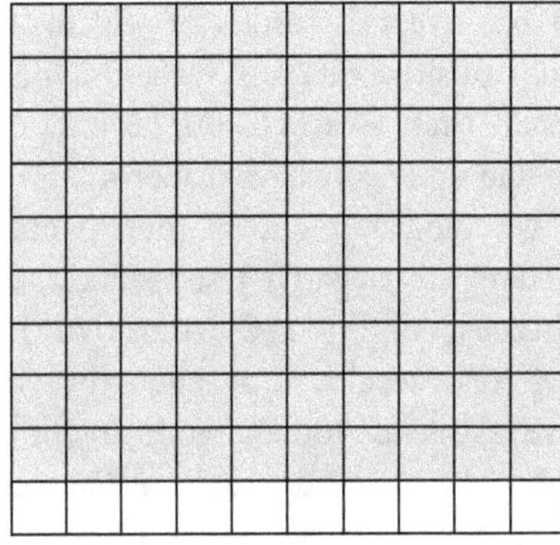

FIGURE 1.46.3: Detection easier if more have the disease

> *[Sensitivity > Indicates the probability (% chance) that someone with the disease will receive a positive test result.]*
>
> *[Specificity > Indicates the probability (% chance) that someone without the disease will receive a negative test result is.]*
>
> [Nuance: a test that is positive for the disease might also indicate false positive results for someone who is healthy. A test that is negative for a disease might also be a false negative for someone who has the disease.]

An easier challenge (see FIGURE 1.46.3) is the last scenario where 10% (10,000 – the white squares) of the population of 100,000 has the disease, and 90,000 are disease-free (90,000 – the gray squares), a good example being diabetes.

If the test has 100% sensitivity, it will give a positive result for each of the 10,000 people with diabetes, and there will be no false negative test results.

If the specificity, the other test characteristic, is 94%, the test will correctly label 84,600 (they are true negatives – TN) of the 90,000 without diabetes (the grey squares), indicating they are healthy, and mislabel as sick 5,400 of them who are healthy by indicating that they are sick.

All together, there are 15,400 (10,000 + 5,400) positive test results of which 10,000 are truly positive. If you receive a positive test result, there is a (10,000/15,400) 64.9% chance that you really have diabetes.

As we indicated above, there would be 84,600 correctly negative test results, and zero (0) (because of the 100% sensitivity) false negative test results. Consequently, with a negative test result you and your doctor could be confident that you do not have diabetes.

Those with a negative result could be confident they are ok. The bad news is for the about 35% of the people who receive a positive test result and might become concerned and modify their diet! If the disease were measles, they might quarantine unnecessarily.

Overall, out of the 100,000 tests, 84,600 are true negative results and 10,000 true positive results. For 94,600 of the people, the test results accurately reflect their condition. The chance that any test result is accurate is therefore 94.6%.

The Message

First, realize that in real world testing, we do not know who has the disease we are testing for and who does not. We are blind to that.

Then we need to recognize that all tests have BOTH characteristics, levels of sensitivity and specificity. Very few are 100% sensitive and 100% specific.

We will now apply a more real-world test that is 94% sensitive and 94% specific for the disease.

If we use the example where 10% of 100,000 have diabetes (FIGURE 1.46.3), the following is what we find:

- The test that is 94% **sensitive** will be positive for 94% of the 10,000 people who have diabetes. There will be 9,400 true positive (TP) and 600 false negative (FN) test results.
- With a test that is 94% **specific**, there will be 0.94 x 90,000 = 84,600 true negative (TN) test results and 5,400 false positive (FP) results.
- The total number of positive test results is 9,400 true positive (TP) test results + 5,400 false positive (FP) test results = 14,800. The total number of negative test results is 84,600 true negative (TN) test results + 600 false negative (FN) test results = 85,200.
- The predictive value, the secret weapon of interpreting test, of a positive test result is 63.5% (9,400 true positive results/14,800 total positive results).
- The predictive value of a negative test result is 99.3% (84,600 true negative (TN) results/85,200 false negative (FN) test results.
- 94% of all of the tests give a result that is helpful and not misleading because of the 100,000 tests 9,400 were true positive tests and 84,600 were true negative test results. 94% of the tests were true reflections of the patients status.

The importance of these predictive value calculations is that clinicians will be able to confidently tell patients who receive a negative test result that they almost certainly don't have the disease. If the patient's problems persist, the doctor should look for other causes that might explain the patient's problem. On, the other hand, for people with a positive test result, there a 36% chance they don't have the disease. The doctor must look for additional information to confirm or disprove the diagnosis.

A British Medical Association article[326] describes the important issues related to understanding the meaning of test results – sensitivity, specificity and their relationship to prevalence (how common a disease is in the community).

A REAL PATIENT EXAMPLE

Years ago, one of DZ's patients we will call "Sally", a delightful mother of 4 whose husband had a stressful and busy job, suddenly became very tired and developed several minor infections. Her fatigue was incapacitating. DZ ordered numerous laboratory tests and Sally saw 13 specialists over the course of 3 years. The universal opinion was that Sally was suffering from "depression" because of the stresses of her life. DZ knew the experts were merely using jargon to restate her problem as a diagnosis. However, he could not explain her serious and peculiar problems.

Over the course of her illness, Sally endured many tests, including a test of her electrolytes (bodily chemicals in her blood). The reason for these last tests is that Addison's disease, or adrenal gland insufficiency, is a rare explanation for chronic fatigue that can cause electrolyte levels – potassium in particular – to become abnormal. It materialized that Sally's electrolytes were normal according to the results of the tests. Unfortunately, it turned out that this was a false negative (FN) test result for Addison's disease. Sally's reported normal potassium level suggested that she did not have Addison's disease.

Later investigations, though, showed that her problem was, in fact, Addison's disease and DZ learned that many cases of Addison's are not associated with abnormal electrolyte levels, especially in their early stages. The normal electrolyte test gave false and distracting reassurance.

Oddly, her mother, who lived in another city, eventually noted something that led DZ to order a specific test – cortisol level – for Addison's disease. What her mother had noticed was that Sally had brown patches on her arms. This was a sign that her pituitary gland – a gland in the skull that tells the adrenal glands to produce more hormones – was overactive. The hormone that stimulates the adrenal gland (ACTH) is similar to the hormone (MSH – melanocyte stimulating hormone) that stimulates the skin to produce pigment (melanin). Hence the brown patches!

Consistently low cortisol levels always indicate something is wrong, and low cortisol is the sine qua non of Addison's disease, which is always a medical problem. However, electrolyte disturbances are not always present, and normal levels of electrolytes (like sodium and potassium) should not have reassured DZ that his patient did not have Addison's disease.

If we had recognized that a test for low potassium has only 80% sensitivity (potassium levels are low in 80% of people with Addison's – 20% have normal potassium), he would have ordered a cortisol blood level much earlier and saved the patient at least 20 months of discomfort and unnecessary anxiety.

Dealing with Real Populations and Real-Tests

Our final step is to define a useful measures: The Positive Predictive Value (PPV) and its Negative Predictive Value.

We included in our examples the chance that a person with a positive test result has the disease. The formal definition of the PVs is simple:

> The PPV is the Total Number of True Positive (TP) test results divided by the sum of the Number of True Positive (TP) test results + Number of False Positive (FP) test results. So, the PPV=TP/(TP+FP).

326 Loong, T, Understanding Sensitivity and Specificity, BMJ 327: 716 doi: 10.1136/bmj.327.7417.716 (Published 25 September 2003). http://www.bmj.com/content/327/7417/716.full. Accessed July 19, 2022.

> The negative predictive value of a test is the proportion of true negative tests divided by the total number of negative tests (TN + FN), The NPP=TN/(TN+FN).

The table below summarizes all the measures.

SUMMARY OF KEY TERMS WE NEED TO KNOW

We will start by assuming that, after doing a test, we do research and learn the truth, i.e., which people tested did actually have the disease and which actually did not have the disease. This means that we will know which people got a result that was a True Positive (TP: positive result was correct) or a True Negative (TN: negative result was correct). This will then inform us which result was a false positive (the positive result was false: FP) or a false negative (the negative result was false: FN).

TOTAL POSITIVE TESTS (TTP)

Number of True Positive (TP) test results + Number of False Positive (FP) test results: TTP=TP+FP.

TOTAL NEGATIVE TESTS (TTN)

Number of True Negative (TN) tests + Number of False Negative (FN) tests: TTN=TN+FN.

PREDICTIVE VALUE

The predictive value of a positive test result reflects the proportion of all positive tests that correctly identify the presence of disease:

- ***Positive Predictive Value** of a test is the Total Number of True Positive (TP) test results divided by Total Number of True Positive (TP) test results + Total Number of False Positive (FP) test results: PPV=TTP/(TTP+TFP).*
- ***Negative Predictive Value:** The negative predictive value of a test is the proportion of true negative tests divided by the total number of negative tests (TN + FN).*

Predictive Value of a Test and Relationship to Prevalence[327]

Our examples illustrate that the less often a condition is present in a community (the fewer people affected), the greater the chance that a **positive** test result will be a False Positive. This means that a positive test result for a **common** condition is more likely to be an accurate reflection (a True Positive) of the presence of a disease than a positive test result for a rare condition. The examples also show the significant impact of less-than-perfect tests. They raise a flag that being tested may be less informative than we have believed.

A Final Example: Actual Test for Diabetes

FIGURES 1.46.4 and 1.46.5 below give yet another example. This time they also show the difference between the US and Canada for a test with lower specificity and sensitivity. The overall rates are shown, they are approximate, and the frequency varies according to age. Older people are more likely to have diabetes. The purpose of these tables is to demonstrate that the predictive value of the same test is different depending on the prevalence of the disease.

Sensitivity= =83.4% Specificity = 84.4%
Prevalence USA = 10% (100 people in 1000)
Prevalence CAN= 6.84% (68.4 in 1000

TEST	POSITIVE	NEGATIVE	TOTAL
TRUE POSITIVE	57 (68 *.834)		57
FALSE POSITIVE	145 (932-787)		145
TRUE NEGATIVE		787 (932*.844)	787
FALSE NEGATIVE		11 (68-57)	11
TOTAL	202	788	1000

POSIT PRED VALUE = 57/202= 28% NEG PRED VALUE =787/798 =98.6%

CANADA

FIGURE 1.46.4: Detecting diabetes in Canadian population

327 Loong, T, Understanding Sensitivity and Specificity, BMJ 327: 716 doi: 10.1136/bmj.327.7417.716 (Published 25 September 2003). http://www.bmj.com/content/327/7417/716.full. Accessed July 19, 2022.

Sensitivity= =83.4% Specificity = 84.4%
Prevalence USA = 10% (100 people in 1000)
Prevalence CAN= 6.84% (68.4 in 1000

TEST	POSITIVE	NEGATIVE	TOTAL
TRUE POSITIVE	83 (100* 83.4)		83
FALSE POSITIVE	56 (900-844)		56
TRUE NEGATIVE		844 (900 * 84.4)	844
FALSE NEGATIVE		17 (100-83)	17
TOTAL	139	861	1000

POSITIVE PREDICTIVE VALUE 83/139= 59.7% NEGATIVE PRED VAL 844/861=98.2%

USA

FIGURE 1.46.5: Detecting diabetes in US population

Most recent prevalence of diagnosed diabetes in the USA is about 10%, with more in older people.[328] In Canada it has increased to 8%.[329]

Why We Need to Understand Test Results

This should be clear by now, but a few further thoughts follow.

Understanding what tests mean is particularly important when agencies and communities decide to start screening programs to detect early disease. Too many false alarms would mean that people may feel they must undergo unnecessary additional investigations, with the upshot that more time and money is spent to determine how serious a non-problem is, and these people may expose themselves to harmful interventions. The other bad outcome, failing to detect disease that is there, means that people who received a negative test result are falsely reassured and may not assertively seek appropriate treatment.

The reality is, though, that some people who feel well just want to know if they are at risk of developing a disease. They want to know what they can do to maintain and improve their health. Clinicians and researchers sometimes screen seemingly normal people to look for factors that are early signs or risk factors of disease. If they do that, the accuracy of testing becomes crucial, especially related to relatively rare conditions. Folks who feel well and do not have symptoms are unlikely to have a disease. Therefore, screening them is like the case above where we seek to identify a rare condition in a large population. That is a situation fraught with potential error! The chance of finding something that is actually wrong is minimal; the chance of causing unnecessary worry is quite high.

When to Avoid Screening

Because testing can generate so many false alarms or miss rare problems, it may be better to eschew some screening programs and to do 'self-screening' instead of the sophisticated physician-assisted, lab-type testing.

We already have a good idea of factors, including happiness, that predict a longer life,[330] wwhile other factors (obesity, sedentary lifestyle for example) predict a shorter life. People with poor personal habits or risk factors or who receive a report of an abnormal lab test result are more likely anyway to become ill than others are. We have mentioned how easy it is for everyone to self-monitor for the most important risk factors for disease – including poor diet, poor lifestyle habits, obesity and reduced exercise. All put a person at risk for sickness and death. Assessing if any of these is present does not require testing by skilled doctors and labs – anyone can do it, and most people can understand their importance.

If, however, people feel compelled to have lab screening, some pharmacies and Public

328 National Diabetes Statistics Report 2020. https://www.cdc.gov/diabetes/pdfs/data/statistics/national-diabetes-statistics-report.pdf. CDC. Accessed August 3, 2022.

329 https://www.canada.ca/en/public-health/services/publications/diseases-conditions/diabetes-canada-highlights-chronic-disease-surveillance-system.html. Accessed July 19, 2022.

330 Frey, B.S., Happy People Live Longer, Science, Feb 4, 2011, vol. 331 pg. 542-543. http://science.sciencemag.org/content/331/6017/542.full. Accessed July 19, 2022.

Health agencies provide screening tests so that people can be reassured or warned without necessarily having to make a visit to the doctor.[331]

We will share with you that this was a challenging chapter to get both correct and clear. As we all may find it difficult to keep this material in mind, consider looking at the following material: Sensitivity and Specificity Simplified: https://www.youtube.com/watch?v=psELBu7muNY; and trying the Sensitivity and Specificity Calculator: https://www.omnicalculator.com/statistics/sensitivity-and-specificity. Thank you for sticking with us at it!

331 Pharmacies, e.g., CVS in the United States, provide screening services and the results may or may not be sent to the client's family doctor. Some pharmacies often make an effort to communicate. http://www.cvs.com/minuteclinic/services/screenings-and-monitoring/N-d8Z3a3jmZd5. Accessed July 19, 2022.

Chapter 47: Clinical Rationales for Testing and Screening

KEYWORDS: Rationale for Screening, Cholesterol, False Positives From Poppyseed Bagels, All Cause Mortality And Morbidity, Prostate Cancer Screening, Colon Cancer Screening, Breast Cancer Screening, Screening For The Elderly, Self Screening

ABSTRACT: Screening is worthwhile when there is a good chance that the screening test will not harm many people because of false alarms, and when accurately detecting the disease will help people assuming treatment will make a difference. The chapter discusses controversies in screening for prostate cancer, breast cancer and colon cancer. The tragic consequence of a false positive test from a poppyseed bagel is a sad example of a serious consequence from a false positive test.

There are many reasons for testing, the most important being to confirm a diagnosis. Here we will present clinical situations wherein screening – the case-finding-type of testing – is useful and even essential.

Clinical Reasons for Screening: Cholesterol Management

Patients ask for and doctors suggest cholesterol screening because they believe, based on research evidence, that high cholesterol increases the chances that a person will have a heart attack or stroke.[332] The screening is the means of discovering if that may be the case and if the cholesterol is high enough to warrant concern even though the patient may be symptom-free.

It is important to realize that high cholesterol is not a disease in itself. Rather, it is a risk factor for conditions including vascular disease, heart attacks and stroke. Cholesterol is good stuff. Some organs, such as the brain, use large amounts of cholesterol and depend on it for cellular development and their function. So, there is a positive side of cholesterol; it is an important bodily constituent and building block. This is illustrated by the fact that research suggests that people with the lowest levels of cholesterol are more likely to die violent deaths or suffer from accidents.[333]

---

332 D.R. Jacobs, Jr., I.L. Mebane, S. I. Bangdiwala, M.H. Criqui, H.A. Tyroler, for the lipid research clinics program; High density lipoprotein cholesterol as a predictor of cardiovascular disease mortality in men and women: the follow-up study of the lipid research clinics prevalence study Am. J. Epidemiol. (1990) 131 (1): 32-47. https://pubmed.ncbi.nlm.nih.gov/2642759/. Accessed Sept. 8, 2023.

333 Repo-Tiihonen E, Halonen P, Tiihonen J, Virkkunen M Total serum cholesterol level, violent criminal offences, suicidal behavior, mortality and the appearance of conduct disorder in Finnish male criminal offenders with antisocial personality disorder. Eur Arch Psychiatry Clin Neurosci. 2002 Feb;252(1):8-11. http://www.ncbi.nlm.nih.gov/pubmed/12056583. Accessed July 19, 2022.

SOME PERSONAL WORK ON CHOLESTEROL

DZ was able to arrange introductions between 2 psychologists (Pat McGrath and Karina Davidson) and an endocrinologist Sethu Reddy, now at the Cleveland Clinic). The result was several articles examining the effect of cholesterol levels on mood and memory.[334 335] *These pieces suggested that lowered cholesterol is associated with increases in depression and decreased memory*[336] *capacity especially in older people.*[337] *More recent studies suggest this might not be the case.*[338] *However, there is also evidence that statin use in older people contributes to increases in falls, myopathy (muscle disease), myalgias (muscle pain), muscle weakness, back conditions, injuries, and arthropathies (joint diseases) and overall mortality.*[339]

People who exercise, have balanced diets and are of normal weight are less likely to have abnormal cholesterol levels. Furthermore, they are less likely to die early compared with people at the same cholesterol level who do not exercise.[340 341]

Insurance companies use sophisticated statistical models to predict the likelihood of death. These models go by many names including 'Cox Proportional Hazards Model' and a variety of 'Parametric Proportional Hazards' models. Most readers will not be interested in the details. We just want people to know that scientists who work on the problem of predicting lifespan have access to several models that produce reasonable predictions, as mortality data demonstrate. However, such predictions are not perfect; alterations in behavior can change them.

Other Reasons for Screening

There are other possibly valuable screening tests (see FIGURE 1.47.1 for examples).

The ones that require a visit to the doctor include the formal assessment of possible diabetes as well as other organ damage (usually through blood testing), the cholesterol we already mentioned, imaging to detect breast and prostate cancer, signal analysis to detect and diagnose heart, brain and muscle problems

334 Davidson, K. W., Reddy, S. S., McGrath, P., & Zitner, D. (1996). Is there an association among low untreated serum lipid levels, anger, and hazardous driving? International Journal of Behavioral Medicine, 3(4), 321-336. https://link.springer.com/article/10.1207/s15327558ijbm0304_3. Accessed Sept. 8, 2023.

335 Davidson, K. W., Reddy, S. S., McGrath, P. J., Zitner, D., & MacKeen, W. (1996). Increases in depression after cholesterol-lowering drug treatment. Behavioral Medicine, 22(2), 82-84. https://scholars.cmich.edu/en/publications/increases-in-depression-after-cholesterol-lowering-drug-treatment. Accessed Sept. 8, 2023.

336 Moyer, M.W., Medication: Cholesterol Drugs and Memory: Why Cholesterol Drugs Might Affect Memory Scientific American: Mind, September 1, 2010. http://www.scientificamerican.com/article/its-not-dementia-its-your-heart-medication/. Accessed July 19, 2022.

337 West R, Beeri MS, Schmeidler J, Hannigan CM, Angelo G, Grossman HT, Rosendorff C, Silverman JM. Better memory functioning associated with higher total and low-density lipoprotein cholesterol levels in very elderly subjects without the apolipoprotein e4 allele. Am. J. Geriatr. Psychiatry. 2008; 16:781–785. https://pubmed.ncbi.nlm.nih.gov/18757771/. Accessed August 3, 2022.

338 Samaras K, Makkar SR, Crawford JD, et al. Effects of Statins on Memory, Cognition, and Brain Volume in the Elderly. J Am Coll Cardiol 2019; 74:2554-2568. https://www.acc.org/latest-in-cardiology/journal-scans/2019/11/19/14/05/effects-of-statins-on-memory-cognition. Accessed July 19, 2022.

339 Curfman G. Risks of Statin Therapy in Older Adults. JAMA Intern Med. 2017;177(7):966. doi:10.1001/jamainternmed.2017.1457. https://jamanetwork.com/journals/jamainternalmedicine/fullarticle/2628968. Accessed July 19, 2022.

340 Rosenthal RL. Effectiveness of altering serum cholesterol levels without drugs. Proceedings (Baylor University Medical Center). 2000;13(4):351-355. http://www.ncbi.nlm.nih.gov/pmc/articles/PMC1312230/. Accessed July 19, 2022.

341 Warburton DER, Nicol CW, Bredin SSD. Health benefits of physical activity: the evidence. CMAJ: Canadian Medical Association Journal. 2006;174(6):801-809. doi:10.1503/cmaj.051351. http://www.ncbi.nlm.nih.gov/pmc/articles/PMC1402378/. Accessed July 19, 2022.

and examinations to detect colon and rectal cancers. These are relatively common disorders and, if detected early, it may be possible to eliminate or mitigate their impacts. However, we must recognize that epidemiologists (who study the health and impacts of interventions on populations) often periodically reconsider the value of screening. They try to assess if, how often and which tests are useful, and what the effects on people's lives are of screening for prostate, breast and colon cancer. The reason is that, today, using our existing testing methods and the criteria for evaluating results, these exams lead to large numbers of false positives and unnecessary or questionable follow-up interventions. We are back to the issue of false positive and false negative test results. Existing tests produce large numbers of false alarms and false reassurance!

It is worthwhile or even essential to do screening:

- *If a serious disease is spreading in a population.*
- *If required for employment, insurance, license or certification purposes.*
- *If physicians are unable to determine a diagnosis.*
- *If a patient or a parent are aware of a family history of a problem that might be intervened on early.*
- *If a patient is excessively worried about health status and does not mind that a false alarm might cause further unnecessary worry. (Added with tongue placed firmly in cheek!)*

FIGURE 1.47.1 Good reasons for screening

THE SAD STORY OF A MOM

A recent article in the Washington Post provides an excellent example of a false positive result and its untoward effects.

A woman ate a poppyseed bagel before giving birth to her child. A blood test just before her child was born indicated that she was on opiates – a finding that had to be reported to the authorities. She even told the doctor that she had eaten the bagel, as she was aware of the possibility of mistaken detection of a controlled substance. Poppyseeds cause the test for opiates to falsely indicate the presence of an opiate and she knew it.

Her 3-day-old child was taken away from her and spent 5 days in a foster home until the truth was discovered. This has happened many times and is a well-known problem. The hospital eventually awarded our mom over $140,000 but the experience was traumatic.

We sincerely hope that she did not name her child 'Poppy'!

The good news is that some screening can be done at home and without professional involvement. Urine test strips are commercially available and inexpensive. Other types of strips for testing urine can give a basic assessment of protein, bilirubin (a biproduct of the liver), blood cells or other substances in the urine. Of course, it would be wise to see a professional if self-screening raises any concerns.

We have mentioned other screening tests that do not require a doctor. Checking one's pulse rate, body weight and blood pressure is easy and smart. If anything gets out of hand, that also may be a reason to follow up with a professional.

What People Should Consider Before Enrolling for Screening-Tests

Health care is always a social transaction and economic transaction. In North America, patients, insurers, government or employers pay care professionals for their services. Laboratory technicians and companies provide services to generate an income. Drug companies need consumers – patients – for their own economic survival. Though we generally recognize that health workers are motivated by their professional achievements in providing care, it is realistic to also recognize that financial incentives are also at play.

These incentives, both professional achievements and financial rewards, are usually to do something rather than nothing. In other words, they dictate action. On the other hand, while healthcare workers pursue their professional exigencies, patients are only interested in remaining or getting healthy. They are not motivated to spend time and their hard-earned money to do things that waste time or money or that may harm them. Consequently, most people are or should be interested in avoiding unnecessary tests and procedures. The problem is that few people have the knowledge needed to evaluate critically which screening tests might be harmful and which might be helpful.

Cholesterol Screening: No Difference in All-Cause Mortality in People Treated or Not[342, 343, 344]

We will come back to cholesterol, as people with high cholesterol serve as an excellent example. Research informs us that they are more likely to develop heart attacks and strokes. For some people, the increased risk of heart attack or stroke is very small because they lack other risk factors. Therefore, treating these patients with cholesterol-lowering drugs, given that they are at minimum or no risk of heart disease or stroke, exposes them to the risk of other problems without the promise of meaningful benefit. It is sort of like buying flight insurance that pays out if you are killed in a crash. For 99.9999% (in the US, about 1 billion fly per year and fewer than 1,000 die in crashes: 0.0001%) of flyers, which is a waste of money, except if it covers delay, cancellation or rescheduling of flights or loss of baggage... that is a much more common 'disease'!

Remember that high cholesterol is not a disease but rather a risk factor for other problems. We have pointed out elsewhere that the makers of Lipitor (a 'statin' – a cholesterol-lowering drug) themselves report that 5 years of treating 100 people with – note – risk factors, avoids one heart attack or stroke. In the case of these 100 high-risk patients, if they were untreated, 3 would have a heart attack or stroke. If they are treated, though, 2 would have a heart attack or stroke. There is, sure, a 33% reduction in risk, but only 1 person in 100 experiences a benefit. The 'relative risk reduction' is 33% (1/3 fewer people on Lipitor have a heart attack or stroke). However, there is only 1 fewer heart attack or stroke. So, only 1 person in 100 (1%) actually benefits! This in the face of the fact that many more people will have adverse effects of the medication, including muscle problems and diabetes.[345]

This raises questions regarding the screening for and treatment of elevated cholesterol. By screening, we may be detecting a problem that is not there. With the exception of very

342 The NNT.Com citing the following: Taylor F, Huffman MD, Macedo AF, et al. Statins for the primary prevention of cardiovascular disease. Cochrane Database Syst Rev. 2013 Jan 31;1:CD004816. http://www.thennt.com/nnt/statins-for-heart-disease-prevention-without-prior-heart-disease/. Accessed July 19, 2022.

343 Thavendiranathan P. Primary prevention of cardiovascular disease with statin therapy. Arch Int Med. 2006; 166: 2307-13. https://www.thelancet.com/journals/lancet/article/PIIS0140-6736(05)67394-1/fulltext. Accessed July 19, 2022.

344 CTT Collaborators. Efficacy and safety of cholesterol-lowering treatment: prospective meta-analysis of data from 90 056 participants in 14 randomised trials of statins. Lancet. 2005; 366: 1267-1278. https://www.thelancet.com/journals/lancet/article/PIIS0140-6736(05)67394-1/fulltext. Accessed July 19, 2022.

345 The Number Needed to Treat Mizuno K, Ray KK, Ford I. Statins and risk of incident diabetes: a collaborative meta-analysis of randomised statin trials. Lancet. 2010 Feb 27;375(9716):735-42. Epub 2010 Feb 16. PubMed PMID: 20167359. http://www.thennt.com/nnt/statins-for-heart-disease-prevention-without-prior-heart-disease/. Accessed July 19, 2022.

elevated cholesterol, there may be no point in treating it. Furthermore, evidence of very high cholesterol is often obvious on physical exam or through patients' complaints. If those cases are tested, the likelihood of detecting the problem is much increased – it isn't a rare disease among that group. Unfortunately, many are tested, people with less than significant problems are treated and even those few with risk factors benefit! What the heck! Oh, and the pharm companies get rich on those afraid they might buy the farm. Now we get it! It's not medicine; it's economics!

BMJ Suggests No Reduction in Overall Likelihood of Dying

The relative reduction in risk from the use of lipid- (cholesterol-) lowering drugs is, as we have said, about 33%. If people are not likely to have heart attacks because they are fit, not overweight, non-smokers and no have family history of either stroke or heart disease, then the number who benefit is very small. An article in the British Medical Journal[346] (BMJ) suggests that treating people taking cholesterol-lowering drugs for 5-7 years reduces death from heart disease but not death from all causes. Meaning that people on cholesterol lowering drugs had an increased risk of death from non-cardiac conditions. Because lifestyle and behavior contribute to the risk of certain conditions, check-ups normally include questions about them. That is the useful screening!

Then There is Colon Cancer

It is worth touching on colon cancer again. Many conditions that might otherwise cause serious problems, when detected early and treated early, become a minor inconvenience.

Colon screening by colonoscopy is definitely recommended for people at high risk (for example, having a family history of colon cancer, inflammatory bowel disease, having observed bleeding from the bowel or having a history of polyps). Some doctors advocate colon screening as a routine but, as with other tests, it seems best reserved for those who would most likely benefit. For people who do not have risk factors "*USPSTF recommends screening for colorectal cancer (CRC) using fecal occult blood testing, sigmoidoscopy, or colonoscopy, in adults, beginning at age 50 years and continuing until age 75 years.*"

A September 2010 study in the Canadian Medical Association Journal states that colonoscopy every 10 years or a yearly stool test to check for blood in the feces seems to save lives. That is not exactly a great yield. Some have pointed out that screening is not without risks. When colonoscopies are done without a biopsy, serious complications (caused by bowel perforation from the colonoscope) occur in about 1 in 1,000 colonoscopies; with a biopsy, serious complications occur in about 7 cases per 1,000. In one study of approximately 16,000 patients having colonoscopy, 10 died as a result.[347] Colonoscopy for screening is worthwhile if you are in a high-risk group. However, for people at low risk, it might be better to wait.

Other Examples: Prostate and Breast Cancer

Sometimes, conditions have a frightening label, like 'prostate cancer', but they are not so serious and early intervention might be worse than the problem. Many prostate

346 M. Pignone, C. Phillips, C., Mulrow, Use of lipid lowering drugs for primary prevention of coronary heart disease: meta-analysis of randomised trials, BMJ October 21, 2000; 321: 983. http://www.bmj.com/content/321/7267/983.abstract?sid=d1f24689-e7ef-432c-9217-9faeebd2d8ea. Accessed July 19, 2022.

347 Levin, T. et. el., Complications of Colonoscopy in an Integrated Health Care System, Annals of Internal Medicine, December 19, 2006 vol. 145 no. 12 880-886. http://www.annals.org/content/145/12/880.short. Accessed July 19, 2022.

cancers grow very slowly and do not present a person with more than minor inconvenience. Furthermore, they do not usually result in death. Asymptomatic people who enroll for prostate screening should know the chances they might have prostate cancer, should know how many people have been treated in the near past and must know how they fared.

Screening for early disease, as we have shown, is not without risks. Danger lurks because some tests produce false alarms leading to unnecessary fear and harmful and unnecessary treatment.

Prostate cancer and breast cancer (see below) are two conditions where screening has become contentious. Whom should we screen and when? If we examine these conditions, we can understand the important principles that we must apply when considering screening for ourselves or becoming involved in the development of a screening program.

Controversies in Screening for Prostate Cancer

Let's start with prostate cancer screening. Recently the United States Preventive Services Task Force (USPSTF)[348] [349] reaffirmed that there is little evidence that routine prostate screening has value. It further stated that there is some evidence that it does harm. Consequently, they do not recommend routine prostate specific antigen (PSA) screening for this cancer.[350]

The American Cancer Society and USPSTF (see also the A and B recommendations[351]) do recognize that prostate cancer is the most common cancer in men. However, a 2008 report by them determined "*The USPSTF concludes that the current evidence is insufficient to assess the balance of benefits and harms of prostate cancer screening in men younger than age 75-years. The USPSTF found convincing evidence that treatment for prostate cancer detected by screening causes moderate-to-substantial harms, such as erectile dysfunction, urinary incontinence, bowel dysfunction, and death. These harms are especially important because some men with prostate cancer who are treated would never have developed symptoms related to cancer during their lifetime.*"

We do know that men who have symptoms of prostate disease including frequent urination, waking up to urinate through the night or discomfort, must see their doctor and they should consider a test for prostate disease to help explain the symptoms. Men at higher risk, including those with a family history of prostate disease, are more likely to benefit from prostate screening because they are more likely to have an abnormality that should treated. This makes it important for all mature men to at least discuss the issue with their doctors. The important point is that it only makes sense to consider prostate testing if these conditions exist – otherwise it is like looking for the rare disease we previously considered, and the testing is not highly specific or sensitive. Screening just in case will yield many false positives and negatives.

Controversies in Breast Cancer Screening

The USPSTF recommends "biennial screening mammography for women aged 50 to 74 years." Women at higher risk, for example because of family history, should start earlier. If an imaging study indicates a possible problem, the next step is to surgically remove a piece of the suspicious area (termed a 'biopsy') The risk of excessive screening is that people will have unnecessary biopsies and receive unnecessary treatment of false positive results, which mistakenly suggests

348 http://www.uspreventiveservicestaskforce.org/. Accessed July 19, 2022.

349 http://www.uspreventiveservicestaskforce.org/uspstf/uspsprca.htm. Accessed July 19, 2022.

350 http://www.uspreventiveservicestaskforce.org/uspstf12/prostate/draftrecprostate.htm. Accessed July 19, 2022.

351 http://www.uspreventiveservicestaskforce.org/uspstf/uspsabrecs.htm. Accessed July 19, 2022.

having the condition. This, in turn, may be followed up with further surgery or other treatment. However, an article in the September 23, 2010 issue of the New England Journal of Medicine reported that mammography screening, in association with a well-developed healthcare system, produces only a modest reduction in deaths from breast cancer. A Journal of Medical Screening report in 2001 suggested that for every 781 women screened, one death from breast cancer was avoided.[352] Of course, unnecessary treatment does no good whatever.

Of course, every woman with breast problems, including a lump, discomfort, change in skin tone, skin induration (thickening) or nipple discharge should see a physician to discuss a diagnostic mammogram (breast imaging). Again, this is a person with objective reasons for testing; it is not screening.

BREAST CANCER SCREENING – A PERSONAL EXPERIENCE

CT, the late spouse of DC, was a diagnostic radiologist who specialized in Mammography and Ultrasound. For many years she debated with confreres and backers of early breast cancer screening, noting the very poor yield in terms of cancer detection versus numerous false positives. At times, this debate became a bit 'edgy', as there was almost propagandistic publicity and personal involvement among promoters of screening. On reaching age 50 (incidentally also called age 35), CT had her own mammogram and, sure enough, it suggested a biopsy that, based on her experience, she believed was unwarranted, as she had relatively dense breasts. Being a good camper, however, she submitted to the procedure and the tissue proved to not be cancerous. She found the procedure painful and, more than anything, infuriating – with herself for following through. That was the last time for screening in her life. She died over 20 years later of unrelated causes.

Screening for the Elderly

How to investigate and treat elderly people has become a contentious issue. Sometimes, children are asked to make choices for aging parents but lack a framework for choice and are forced to make decisions based on intuition alone. Often, they and other relatives don't even know which questions to ask and they are often unsure about what the answers they get mean. Doctors, who are naturally motivated to help people, may also lack a useful framework for deciding why and when to test and treat elderly people. Finally, older people themselves rarely have a framework to guide their own medical choices.

The key is to think things through before starting down the screening pathway. The problem is that one can get bogged down pretty quickly. The worst is in the case of screening where there are no initial symptoms, findings or family history. Then one is searching for a problem that may not be there and the possibly turning up false positives. A wag defined a mathematician as a blind person searching in a dark room for a black cat that isn't there. Well, it may be that the test reveals something fuzzy that isn't a cat!

However, for the elderly, especially the very elderly, there is another problem. It may be that there isn't anything that can or should be done even if a real problem might be there.

We told the story elsewhere about a patient discovered to have a small kidney cancer. The treatment in this case is surgery, called a 'nephrectomy' (the removal of the kidney). We know that every patient who has surgery has an immediate postoperative reduction in comfort and function and that the average postoperative time in hospital after a nephrectomy was 11 days.[353] In other words, this patient was almost

352 Beral V, Alexander M, Duffy S, et al. The number of women who would need to be screened regularly by mammography to prevent one death from breast cancer. J Med Screen. 2011;18(4):210-212. doi:10.1258/jms.2011.011134. https://www.ncbi.nlm.nih.gov/pmc/articles/PMC3266234/. Accessed July 19, 2022.

353 Arnaud Mejean, Benoit Vogt, Jean Emile Quazza, Yves Chretien, Bertrand Dufour. Mortality and Morbidity after Nephrectomy for Renal Cell Carcinoma Using a Transperitoneal Anterior Subcostal Incision, European Urology, v.34, 4, 1999. https://pubmed.ncbi.nlm.nih.gov/10473988/. Accessed August 3, 2022.

guaranteed to be worse off in terms of comfort and function after surgery, and the likelihood of benefit was unknown and at best very small. We also know that older people, even if they are healthy, are less resilient and more likely to be harmed and suffer from traumatic events from such a procedure. This patient did not do well, dying soon after.

An elderly person or a responsible caretaker, in order to decide whether a treatment is worthwhile or not, should consider if the treatment will enable their being able to do more, feel better or live longer than without the treatment or using less invasive alternatives. The important questions to consider include:

- What is the best result that one can hope for, with and without intervention?
- What's the worst result that might avail? And do not forget psychological impacts.
- What are the harms usually associated with the treatment?
- What are the chances of the various outcomes?
- Usually there is a lot that modern medicine can do to improve comfort while avoiding the bad stuff, but is this likely to be the case with an elderly person?
- If the person is not fully cognitively capable, what would the person have likely wanted when so?

Sometimes, we get tests because we are afraid of a condition where late detection would lead to serious consequences and early detection would be at most an inconvenience. However, how does this apply to a person nearing the end of their natural life?

Screening the elderly is fraught with problems and needs to be engaged seldom and with serious consideration of the consequences. We cannot allow our own curiosity, fear of death or youthful sense of immortality drive decisions when we or our family members are of advanced years.

How Behavior Influences Your Health

Certain personal behaviors influence the decision regarding screening, as they increase the likelihood of becoming sick. We have again and again reiterated health-affecting lifestyle factors including diet, exercise, sexual habits, smoking, family history and even how food is prepared (e.g., by barbecuing). Considering these has properly become an important part of making the decision about how to proceed.

If there is a negative factor, it helps justify the decision to screen. Those with genetic dispositions to certain diseases may be able to avoid or mitigate the effects of those diseases by modifying other factors that contribute to illness.[354] What one eats and drinks are of particular importance as "*Most carcinogens that are ingested, such as nitrates, nitrosamines, pesticides, and dioxins, come from food or food additives or from cooking.*" [355] However, obesity, infections, radiation and environmental pollutants also damage our bodies.

For those of us who experience factors like these, screening has also the potential of providing false reassurance that we are and will

354 Anand P, Kunnumakkara AB, Sundaram C, Harikumar KB, Tharakan ST, Lai OS, Sung B, Aggarwal BB. Cancer is a preventable disease that requires major lifestyle changes. Pharm Res. 2008 Sep;25(9):2097-116. Doi: 10.1007/s11095-008-9661-9. Epub. 2008 Jul 15. Erratum in: Pharm Res. 2008 Sep;25(9):2200. Kunnumakkara, Ajaikumar B [corrected to Kunnumakkara, Ajaikumar B]. PMID: 18626751; PMCID: PMC2515569. http://www.ncbi.nlm.nih.gov/pmc/articles/PMC2515569/. Accessed July 19, 2022.

355 Anand P, Kunnumakkara AB, Sundaram C, Harikumar KB, Tharakan ST, Lai OS, Sung B, Aggarwal BB. Cancer is a preventable disease that requires major lifestyle changes. Pharm Res. 2008 Sep;25(9):2097-116. doi: 10.1007/s11095-008-9661-9. Epub 2008 Jul 15. Erratum in: Pharm Res. 2008 Sep;25(9):2200. Kunnumakkara, Ajaikumar B [corrected to Kunnumakkara, Ajaikumar B]. PMID: 18626751; PMCID: PMC2515569. http://www.ncbi.nlm.nih.gov/pmc/articles/PMC2515569/. Accessed July 19, 2022.

remain ok despite them. People with seemingly minor problems can go on to unnecessary suffering because the false negative led them to avoid finding a resolution to the problem.

Screening and the annual regular "check-up" have become big business in North American. Health boutiques provide regular checkups to senior executives who regard these checkups as a benefit of employment. Some law firms have contracted with testing firms to provide routine check-ups as a benefit of partnership and people use this benefit whether or not they are at high risk of illness. People at low risk are subjecting themselves to a serious risk of false alarms. And in some jurisdictions, it is a taxable benefit.

Screen Yourself

We have recommended 'self-screening', an easy, inexpensive and routine process. Everybody can monitor their own health and recognize without a doctor or a laboratory what to do to preserve their comfort and energy and to reduce the likelihood of the common diseases that plague North Americans.

So, people can safely do their own screening. We can learn to check our heart rates – the pulse you feel in your wrist – a lower resting heart rate usually signaling health and being associated with a longer lifespan. A recent, study in the Canadian Medical Association Journal reported that grip strength is a simple measure of overall muscle strength; a stronger grip is also associated with a longer life and fewer early deaths from any cause. Other simple measures we mentioned earlier. Anyone can discuss with their own doctor what they should aim for in terms of muscle strength, weight, waist size and resting pulse rate and then they can monitor and maintain their own health.

Other tools to monitor health and find disease before much damage is done need periodic collaboration and discussion with a health professional because they require blood tests, x-rays or other analyses that may only be done by a health professional.

The FIGURE 1.47.2 below shows the 10 most common causes of death in Canada in all age groups according to Statistics Canada.[356]

Personal health habits are known to influence each of these causes. This suggests that people who have healthy personal habits, who don't smoke, who eat well and who undertake regular exercise can delay the discomfort, disability and death that eventually afflicts each of us.

	Rank	Number	%
Total, all causes of death		**284,082**	**100.0**
Cancer	1	80,152	28.2
Diseases of heart	2	52,541	18.5
Accidents (unintentional injuries)	3	13,746	4.8
Cerebrovascular diseases	4	13,660	4.8
Chronic lower respiratory diseases	5	12,823	4.5
Diabetes mellitus	6	6,912	2.4
Influenza and pneumonia	7	6,893	2.4
Alzheimer's disease	8	6,166	2.2
Suicide	9	4,012	1.4
Kidney diseases (Nephritis, nephrotic syndrome and nephrosis)	10	3,767	1.3
All other causes of death	-	83,410	29.4

Source(s): Table 13-10-0801-01.

FIGURE 1.47.2: Causes of death in Canada in 2019

A cursory look at the table stimulates several immediate thoughts on what people can do to avoid or delay these serious problems. Clearly, personal behaviors and where we live have important influences on each of the top 10 fatal diseases.[357] [358] For instance, there are lots of things a person can do to get cancer. These include smoking, using lots of alcohol,

356 Leading Causes of Death for Both Sexes, Statistics Canada, 2019. https://www150.statcan.gc.ca/n1/daily-quotidien/201126/t001b-eng.htm. Accessed August 24, 2022.

357 Armstrong, B.K. THE Epidemiology and Prevention of Cancer in Australia, Ausf. N.Z J. Surg. 1988,58, 179-187. http://onlinelibrary.wiley.com/doi/10.1111/j.1445-2197.1988.tb01035.x/pdf. Accessed July 19, 2022.

358 Anand P, Kunnumakkara AB, Sundaram C, Harikumar KB, Tharakan ST, Lai OS, Sung B, Aggarwal BB. Cancer is a preventable disease that requires major lifestyle changes. Pharm Res. 2008 Sep;25(9):2097-116. http://www.ncbi.nlm.nih.gov/pmc/articles/PMC2515569. Accessed July 19, 2022.

living or working in a polluted environment, living a sedentary lifestyle, eating too much food or eating food that contains carcinogenic substances such as lots of red meat, especially if it is barbecued or contains nitrates or nitrites.

Some other examples of the relationships of these with problems, include alcohol, which can cause diseases of the liver, pancreas, mouth and breast. Poor diet can cause colorectal cancer related to additives and barbecuing. Obesity can cause diseases of the colon, breast, endometrium, kidneys, stomach, pancreas, gall bladder and liver. Infections, environmental pollutants and radiation can have similar effects. (See Anand reference for more detail).

CANCER AS A PREVENTABLE DISEASE

Preetha Anand, Ajaikumar B. Kunnumakkara, et al. in their article "Cancer is a Preventable Disease that Requires Major Lifestyle Changes" in 2008 stated: "This year, more than 1 million Americans and more than 10 million people worldwide are expected to be diagnosed with cancer, a disease commonly believed to be preventable. Only 5–10% of all cancer cases can be attributed to genetic defects, whereas the remaining 90–95% have their roots in the environment and lifestyle. The lifestyle factors include cigarette smoking, diet (fried foods, red meat), alcohol, sun exposure, environmental pollutants, infections, stress, obesity, and physical inactivity. The evidence indicates that of all cancer-related deaths, almost 25–30% are due to tobacco, as many as 30–35% are linked to diet, about 15–20% are due to infections, and the remaining percentage are due to other factors like radiation, stress, physical activity, environmental pollutants etc. Therefore, cancer prevention requires smoking cessation, increased ingestion of fruits and vegetables, moderate use of alcohol, caloric restriction, exercise, avoidance of direct exposure to sunlight, minimal meat consumption, use of whole grains, use of vaccinations, and regular check-ups. In this review, we present evidence that inflammation is the link between the agents/factors that cause cancer and the agents that prevent it. In addition, we provide evidence that cancer is a preventable disease that requires major lifestyle changes." [359]

Lifestyle Diseases, Affluenza: Diseases of Choice.

Communities strive for affluence not sickness, yet, as societies become increasingly wealthy, they suffer from increases in major disease like diabetes, heart disease[360] and cancer[361]. These are diseases that seem to be linked to changes in how people behave and eat as their wealth increases. So, both affluence and poverty are risk factors for some medical conditions. That is counter-intuitive but true! The fact is that "*Obesity increases the risk of cancers in the (throat) esophagus, bowel (colorectal), breast, endometrium (lining of the uterus), and kidney. Alcohol causes cancers of the oral cavity, pharynx, larynx, esophagus, and liver, and causes a small increase in the risk of breast cancer.*" [362] It seems

359 Anand P, Kunnumakkara AB, Sundaram C, Harikumar KB, Tharakan ST, Lai OS, Sung B, Aggarwal BB. Cancer is a preventable disease that requires major lifestyle changes. Pharm Res. 2008 Sep;25(9):2097-116. http://www.ncbi.nlm.nih.gov/pmc/articles/PMC2515569/. Accessed July 19, 2022.

360 Lee DS, Chiu M, Manuel DG, Tu K, Wang X, Austin PC, Mattern MY, Mitiku TF, Svenson LW, Putnam W, Flanagan WM, Tu JV. Canadian Cardiovascular Outcomes Research Team. Trends in risk factors for cardiovascular disease in Canada: temporal, socio-demographic and geographic factors. CMAJ. 2009 Aug 4;181(3-4): E55-66. Epub 2009 Jul 20. PubMed PMID: 19620271; PubMed Central PMCID: PMC2717674. http://www.cmaj.ca/cgi/content/full/181/3-4/E55?maxtoshow=&hits=10&RESULTFORMAT=1&author1=Lee%2C+ds&andorexacttitle=and&andorexacttitleabs=and&andorexactfulltext=and&searchid=1&FIRSTINDEX=0&sortspec=date&resourcetype=HWCIT,HWELTR. Accessed July 19, 2022.

361 Key TJ, Allen NE, Spencer EA, Travis RC. The effect of diet on risk of cancer. Lancet. 2002 Sep 14;360(9336):861-8. Review. PubMed PMID: 12243933. http://www.chiroonline.net/_fileCabinet/cancerdiet.pdf. Accessed July 19, 2022.

362 Key TJ, Allen NE, Spencer EA, Travis RC. The effect of diet on risk of cancer.
Lancet. 2002 Sep 14;360(9336):861-8. Review. PubMed PMID: 12243933. http://www.chiroonline.net/_fileCabinet/cancerdiet.pdf. Accessed July 19, 2022.

that we put our money not just into our pockets but also into our mouths!

People who rarely exercise, over-eat and become overweight are much more likely to limit both the length and their enjoyment of life. This is not only because activities of daily living become tiresome for people who aren't fit, but also because people who are not fit are more likely to develop these diseases. It is a paradox, however, that the poorest communities also seem to suffer from an increased number of diseases related to their poor diets and obesity. This may be because poor people have less access to recreational activities and seem to have less knowledge about nutritious eating. In North America, some types of sickness increase with the wealth of the community, although poor North Americans are more likely to have shorter and less healthy lives "*Logistic regression models showed that higher wealth index was associated with higher prevalence of hypertension, hyperlipidemia, and allergy, while lower wealth index was associated with higher prevalence of rheumatism/arthritis.*[363] Some believe that poor people have shorter and less healthy lives because they receive different health care and are investigated differently.[364]

On the other hand, healthy people function better and therefore are more likely to do work that generates wealth and become richer[365] so it is difficult to know if increased wealth predisposes to improved health, or if better health enables you to become wealthier, or some combination of both factors.

363 Vuković D, Bjegović V, Vuković G. Prevalence of chronic diseases according to socioeconomic status measured by wealth index: health survey in Serbia. Croat Med J. 2008 Dec;49(6):832-41. https://pubmed.ncbi.nlm.nih.gov/19090609/. Accessed August 26, 2022.

364 Sheldon M. Singh, L.F. Paszat, C. Li, J. He, C. Vinden, and L. Rabeneck Association of socioeconomic status and receipt of colorectal cancer investigations: a population-based retrospective cohort study.

365 Health and Wealth Issues-The Health and Wealth of Nations, Bloom and Canning http://www3.pids.gov.ph/popn_pub/full_papers/DBloomCanning.pdf. Accessed July 19, 2022.

VOLUME 1

Section 8

IN CLOSING

We have arrived at our destination! Is it fateful that this is 'Section 8'? Isn't that what Klinger was always bucking for in MASH? Therefore, a therapist joke would seem highly relevant.

There was a man who was unable to sleep because he believed that there was a monster under his bed, and he had to do something about it, as he was exhausted! He decided to go to a therapist to try to address the problem.

The therapist said that she could help, but that it was a serious problem, might take a year to address, and the fees would probably be about $20,000 – steep but worth it.

The man decided to go get a drink and think over how to proceed.

About a year later, the man ran into the therapist when out walking. The therapist was surprised to see him and asked why he hadn't come to see her.

The man told the therapist that he had solved the problem with the help of the bartender on that first night after they had met and had since used the money he saved to buy a new truck. When he said that, the therapist expressed surprise and disdainfully asked him about the obviously inexpert advice of a bartender.

The man responded that the bartender suggested just cutting the legs off his bed so there'd be no room for the monster! Sure enough, it worked!

Based (loosely) on: https://news.amomama.com/199658-daily-joke-a-man-goes-a-psychiatrist-bec.html. Accessed August 26, 2022.

Chapter 48: Final Comments and Summary

We hope that you have found this book to be interesting and full of ideas that make health, health care and related matters both clear and actionable.

We have focused on physical medicine and presented the crucial concepts underlying clinical care. This is a summary of the most important concepts we addressed.

This material is crucial as patients, clinicians and others associated with health care must understand it to be able to meaningfully participate in, work with or deal with the professionals, information and processes of health care. The concepts we told you about embody the essence of clinical practice. Understanding them enables those who absorb them to comprehend and critically assess clinical activities and to contribute to their and others' knowledge about clinical care.

However, we can go a step further by noting that someone armed with these concepts and having access to the full range of health information available on the Internet, will be able to understand and solve many clinical problems and evaluate proposed treatments they or their families may encounter.

Let's review them.

The Purposes of Health Care and Medical Visits

People visit doctors for only four reasons. They want to (1) feel better, and/or (2) be able to do more, and\or (3) be able to live longer, and/or (4) to learn about their own health. In the latter case, they may wish to get recommendations on how to maintain and improve their health, or to address some administrative purpose, such as getting a doctor's note for insurance, for absences from work, for having missed school, or for immigration or travel documentation.

At every visit, doctors collect information about a patient's comfort and function and may do laboratory investigations to get an estimate of how sick a person is and what their likely longevity is. Based on this information they may intervene if a patient is sick. Health informaticians (professionals who specialize in the creation, management, analysis and use of medical information) and researchers use information management techniques to learn if people are better or worse off after treatment or which types and groups of patients are most likely to benefit or be harmed, feeding this back into clinical care process.

Knowing the purposes of care enables participation in or assessment of the actions of healthcare teams. This enables answers to important questions. For example: Do the processes and interventions help patients feel better, do more, or live longer? What are the trade-off patients are prepared to make, such as preferring to avoid cancer chemotherapy because they might prefer a more comfortable life, even if it means shorter survival? When patients are clear about what they expect in terms of changes in comfort, function or life expectancy, clinical teams can design interventions that address patients' personal goals.

Measuring Health

Over the years, experts have developed measures of health. These measures, together with information about a patient's comfort, function, laboratory and imaging findings, help evaluate health status and point to appropriate treatment.

Clinicians, during a visit use these measures, which include qualitative and quantitative information, including symptoms (what a person feels), signs (objective measures from observing a patient or doing tests such as knee reflexes or walking speed) and findings (results from laboratory tests and diagnostic imaging), along with information about an individual's surroundings, to estimate a person's current and future health and the likelihood an intervention will succeed.

There are many health rating scales. 'Measuring Health' by Ian McDowell provides a timeless guide to rating scales and questionnaires that includes some of the many formal systems clinicians use to measure comfort, function and longevity. Knowing how to measure health enables experts on healthcare teams to evaluate the outcomes of care for individual patients. It also supports clinicians and researchers in developing and using information systems to evaluate clinical care.

Outcomes of care are measured by considering the qualitative and quantitative descriptions of patients before, during and after interventions and using that information to link clinical care to results.

Making a Diagnosis

A diagnosis is an explanation or interpretation of the cause of a problem. Most problems have many possible diagnoses or interpretations. For example, there are at least 3,000 possible diagnoses associated with fatigue. The challenge for clinicians is to develop strategies that enable them to recognize not only common causes for a condition but also rare ones. About 10% of patients have a rare affliction – often ones that are not top of mind for clinicians.

Clinicians must use many techniques to make sure that they have considered all possible causes of a problem before giving up the search. Easily accessible information sources indicate the possible causes of any problem, the additional information necessary to confirm or disprove a diagnosis, and the most effective strategies, questions, examinations and laboratory findings, to pinpoint the correct diagnosis.

DXplain is a medical information system that can help a physician determine the cause (a diagnosis) of a patient's symptoms and findings. Professors use it to teach students about diseases and the strategies they can use to make a diagnosis. DXplain, developed by Dr. Octo Barnett at Massachusetts General Hospital (now part of Mass General Brigham), is only available to credentialed professionals. A simpler one, Symptomate (https://symptomate.com/), can be tried online.

Anyone, including patients, who know what diagnosis is about, can cooperate with a healthcare team to produce more complete lists of possible causes of patient problems and help to identify the information necessary to confirm or refute a diagnosis. This is especially important when reaching a diagnostic conclusion proves challenging. Patients who work with their healthcare team will feel more confident about abiding medical advice and will recognize when advice might not be appropriate for what they desire or will work in their circumstances.

Evaluating the Usefulness of Tests – False Reassurance, False Alarms, Early Detection and Screening

Physical examination and findings from laboratory tests and medical images produce signals indicating a person's health. Usually, these signals are easy to interpret and suggest a particular health condition or diagnosis. However, occasionally, test results provide false reassurance or incorrectly suggest the presence of a condition that the patient does not have.

False alarms in health care are similar to false alarms for detecting fire: there may be smoke and no fire. False alarms cause needless anxiety and might also produce harm. Just as a fire truck responding to a false fire alarm can be involved in an accident, so a patient can suffer harm when a doctor follows up on a false medical test result alarm. For example, a doctor performing colonoscopy to examine the bowel to follow up on a positive result of stool test (showing blood, a sign of possible colon cancer), might perforate the bowel. Not a good thing if the patient has no disease!

Similarly, men who have a false positive PSA test result for prostate cancer may receive unnecessary and invasive further investigation and intervention, leading to their becoming impotent or incontinent, when the prostate cancer itself would not have harmed them. This is because some prostate cancers grow slowly and will not alter the patient's life expectancy, comfort or function.

The chances of false reassurance or false alarms relate to the characteristics of the tests (sensitivity and specificity, discussed in detail in Section 7) and to the prevalence (frequency of occurrence) of the condition in the population tested. A smoke alarm is more likely to correctly signal for fire in an area with combustible materials. The same is true of a positive test result in people living in an area with a high prevalence of a disease. This means that evaluating the predictive value (accuracy) of a test, we must know not only the characteristics of the test, but also the frequency of the condition in the population being tested. For example, a positive test result for an uncommon disease is more likely to be a false alarm than a positive test for a common disease. The predictive value of a test is based on the prevalence (frequency of the condition in the community tested) of the condition, in addition to the test's sensitivity and specificity, as well as other factors, including the methodology used by the testing laboratory.

Based on all this, it is easy to understand why certain investigations suggesting the presence of an illness must be repeated to make sure the test result was meaningful, and why some tests must be followed with other tests that are more specific to an illness. It also makes clear the issues associated with disease screening, which sometimes tests for diseases unlikely for the person's age or situation.

Informaticians track the outcomes of people who have had positive or negative test results in order to produce information about the specificity and sensitivity of tests done by each laboratory.

Biomarkers

Biomarkers are objective (distinct and measurable) findings that provide information about health, illnesses and future health status. Publications have extensive lists of biomarkers and their meanings.

Drugs, both prescription and non-prescription, may also be markers or risk factors predicting the future health of a person. For example, cholesterol lowering drugs may be associated with increased risk of diabetes, and certain antidepressant medications may increase the risk of weight gain, fatigue, or reduced libido.

Issues in Treatment

NNT + NNH

Whenever patients accept treatment recommendations they are making a wager that an intervention is more likely to be helpful than harmful. Almost every treatment helps many people but also harms some.

The standard way of portraying the risk of an intervention, one hardly ever revealed to patients, is a description of The **Numbers Needed to Treat** and of **The Numbers Needed to Harm**. In other words, how many people must receive a treatment for, on average, one person to benefit (NNT), and how many people who receive a treatment for, on average, one person to be harmed (NNH)?

Relative Risk Reduction

Doctors and patients must also understand the difference between relative risk reduction and absolute risk reduction. Everyone has encountered advertisements claiming that a drug produces a 35% reduction in the risk of harm. Yet, few people understand what this means, and fewer yet understand how the 35% reduction in risk applies to their own circumstance.

One way to understand the difference between absolute and relative risk reduction, is to consider pedestrians crossing a street. People can cross at an intersection or they can jaywalk. The chance of a pedestrian being hit be a car is normally very low regardless of whether the person uses a crosswalk or jaywalks. However, in some cities, a person might be twice is likely to be hit when jaywalking. So, the relative risk reduction by using the crosswalk is 50%; a person is 50% less likely to be hit by a car there. However, this might mean that for every 100,000,000 crossings in crosswalks, vehicles will kill one person, while for every 100,000,000 people jaywalking, vehicles will kill two people. Based on these odds, most people would be unlikely to change their behavior. The lifetime risk of being killed as a pedestrian-car accident is quite low: https://www.tnklaw.com/blog-odds-dying-pedestrian-collision/.

Interventions and Consequences

Doctors may prescribe drugs, but at least a few people experience unintended, moderate to serious consequences. Therefore, measures of the effectiveness of treatments must include an estimate of how the treatment influences sickness or death from any cause, not just the condition the doctor is trying to treat. Consider a treatment to ablate a headache but induces drowsiness. This might or might not be worthwhile for a patient. Knee surgery that successfully cures a knee problem but is associated with a stroke or brain problems from the operation or anesthetic is not necessarily worthwhile.

Accordingly, in evaluating interventions it is important to measure the impact of the treatment on overall health, as well as on the targeted condition, and to have a reasonable estimate of how many people are likely to be helped or harmed.

The Art of Medicine

Some treatment recommendations are based on objective evidence (e.g., studies and statistics) showing how likely the intervention will benefit or harm a patient. Other treatment recommendations are based on the doctor's knowledge of Biology, Pharmacology and Physiology and represent a 'guesstimate' about which treatment will help. This represents the art of Medicine. Unfortunately, some equally knowledgeable, conscientious and caring clinicians might reach differing conclusions about which intervention is the best, leaving patients and care team members wondering how to resolve the differences in opinion. Reality is that not everything is known or 'computable.' The key is to keep track of what worked and didn't over large numbers of patients.

Another aspect of the art of Medicine is based on the recognition that patients are humans and have needs and feelings. The physician delivers on that by demonstrating listening, caring, empathy and other signs that support patients in their dealing with problems and facing realities.

Other Major Topics

It is challenging to touch on all of the major content of Volume 1 – only through reading it can one get all of the messages. Here, though, we mention a few of the other topics to give readers some idea of what awaits them when they decide to read Volume 1.

A major issue today, in addition to dealing with biologically based disease, is addressing what can be classed as a sociological disease: Misinformation Disease. Our world is polluted with ideas from misinformed or misogynist individuals who seek either profit or the opportunity to manipulate others. Our approach has been to provide a reasonably good description of what misinformation and disinformation are and how we can protect ourselves from them. We emphasize that the important tactics are to become knowledgeable, seek reliable sources and remain skeptical.

In addition to proffering information about health and health care, we have provided advice on how to go about learning about health. This can be challenging because those who provide care have their own vocabulary and may find it difficult to communicate using terms understandable by patients. Our overall advice regarding the information in these books is to focus on key ideas while leaving the details to when knowing them becomes important to the reader. Towards this objective, we have distinguished between 'Just in Case' learning, typical of how schools approach teaching – where detailed knowledge is jammed into learners' heads just in case they may need it. We have suggested, instead, 'Just in Time' learning, where crucial ideas are the initial focus and learning the details is addressed when people find that important in their own circumstances.

Throughout the text we have emphasized the importance of evidence: evidence of the various levels of the quality of the information we get. In Medicine, sometimes all that is available is the result of treating a small group of patients with a specific problem. Other times, researchers have done more formal studies that involved carefully selecting groups of patients and carefully intervening in controlled ways. Interventions not based on evidence of their effectiveness are just shots in the dark and one must rely on luck in terms of outcomes. We point out that the ultimate evidence is what are called systematic reviews (or meta-analyses). In this latter case, the results of many well structured and carefully executed (randomized and controlled) clinical trials with significant numbers of patients are examined, analyzed and their results combined to tell us what overall will work.

Throughout the text we mention Health Informatics, the discipline that focuses itself on improving health care and the health system, particularly through the use of information, formal processes and computer systems. One of the emphases in Volume 1 is on what Health Informatics has contributed to the development of usable medical records. Regarding those records, we emphasize that their purpose is not just to provide a repository for patient information, but also to serve as the informational basis for analysis and evaluation to ensure that what we do in the health system is worth its substantial cost.

The final matter we will mention related to Volume 1 is that it provides an understanding of the nature of the human beings involved in patient care, including their biases and the possibility of errors. We cite several studies of errors in health care that have shown that patients are injured through misadventures that sometimes were preventable. We show how relatively simple processes can potentially reduce errors and the impacts of human bias, thereby minimizing injuries and saving lives.

Through all of this we emphasize that clinical care is intended to help patients, not harm them. Carefulness, mindfulness, critical thinking and acting based on the best evidence available are crucial ways for both physicians and patients to assure that.

Now It is on You!

We leave you with all of this and plus the challenge to use it in your own care and that of your family and friends. For those of you who are in or entering a career that relates to health care, we are confident that this material has prepared you well to really understand clinical care and to use your knowledge as you endeavor to serve!

Chapter 49: What You Can Look Forward To

Introduction

This compendium comprises three volumes and that is what awaits you next! We move through the three by first concentrating on the health and sickness of the body, then taking on the health and problems of the mind and then tying up the material by thinking about crucial issues that affect us and the health system.

You have now powered though the first Volume and here you can get a taste of what you can delve into next. We wish you godspeed and much benefit!

Volume 2: Mental Health and Public Health

Most of Volume 1 dealt with the health and sickness of the body, largely ignoring the issues associated with the mind. However, it is likely that the total impact of mental health problems is substantially greater than the problems that confront the body.

In Part 1 of Volume 2, we define the true nature of mental health problems, clarifying that they are most often not 'illnesses' – biological diseases of the brain – but rather disturbances in thoughts, feelings and behaviors that beset many of us. This is a crucial distinction, as many treatments make the assumption that mental health problems have a medical basis – are caused by a biological problem with the brain. Some, in fact, are caused by problems with the body's organs or its biochemistry, which secondarily affect the mind. One of the most significant responsibilities of those who deal with mental health problems is first assuring themselves that there is not an underlying biological problem and avoiding treatment of the patient as if there were one.

We discuss the nature of psychoactive drugs, those that have an impact on the function of the mind, and the general issues associated with pharmaceuticals in mental health care. In choosing a treatment, one must first diagnose what the cause may be. If the cause of the person's mental disturbance is not biological, then the treatment is typically one of the verbal therapies, which have demonstrated significant success. Even when psychopharmaceuticals are used, these verbal therapies are valuable, if not essential, adjuncts in returning the patient to a comfortable and functioning state.

We make our best efforts to describe the body and the brain related to the function of the mind. We emphasize that everything we think, feel, remember and do is determined in our brain that gives birth to our mind. The mind cannot exist without that brain.

We elucidate some of the major psychotherapies and what we as individuals can do in our and others' lives to improve their mental state. We also try to make clear the nature of the complexity of the mind and how things can go wrong within that complex entity.

In its final chapter on mental health, we include some of the views of a psychiatrist regarding how he deals with people with mental health issues.

Part 2 of Volume 2 focuses on the nature of Public Health, the care of the populace as a whole. It notes that Public Health has likely made the greatest contributions to the lives of human beings. It accomplished this through centuries of the efforts of key people who found ways to prevent disease and to improve the environment to make it less likely to sicken or even kill us.

At the end of volume 2, we reflect on the COVID-19 Pandemic to illustrate what Public Health is all about.

Why this material is so important, is the fact that we have allowed the system for public health to wither. We present this in the form of a story about Dr. Methuselah and how societal attention can drift. We also define the concept of the Humongous Body – the body of bodies of all people – and the Humongous Mind – the reality that we all, to some degree, think and believe together with many others. Interestingly, this work brings us back to the issues of misinformation and disinformation and the dangers they pose for communities, countries and even the world.

Volume 3: Personalizing Health Care

Among the most interesting and thought stimulating of the three volumes is Volume 3, which addresses crucial knowledge to assist in personalizing the healthcare experience, healthcare problems and solutions and outstanding issues.

This Volume lays out the nature of what occurs, or should occur, when a patient and the doctor meet for the patient's care. It makes it clear that, for this encounter to be successful, trust must exist between the parties, as well as a high degree of intimacy and acceptance, if we are to realize the full value of the engagement.

We review the differing levels of seriousness of medical problems and suggest how to go about dealing with them, including some advice about how and when to get advice.

We discuss many medical issues in the volume. These include how to avoid overprescribing, the ethics and principles that must be in place to protect the patient and how to get good information and make rational decisions.

There is a very interesting chapter on death and dying and, though it may sound weird, on how to get sick – primarily so we can all avoid that. We also provide information how the body deals with medications.

Finally, we describe the nature of anesthesia, and include a collection of brief topics that we believe readers will find quite interesting and informative.

Volume 3 is we collected our thoughts about issues in Medicine. We include what it means to be an expert, and how to confront Medicine – which usually seems to be very challenging area with its own secret language, its own culture and its own cult of high priests.

The overall objective of volume 3 is to help all of us think more deeply about Medicine, health care and the people who attempt to help us.

Chapter 50: Authoring these Books

Reflections by David (See FIGURE 1.50.1)

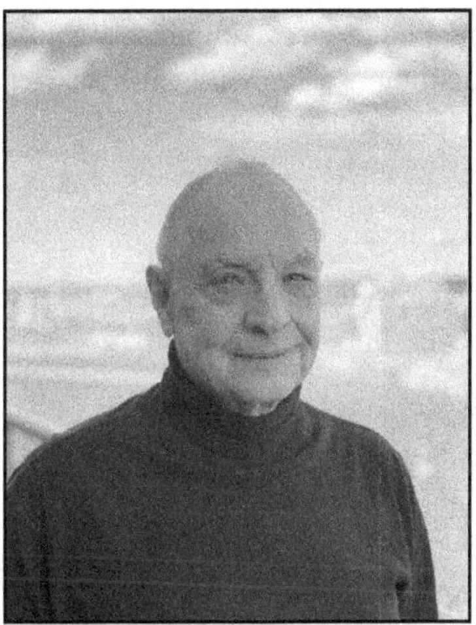

FIGURE 1.50.1: David Zitner

The headlines read "IBM Watson Supercomputer Beats Two Humans at Jeopardy (Feb 2011)".

Computers can record, store and retrieve the world's information. Why wouldn't we expect a thoughtful person using a computer with the world's knowledge at hand to be more effective than people trying to solve problems using only the knowledge in their head? Every thoughtful and empathetic person with access to the world's knowledge can participate in health care – their own and the community's – and contribute to improved health outcomes.

Knowing the essential ideas in clinical care and health services enables each of us to diagnose most problems, evaluate the benefits and harms of proposed remedies, and evaluate and suggest improvements to the proposals of politicians who regulate health care.

Over years of family medical practice, I was startled that even the most sophisticated patients, some with international academic credentials, rarely asked pertinent questions about the care I recommended. They usually accepted my suggestions and did not enquire, even when my recommendation was based on a shaky foundation. They accepted statements without reflection that they would not have accepted in the course of their academic work. On the other hand, a few patients were totally engaged. Even before the Internet, some non-clinicians read the current medical literature and brought me up to date on the recent literature related to their diseases.

Knowledge about health services is becoming increasingly important as each of us becomes more involved in the health services controversies routinely headlined in print and on TV. This book is dedicated to helping people think about health and health care so they can participate in healthcare decisions and become the Chief Executive Officer of their own health care.

I am a retired family doctor, a retired professor in the Division of Medical Education and the founding Director of Medical Informatics at Dalhousie University Medical School, in Halifax, Nova Scotia, Canada. Along with colleagues in Computer Science, I organized and implemented the first Canadian graduate program in Health Informatics.

Half of the students in our graduate program were doctors, nurses, dentists, pharmacists or health educators. The others come from varied backgrounds including Computer Science, Law, Management, and Engineering and had minimal healthcare experience.

I developed two graduate courses. One, "Health Information Its Flow and Use", tracked the use of information in health care, and addressed how information normally collected during care could be used to inform health policy and future healthcare decision-making. We dealt with topics, such as what happens to the information collected during clinical encounters and the uses of that information; what happens to the information collected when a doctor examines a patient and recommends treatment; and what happens to the information when a drug either helps someone to heal or when it provokes a serious adverse reaction.

This book is based on another course, "Clinical Care Fundamentals for Non-Clinicians", also known as "learn to think like a doctor and solve medical problems in three months". I developed this course for students who entered the graduate program without any previous healthcare experience. The course was developed so that students could learn how doctors and other health professionals make decisions and which information clinicians need to support their choices.

I was surprised – and so were our students – to find that after 3 months the students were able to solve many medical problems using their brain and a computer, including difficult problems suggested by my doubting clinical colleagues.

Several times a year, students in the course inquired about a diagnosis, test or treatment that doctors prescribed to them, a friend or a family member and they wondered why it had been suggested and if it was appropriate.

However, it went beyond that when our inexperienced, "three-month doctors" offered interpretations that were more consistent with modern thinking than the ones the practicing physicians offered. We were especially surprised to find that, in a three-month course, students learned how to choose from various diagnostic and treatment possibilities and made thoughtful speculations about the causes and treatment of disability and discomfort.

Colleagues at other universities, who heard about our course, including those teaching in other Health Informatics programs, asked for a textbook. Ultimately, this led to these 3 volumes. The material has been adapted to help health services administrators, anyone else pursuing a career in health services, and the general public:

- To understand the purposes of health care
- To consider the many uses of health information
- To consider health policy
- To develop an approach to clinical problems.

Medicine is all about information and knowledge. We all need to ask: Why do I feel sick? Why can't I walk up a flight of stairs? What can I do to prevent and deal with aches, pains, disabilities and the diseases that lead to discomfort, disability and death? Are politicians proposing worthwhile health policies? Are journalistic reports of clinical breakthroughs reasonable or premature?

Those not in health care will benefit from this book because they will learn how doctors make decisions, the questions patients should ask in order to make informed decisions about their own health care, and what we all can do to avoid harm from inappropriate recommendations and medical mistakes.

Graduates of the course understood the purpose of health care; they learned how to diagnose problems, and how to evaluate prospective treatments. You will to!

We expect students, after three months, to use readily available information to understand and solve medical problems. It was a surprise to me that most of our students are able, with the help of a computer, to solve simple and complex medical problems, including dermatology images.

In their final exams our students showed they understood which blood or x-ray tests to use and why, where to find information to tell them all of the possible causes for a particular ache, pain, dysfunction or disability, how to decide what is the most likely cause of a problem, and how to find the right treatment. Our graduates did that, and you, armed with this material, have that potential too.

OUR TARGETS FOR THIS BOOK

1. **The public to help them understand important ideas related to:**
   - *The purposes of health care.*
   - *How the results of care – benefits and harms – are measured.*
   - *Issues around Preventive Medicine and screening for undiagnosed problems such as breast cancer, cervical cancer (pap smears).*
   - *Deciding if a person has a disease, including how to assess the value of diagnostic tests and procedures. People are surprised to learn that often a positive or negative test result for a disease does not necessarily mean they have or do not have the condition tested for because many tests produce false alarms or false reassurance.*
   - *Assessment of the value of specific treatments, like medications and surgical procedures.*
   - *How interventions can be used to prevent conditions.*
   - *Error prevention and types of errors that can be minimized or avoided.*
2. **Ministries of Health, health services administrators, insurance companies regarding:**
   - *Evaluating health interventions.*
   - *Healthcare resource allocation, including how to measure results and elect among competing demands for resources.*
3. **People working on teams with doctors so that they:**
   - *Have shared and compatible ideas around the purposes of care.*
   - *Can converge on the general and particular approaches to clinical problems.*
   - *Develop ways to resolve differences of opinion among members of healthcare teams.*

Reflections by Dominic (See FIGURE 1.50.2)

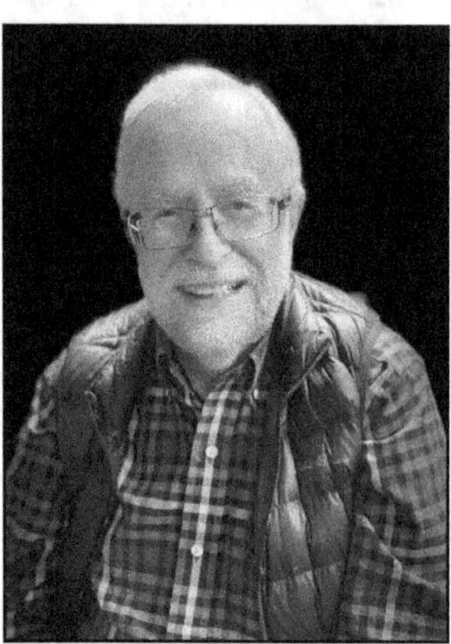

FIGURE 1.50.2: Dominic Covvey

"It's the Journey, not the destination." Stating this often punctuates a disappointing or failed enterprise... sometimes not carried out in one's office! In this case, though, it is a very positive statement about a long writing venture.

David first contacted me over 7 years ago (in December 2016) and asked if I wanted to work with him on his interesting and exciting Magnum Opus, his having already put several years into it. He had begun writing a book as a text for his Health Informatics course. I agreed that this might be an interesting way to spend a few months – dramatically misjudging what I faced – as has been most of my life. We began working and soon mutated and evolved the nature of the end product into something that we hope will have far deeper and broader impacts.

We spent many, many days since that time, writing, editing, repurposing, refining, augmenting and altering the emphasis on many different ideas. The greatest reward in all of this, at least for me, was our communication. We carried out our discussions by telephone across the thousands of kilometers and four hours separating us – we quite literally reach from sea to shining sea! In our discussions, we posited ideas, critiqued them, debated them and both frustrated and delighted each other.

I am not a physician, having started in the areas of Physics, Astrophysics and Medical Biophysics. In the course of my decades of postgraduate study and research in Medicine and immersion in the healthcare system, particularly in cardiovascular research, I picked up a fair amount of medical knowledge. My experience with Medicine was grandly augmented by my wife, Carol Thompson, a diagnostic radiologist and ultrasonographer. Regretfully, she exited this mortal coil in 2011, an unendurable loss of the genre the Japanese Emperor said we must endure, when he accepted defeat at the end of WW2.

Carol taught me a great deal over more than four decades. Some lessons were overheard by my daughter Beth's dinner guests, turning them disturbingly green! However, being cooked in the soup of Medicine just is not the same as being a clinician who sees patients and diagnoses and treats them. Since my early research endeavors, I transformed into a health informatician and had the opportunity to work for over 30 years with many different clinicians (including David) and medical groups, as well. Even if you put all that together, clinical medicine is a whole other world. David has been very tolerant of what I claim to know versus what I actually knew. Through discussion, we somehow were able to jointly clarify and even develop novel explanations for some tricky areas, like the nature of health and the mind-brain dichotomy. We also managed to do this despite at times having significant initial disagreements about certain ideas and nuances.

Despite all my limitations, we managed to have what has been one of the most enjoyable intellectual exercises of my career. I have written books previously, back in the 1980s on computer literacy and more recently on esoteric topics like Health Informatics competencies. The latter contribution was completed in the early 2000s with David and with Bob Bernstein, also a physician (Pointing the Way: Competencies and Curricula in Health Informatics: http://www.nihi.ca/nihi/ir/Pointing%20the%20Way%20MASTER%20Document%20Version%201%20Final.pdf). Relatively speaking, those more recent efforts were intellectually easy and just a lot of hard work. They produced material of interest to only a few thousand people on the planet and, although they have been cited as a contribution, bore none of the satisfaction of the material we share with you.

It has been said that the only way to truly understand a topic is to be required to teach it. When we prepare to teach, we often discover that our ideas are ambiguous, incomplete, confused, based on inadequate foundations or just plain wrong. Writing these books has been an exercise like teaching hundreds of classes on the topics of health care and the nature of Medicine. The effort involved in getting the ideas clear enough (albeit never perfectly so – we are mere humans), was enormous and sometimes temporarily insuperable. I hope the effort, with all its near headache-producing intensity, has been worth it for you.

Finally, I wonder if you will be able to extend into your own lives the incredible experience we had. It is my wish that you will read our books and discuss them with your friends, considering, parsing, critiquing and debating the many points we have raised. Book writers probably always hope that people will read what they have written. My hope is that these books will go further and cause you to think about things and explore far beyond what you will find in their pages.

So, I wish you many enjoyable discussions with friends and acquaintances that help you arrive at a place where health, health care, and the practice of Medicine can be seen for their value and recognized for their dangers. That will make our effort worth it!

INDEX

Symbols

A

B

C

D

I

J

K

L

M

N

O

P

R

S

T

U

V

W

Compendium on The Nature of Clinical Care

Volume 1: A Gentle Introduction –

Section 1 – Introduction

Section 2 – The Meaning of Health

Section 3 – The Nature of Diagnosis

Section 4 – Measuring Health

Section 5 – Health Prevention and Maintenance

Section 6 – The Nature of Treatment

Section 7 – The Challenge of Testing

Section 8 – In Closing

Compendium on The Nature of Clinical Care

Volume 2: Mental + Public Health Care

Section 1 – Introduction

Chapter 1: A Preface
Chapter 2: Welcome to Our Readers
Chapter 3: Our Promises and Overview

Section 2 – Mental Health

Chapter 4: Am I Crazy?
Chapter 5: Thinking About Mental Health Problems
Chapter 6: Mental Health Treatment
Chapter 7: The Nature of Psychoactive Drugs
Chapter 8: More on Non-Pharmaceutical Interventions
Chapter 9: Measuring and Categorizing Mental Health
Chapter 10: The Diagnostic and Statistical Manual (DSM)
Chapter 11: Predicting and Treating Dangerousness
Chapter 12: Thinking More About Psychotherapy
Chapter 13: Major Varieties of Psychotherapy
Chapter 14: There and Care – A Call to Ears
Chapter 15: Further Thoughts Mental Health and Dysfunction
Chapter 16: Interview with a Psychiatrist
Chapter 17: Understanding Mind Versus Brain

Section 3 – Public Health

Chapter 18: Introduction to Public Health
Chapter 19: The Pandemic as Lens

Section 4 – In Closing

Chapter 20: Final Comments
Chapter 21: Summary of Volume 2
Chapter 22: What You Can Look to Learn in Volume 1
Chapter 23: What You Can Look Forward to in
Chapter 24: Writing these Books

Volume 3: Personalizing Health Care

Section 1 – Introduction

Chapter 1: A Preface
Chapter 2: Welcome to Our Readers
Chapter 3: Our Promises and Overview
Chapter 4: Introduction to This Volume
Chapter 5: Learning About Health

Section 2: The Medical Office and Medical Care

Chapter 6: The Office Visit Conversation
Chapter 7: Understanding the Health System
Chapter 8: Considering When to Get Advice
Chapter 9: Advice for Usually Mild Problems
Chapter 10: Advice for Less Common but More Serious Problems
Chapter 11: Advice for More Serious Problems
Chapter 12: Mnemonics That Help in Diagnosis

Section 3 – Medical Issues

Chapter 13: How Measurement Helps Choices About Treating the Elderly
Chapter 14: Avoiding Overprescribing
Chapter 15: Complexity... Beyond Complicated
Chapter 16: How to Get Sick
Chapter 17: Records and Computers
Chapter 18: Ethics and Medicine
Chapter 19: On Death and Dying
Chapter 20: On the Nature of Expertise
Chapter 21: Data, Information, Knowledge and Decisions
Chapter 22: About the Body and Drugs

Section 4: Potpourri

Chapter 23: Anesthesia
Chapter 24: Search and You Will (Possibly) Find
Chapter 25: Brief Topics

Section 5: Final Comments

Chapter 26: Final Comments
Chapter 27: Writing These Books

www.ingramcontent.com/pod-product-compliance
Lightning Source LLC
Chambersburg PA
CBHW080903170526
45158CB00008B/1977

* 9 7 8 1 0 3 9 1 8 0 0 2 4 *